Clinical Cases in Critical Care

Clinical Cases in Critical Care

Editor: Ira Moore

AMERICAN
MEDICAL PUBLISHERS
www.americanmedicalpublishers.com

AMERICAN
MEDICAL PUBLISHERS
www.americanmedicalpublishers.com

Cataloging-in-Publication Data

Clinical cases in critical care / edited by Ira Moore.
p. cm.
Includes bibliographical references and index.
ISBN 979-8-88740-627-5
1. Critical care medicine. 2. Emergency medicine. 3. Intensive care units.
4. Medical emergencies. I. Moore, Ira.
RC86. 7 .C75 2023
616.028--dc23

American Medical Publishers,
41 Flatbush Avenue,
1st Floor, New York,
NY 11217, USA

ISBN 979-8-88740-627-5 (Hardback)

Contents

Preface IX

Chapter 1 **Clinical and Imaging Resolution of Neonatal Hemochromatosis following Treatment** 1
Ayelet Machtei, Gil Klinger, Rivka Shapiro, Osnat Konen and Lea Sirota

Chapter 2 **A Rare Clinical Course of Seronegative Pulmonary-Renal Syndrome** 5
M. Fröhlich-Gildhoff, W. J. Jabs, C. Berhold, M. K. Kuhlmann, U. Ketterer, S. Kische and H. Ince

Chapter 3 **Malignant Catatonia Warrants Early Psychiatric-Critical Care Collaborative Management: Two Cases and Literature Review** 9
Julia Park, Josh Tan, Sylvia Krzeminski, Maryam Hazeghazam, Meghana Bandlamuri and Richard W. Carlson

Chapter 4 **Euglycemic Diabetic Ketoacidosis in the ICU: 3 Case Reports and Review of Literature** 13
Pablo Lucero and Sebastián Chapela

Chapter 5 **Critical Care Management for Novel 2019 SARS-CoV-2 and HCoVNL63 Coinfection in a Young Immunocompromised Patient: A Chicago Experience** 19
Alejandro Sanchez-Nadales, Miguel Treminio-Quezada, Hasan Abad, Jessica Navarro-Motta, Pamela Contreras-Chavez, Anil Kachru and Chae Chu

Chapter 6 **Gastric Emphysema in a Critically Ill Patient Successfully Treated without Surgery** 27
Hiromi Ihoriya, Tetsuya Yumoto, Masaya Iwamuro, Noritomo Fujisaki, Takaaki Osako, Hiromichi Naito and Atsunori Nakao

Chapter 7 **A Critically Ill Child with Gangrenous Appendicitis Masquerading as Hollow Viscous Perforation** 31
Ashish Lal Shrestha, Santosh Maharjan, Anil Dev Pant and Pankaj Bahadur Nepali

Chapter 8 **Gastric Emphysema in a Critically Ill Patient Successfully Treated without Surgery** 35
Hiromi Ihoriya, Tetsuya Yumoto, Masaya Iwamuro, Noritomo Fujisaki, Takaaki Osako, Hiromichi Naito and Atsunori Nakao

Chapter 9 **Complete Heart Block as a Clinical Feature in Critically Ill Coronavirus Disease 2019 (COVID-19) Patients: A Case Series of Three Cases** 39
Farook Ahmad, Priti Gandre, Julien Nguekam, Alanna Wall, ShiYu Ong, Abdul N. Karuppamakkantakath, Konstantinos Tasopoulos, Muhammad Athar Sadiq, Sazzli Kasim and Jeronimo M. Cuesta

Chapter 10 **Massive Pulmonary Embolism Complicating Coronavirus Disease 2019 (COVID-19) Pneumonia** 45
Shruti Hegde, Gemini Yesodharan, John Tedrow and Alena Goldman

Chapter 11 **Acute Pancreatitis Induced by Diabetic Ketoacidosis with Major Hypertriglyceridemia: Report of Four Cases** 50
Karama Bouchaala, Mabrouk Bahloul, Sabrine Bradii, Hela Kallel, Kamilia Chtara and Mounir Bouaziz

Chapter 12 **Liver Transplantation for Acute Liver Failure Attributed to Leptospirosis: A Report of Two Cases** 54
Thibault Lebreton, Fréderic Aubrun, Jean-Yves Mabrut, Laurent Heyer and Camille Perrin

Chapter 13 **Different Outcomes of "Silent Hypoxia" in Patients with COVID-19 Pneumonia** 58
Ashani Ratnayake, Prabhashini Kumarihamy, Sujeewa Gunaratne, Hiranya Abeysinghe, Sahan Perera and Shirley Ekanayake

Chapter 14 **Symmetrical Peripheral Gangrene: Report of Three Cases** 64
Héctor Acosta, Pau Forcada, Marta Bonjorn, Amer Mustafa, Paul Pilares and Jordi Colomina

Chapter 15 **Ultrasound Detection of Portomesenteric Venous Gas is an Early Sign of Bowel Ischaemia in Non-Traumatic Abdominal Pain: Old Dogs, New Tricks—Four Cases Report** 69
Mirko Di Capua, Michela Tonani and Stefano Paglia

Chapter 16 **A Fatal Case of Primary Amoebic Meningoencephalitis from Recreational Waters** 73
Edward Hamaty Jr., Saif Faiek, Minesh Nandi, David Stidd, Manish Trivedi and Hari Kandukuri

Chapter 17 **The Conundrum of Septic Shock Imitators in Patients with Hematologic Cancers: Case Presentation and Possible Differential Diagnoses** 79
Giorgio Berlot, Giulia Moratelli, Martina Tarchini, Katiuscia Battaglia, Paolo Grassi, Nadia Zarrillo, Vincenzo Colella and Rossana Bussani

Chapter 18 **Right Sided Intracardiac Thrombosis during Veno-Arterial Extracorporeal Membrane Oxygenation: A Case Report and Literature Review** 86
Anusha Ganapati Bhat, Armand Golchin, Deepak Kumar Pasupula and Jaime A. Hernandez-Montfort

Chapter 19 **Critical Illness Associated Fatal Hypoglycemia in a Nondiabetic Male** 90
Amit Toor, Anika Toor and Mahesh Krishnamurthy

Chapter 20 **Wanting to Forget: Intrusive and Delusional Memories from Critical Illness** 93
Lauren Doig and Kevin Solverson

Chapter 21 **Critical Care Admission of an HIV Patient with Diabetic Ketoacidosis Secondary to Pembrolizumab** 96
John A. Cuenca, Andres Laserna, María P. Reyes, Joseph L. Nates and Gregory H. Botz

Chapter 22 **Hopeful News for Physicians Who Involved in the Treatment of Critical Aluminum Phosphide (Rice Pill) Poisoning Patients** 99
Fatemeh Vafapour and Moslem Sedaghattalab

Chapter 23 **Tetanus Complicated by Dysautonomia: A Case Report and Review of Management** 102
Nishant Sharma, Si Li, Metlapalli Venkata Sravanthi, Dan Kazmierski, Yichen Wang, Amit Sharma and Pragya Dhaubhadel

Chapter 24 **Life-Threatening Intrapulmonary Hemorrhage due to Vancomycin-Induced Thrombocytopenia: A Case Report** 106
Haneen Abdalhadi, Yazan Fahmawi, Abhijin Das and Brian Fouty

Chapter 25 **COVID-19-Associated Coagulopathy: A Case Report of Thrombosis despite Therapeutic Anticoagulation** 109
Habiba Hussain, Matthew Sehring and Bhagat Singh Aulakh

Chapter 26 **Flecainide Toxicity Secondary to Accidental Overdose: A Pediatric Case Report of Two Brothers** 113
Sarah E. Gardner Yelton, James B. Leonard, Caridad M. de la Uz, Rajeev S. Wadia and Sean S. Barnes

Chapter 27 **Euglycemic Diabetic Ketoacidosis in Pregnancy: A Case Report and Review of Current Literature** 119
Johnny F. Jaber, Matthew Standley and Raju Reddy

Chapter 28 **Coccidioidomycosis of the Vocal Cords Presenting in Sepsis** 124
Curtis Converse, Atish Dey, Samuel Decker, Sarkis Arabian and Michael Neeki

Chapter 29 **Extreme Rhabdomyolysis, Acute Renal Failure and Protracted Ileus in a Case of Legionella Pneumonia** 130
C. Laivier, M.-O. Bleuze, P. Hantson and J. Devos

Chapter 30 **Refractory Paraneoplastic Diarrhea Secondary to Adenocarcinoma of the Lung** 134
Lauren Howdershelt, Michael J. Forte and Rahul G. Sangani

Chapter 31 **Considerations in Neuromuscular Blockade in the ICU** 137
Jessica D. Workum, Stephanie H.V. Janssen and Hugo R.W. Touw

Chapter 32 **A Curious Case of MRSA Bacteremia and Septic Pulmonary Embolism Secondary to Peripheral Venous Catheter** 141
Joshua Twito, Syeda Sahra, Abdullah Jahangir and Neville Mobarakai

Chapter 33 **Super-Refractory Status Epilepticus Treated with High Dose Perampanel: Case Series and Review of the Literature** 145
Christopher R. Newey, Naresh Mullaguri, Stephen Hantus, Vineet Punia and Pravin George

Chapter 34 **Right Sided Intracardiac Thrombosis during Veno-Arterial Extracorporeal Membrane Oxygenation** 152
Anusha Ganapati Bhat, Armand Golchin, Deepak Kumar Pasupula and Jaime A. Hernandez-Montfort

Chapter 35 **Circulatory Collapse due to Hyperinflation in a Patient with Tracheobronchomalacia: A Case Report and Brief Review** 156
Niclas Lundström, Gert Henriksson, Ola Börjesson, Malin Jonsson Fagerlund and Johan Petersson

Chapter 36 **Successful Use of Octreotide Therapy for Refractory Levofloxacin-Induced Hypoglycemia: A Case Report and Literature Review** 161
Matthew R. Watson, Ceressa T. Ward, Amit Prabhakar, Babar Fiza and Vanessa Moll

Chapter 37 **Does Dexmedetomidine Improve or Worsen Restless Leg Syndrome under Sedation: A Case Report and Extensive Review** 166
Sandra Iskandar, Marina Souto Martins, Andrew Hudson, Jason G. Hirsch and Jonathan S. Jahr

Chapter 38 **Dantrolene Administration in the Management of the Prehospital Patient with Methylenedioxymethamphetamine Overdose** 171
Kia Nikoomanesh, Alexander T. Phan, Julian Choi, Sarkis Arabian and Michael M. Neeki

Chapter 39 **Postoperative 'STEMI' in Intracerebral Hemorrhage due to Arteriovenous Malformation: A Case Report and Review of Literature** 177
Ravinder Datt Bhanot, Jasleen Kaur, Shitiz Sriwastawa, Kendall Bell and Kushak Suchdev

Chapter 40 **A Case of Linezolid Toxicity Presenting as a Sepsis Mimic** 182
Rashmi Mishra, Harish Patel, Bindu Goel and Trupti Vakde

Chapter 41 **The Considerations and Controversies in using High-Flow Nasal Oxygen with Self-Prone Positioning in SARS-CoV-2 COVID-19 Disease** 186
Kieran P. Nunn, Murray J. Blackstock, Ryan Ellis, Gauhar Sheikh, Alastair Morgan and Jonathan K. J. Rhodes

Chapter 42 **Use of Continuous Intravenous Anakinra Infusion in Multisystem Inflammatory Syndrome in Children** 195
Abdulaziz Alolayan, Abdullah S. Aldamegh and Azzah Alkhayrat

Chapter 43 **A Rare Cause of a Rare Disorder: *E. coli*-Induced Purpura Fulminans Secondary to Urinary Tract Infection** 199
Jacob Lowry and Edva Noel

Chapter 44 **It is Always Early with Point-of-Care Ultrasound** 205
Zouheir Ibrahim Bitar, Tamer Mohamed Zaalouk, Ossama Sajeh Maadarani and Ragab Desouky Elshabasy

Permissions

List of Contributors

Index

Preface

Critical care is a specialized area of medicine focused on the management and treatment of patients with life-threatening conditions or severe organ dysfunction. It involves providing comprehensive care and monitoring patients in intensive care units (ICUs) or critical care settings. The primary goal of critical care is to stabilize and support vital functions, such as breathing, circulation and organ function, while addressing the underlying cause of the patient's critical condition. Some of the advanced medical interventions which are provided within this field include mechanical ventilation and hemodynamic support. Critical care encompasses a wide range of medical specialties, including cardiology, pulmonology, nephrology, and infectious diseases. This book unfolds the innovative aspects of critical care which will be crucial for the progress of this field in the future. It will provide comprehensive knowledge to the readers.

Various studies have approached the subject by analyzing it with a single perspective, but the present book provides diverse methodologies and techniques to address this field. This book contains theories and applications needed for understanding the subject from different perspectives. The aim is to keep the readers informed about the progresses in the field; therefore, the contributions were carefully examined to compile novel researches by specialists from across the globe.

Indeed, the job of the editor is the most crucial and challenging in compiling all chapters into a single book. In the end, I would extend my sincere thanks to the chapter authors for their profound work. I am also thankful for the support provided by my family and colleagues during the compilation of this book.

Editor

1

Clinical and Imaging Resolution of Neonatal Hemochromatosis following Treatment

Ayelet Machtei,[1] Gil Klinger,[1,2] Rivka Shapiro,[2,3] Osnat Konen,[2,4] and Lea Sirota[1,2]

[1] *Neonatal Intensive Care Unit, Schneider Children's Medical Center of Israel, 14 Kaplan Street, 49202 Petah Tikva, Israel*
[2] *The Sackler School of Medicine, Tel Aviv University, Tel Aviv, Israel*
[3] *Institute of Gastroenterology, Nutrition and Liver Diseases, Schneider Children's Medical Center of Israel, Petah Tikva, Israel*
[4] *Radiology Department, Schneider Children's Medical Center of Israel, Petah Tikva, Israel*

Correspondence should be addressed to Ayelet Machtei; ayelet.malamud@gmail.com

Academic Editor: Ricardo J. Dinis-Oliveira

Neonatal hemochromatosis (NH) is an acute liver disease associated with both hepatic and extrahepatic iron deposition and is a leading cause of neonatal liver transplantation. The concept that NH is an alloimmune disease has led to the emergence of a new treatment approach utilizing exchange transfusion and intravenous immunoglobulin therapy. We present a two-day old neonate with progressive liver dysfunction who was diagnosed with NH. Magnetic resonance imaging confirmed tissue iron overload. Treatment with intravenous immunoglobulins and exchange transfusion led to rapid improvement in liver function. Follow-up physical examination at the age of 8 months showed normal development and near normal liver function. A repeat abdominal magnetic resonance scan at 8 months showed no signs of iron deposition in the liver, pancreas, or adrenal glands. The present report provides further support for the use of exchange transfusion and immunoglobulin therapy in NH and is the first to document resolution of typical iron deposition by magnetic resonance imaging.

1. Introduction

Neonatal hemochromatosis (NH) is a rapidly progressive disease presenting within a few days after birth with fulminant hepatic failure and ensuing multiorgan failure. NH is also known as neonatal iron storage disease or congenital alloimmune hepatitis. For many years the only curative treatment for NH was liver transplantation with survival rates of 50% [1]. Treatment with antioxidants and chelation therapy may improve symptoms but is associated with severe side effects [2]. In recent years the realization that NH is probably an alloimmune disease [3, 4] has led to the emergence of a new treatment approach utilizing exchange transfusion (ET) and intravenous immunoglobulins (IVIG). This has resulted in an improved survival rate and in a dramatic decrease in the need for liver transplantation. The understanding of the pathophysiology of the disease has also led to antenatal treatment with IVIG from 16 weeks' gestation and has been shown to prevent the development of NH in subsequent pregnancies [4]. In the present report we present a full-term newborn with liver dysfunction and multiorgan failure, diagnosed with NH that recovered fully following treatment with IVIG and ET.

2. Case Report

A female neonate was born at 39 weeks of gestation following an uneventful pregnancy. The infant was delivered by vacuum extraction due to a profound deceleration. Apgar scores at birth were 9 and 10 at 1 and 5 minutes, respectively. The infant weighed 2.724 kg (10th percentile) and the initial physical examination was normal. The patient was the first born (and first gestation) to healthy nonconsanguineous Ashkenazi Jews. At the age of two days the mother reported a decreased appetite and subsequently the infant's condition deteriorated rapidly. Physical examination showed pallor, hypothermia (35.9°C), and bradycardia of 70 beats per minute (bpm).

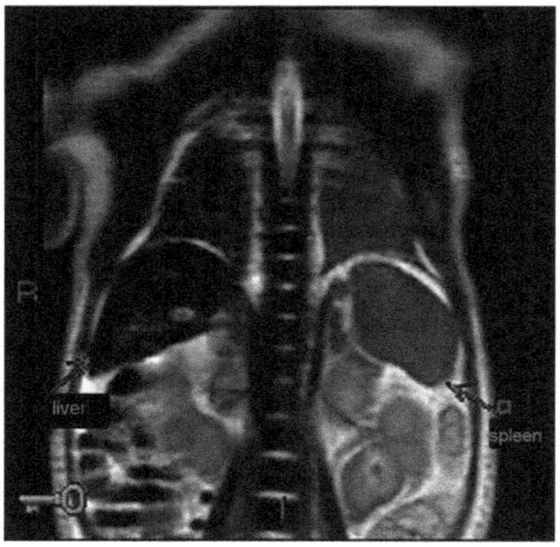

Figure 1: Abdominal MRI, coronal view, on day five of life showing low signal intensity of the liver parenchyma with preservation of the signal intensity of splenic parenchyma (T2WI protocol). Calculations of T2* showed rapid decay consistent with iron overload.

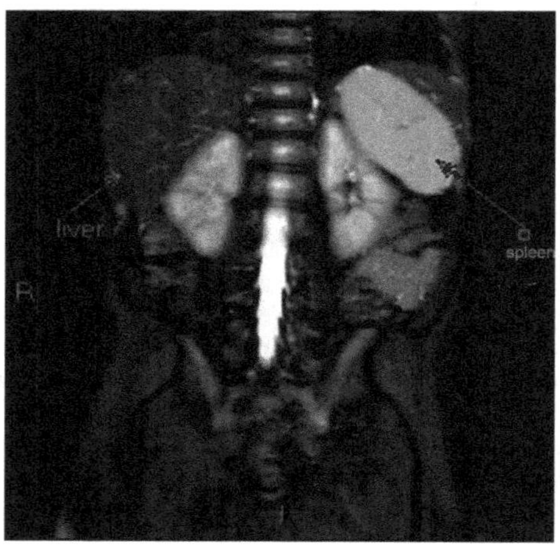

Figure 2: Follow-up abdominal MRI, coronal view, at 8 months showing normal intensity of liver parenchyma on T2WI with fat saturation protocol.

The initial laboratory evaluation showed hypoglycemia of 13 mg/dL (normal lower limit of 40 mg/dL). The patient was treated with intravenous boluses of 10% glucose and normal saline and was transferred to the neonatal intensive care unit (NICU). Upon admission to the NICU the infant's vital signs were as follows: temperature of 35.8°C, heart rate of 116 bpm, breath rate of 51 per minute, and blood pressure of 61/33 mm/Hg. Physical examination showed a lethargic infant with glucose level of 19 mg/dL; thus, a second bolus of 10% glucose was administered. During the hypoglycemic episode a critical blood sample was taken (insulin, cortisol, growth hormone, thyroid function, and lactate) and a full sepsis workup (complete blood count, C-reactive protein level, blood culture, and cerebrospinal fluid analysis and culture) was performed. Additional tests drawn included blood chemistry, a coagulation panel, and tests for possible metabolic abnormalities. Treatment with ampicillin, gentamycin, and acyclovir was initiated. Initial blood tests showed leukocytosis, elevated liver enzymes and creatinine, and evidence of coagulopathy (Table 1). The remaining endocrinological parameters were within normal limits. During the next few days the patient's condition deteriorated. Although she remained normoglycemic, her liver function worsened progressively; coagulation tests showed disseminated intravascular coagulation (DIC) despite treatment with platelets, fresh frozen plasma, and vitamin k. A workup for possible hepatitis causing pathogens turned out negative. The metabolic evaluation was negative (including blood carnitine, acyl carnitine, amino acids, very long chain fatty acids, galactosemia, pyruvate dehydrogenase, E3 deficiency, and congenital disorder of glycosylation). Alpha 1 antitrypsin level was normal, alpha-fetoprotein was high (143,621 ng/mL) compared to normal values [5], iron was 155 μg/dL (normal 40–145), and ferritin was extremely elevated (24,256 ng/mL) compared to standard range (10–291). An abdominal ultrasound showed normal hepatic and bile ducts and a moderate degree of ascites. Because of suspected convulsions the patient underwent a head ultrasound which showed mild cerebral edema and an electroencephalogram that was normal.

Based on the clinical and laboratory findings we suspected NH to be the cause of the infant's condition and performed an abdominal magnetic resonance imaging (MRI) scan and a buccal biopsy. The MRI showed a clear shortening of the T2 signal to 3.5–5.5 ms (normal 25–30 ms) from the liver and pancreas which is characteristic of tissue iron overload (Figure 1). The buccal biopsy was negative for iron staining, as was a repeat biopsy. Treatment was initiated on day 8 with double volume exchange transfusion and IVIG 2 gr/kg as well as with vitamin E 25 IU three times per day. Following treatment, the patient showed rapid clinical and laboratory improvement (Table 1): platelets count (76,000 to 142,000), INR (2.83 to 1.99), ammonia (502 to 149), and creatinine (1.33 to 0.16). The patient was discharged home on day 22 of life.

The infant has continued the follow-up by our Gastroenterology outpatients service. At the age of 8 months the infant was healthy, developing normally, and liver function tests were approaching normal values. A repeat abdominal MRI at the age of 8 months was normal and showed no signs of iron deposition in the liver, pancreas, or adrenal glands as compared to the spleen (Figure 2).

3. Discussion

NH is a rare condition affecting the fetus and newborn that presents during the neonatal period with acute liver failure and ensuing multiorgan failure. Untreated NH is uniformly fatal. No single gene has been recognized as being responsible for the disease [3]. In families with one affected child there is a 70–80% chance of recurrence in subsequent pregnancies [4], a recurrence rate that is not compatible with either an autosomal recessive or dominant inheritance pattern. Mitochondrial inheritance has been suggested but has not been confirmed [1, 2, 6].

TABLE 1: Laboratory values before and after treatment.

	Reference values	Peak value	After treatment
International normalized ratio	0.8–1.20 INR	2.83	1.99
Platelets	150–450 K/micl	76	142
Bilirubin total	0.3–1.2 mg/dL	11	8.4
Bilirubin direct	0.3 mg/dL	3.3	3.8
Aspartate transaminase	25.0–75.0 U/L	727	181
Alanine transaminase	13.0–45.0 U/L	196	114
Albumin	2.8–4.4 g/dL	2.2	2.9
Phosphorus	4.0–6.5 mg/dL	4.3	5.8
C-reactive protein	0.0–0.50 mg/dL	1.552	0.4
Iron	40–145 μg/dL	155	
Ferritin	10.0–291.0 ng/mL	24256	3030
Alpha-fetoprotein	Mean 41,687 ng/mL	143621	94709
Ammonia	0–228 mcg/dL	502	149
Urea	8–26 mg/dL	70	11
Creatinine	0.26–1.01 mg/dL	1.33	0.16

Knisely at al. [7] and Whitington and Malladi [8] suggested that the pattern of recurrence in NH resembles that of gestational alloimmune diseases in which the maternal immune system develops antibodies of the immunoglobulin G class which then cross the placenta and attack the fetal liver (in the current and subsequent pregnancies). In NH this process causes synthetic dysfunction of the different proteins involved in iron homeostasis which results in siderosis.

Patients with NH may present during pregnancy with intrauterine growth retardation, oligohydramnios (or, at times polyhydramnion), and placental edema and are often born prematurely. Within hours or days they develop acute liver failure. Frequently the infants are at first misdiagnosed with overwhelming sepsis. Laboratory abnormalities include hypoglycemia, hypoalbuminemia, and marked coagulopathy. Jaundice with elevated direct and indirect hyperbilirubinemia develops within days. Serum aminotransaminases are disproportionately low for the degree of hepatic injury, while alpha-fetoprotein levels are very high. Characteristic iron studies show low levels of transferrin that is unusually highly saturated and extremely elevated ferritin levels (150–450 K/micl; [9]). The diagnosis of NH can be difficult to establish because other hepatic disorders may cause liver siderosis or high ferritin levels. The diagnosis is made by exclusion of other causes of neonatal liver failure and by demonstrating extra-hepatic siderosis with reticuloendothelial sparing (as seen in hereditary hemochromatosis). Extrahepatic siderosis may be demonstrated by biopsy of the minor salivary glands that are positive in about two thirds of infants with proven NH [9] or by MRI, which demonstrates abnormal iron distribution in about 90% of proven cases. Ferric ions cause shortening of the T1 and, more impressively, of the T2 relaxation times. In NH, tissues that contain iron, such as the liver and pancreas, have a lower intensity signal than that of the normal spleen; although it should be noted that a physiological increase in iron content of the liver (alone) exists during the third trimester and neonatal period. An MRI can therefore be used for third trimester prenatal diagnosis.

Liver biopsy demonstrates nodular cirrhosis, pronounced fibrosis, and typically significant siderosis. Notably there are no signs of necrosis.

Until recently liver transplantation was considered the only curative treatment for NH with survival rates as high as 50%. Use of an ET for treatment of NH was first reported in 2005 by Rodrigues et al. [1]. In their report of 19 neonates, 17 with NH were treated with ET as a supportive measure. All these treated patients either died or needed subsequent liver transplantation. However, one should note that in this report, ET was given as a last measure to severely compromised patients. Whitington and Hibbard [4] described in 2004 a preventive prenatal treatment for pregnant women whose last pregnancy resulted in an infant or fetus with NH (based on the alloimmune theory). Treatment consisted of IVIG 1 g/kg weekly starting at 18 weeks of gestation (at which point maternal IgG antibodies are actively transported across the placenta). They reported 16 pregnancies that progressed uneventfully and resulted in all infants surviving. High dose immunoglobulin therapy during pregnancy for recurrent NH has since become common practice. In 2009 Rand et al. [10] published the largest series to date of neonates diagnosed with NH and treated by ET at twice the calculated blood volume and/or IVIG 1 g/kg. The ferritin levels were as high as 5509 ng/mL. Twelve subjects (75%) had a good outcome following treatment (poor outcome defined as death or receipt of a liver transplant). Since the initial report, additional reports by Lopriore et al. [11] and Babor et al. [12] have confirmed the effectiveness of ET and IVIG for NH.

The present report includes a newborn diagnosed with NH that presented with untypical severe liver failure. As this infant was the firstborn in her family the patient was only diagnosed after birth, thus adversely affecting the severity of the NH. Our report confirms that even when NH is severe, combined treatment with IVIG and exchange transfusion may achieve complete symptom resolution. The reported infant is the first to demonstrate resolution of iron deposition confirmed by follow-up MRI scan. We add our experience to the accumulating data supporting combined neonatal treatment with IVIG and exchange transfusion.

Abbreviations

NH: Neonatal hemochromatosis
IVIG: Intravenous immunoglobulin
ET: Exchange transfusion
NICU: Neonatal intensive care unit
MRI: Magnetic resonance imaging.

References

[1] F. Rodrigues, M. Kallas, R. Nash et al., "Neonatal hemochromatosis—medical treatment vs. transplantation: the King's experience," *Liver Transplantation*, vol. 11, no. 11, pp. 1417–1424, 2005.

[2] D. M. Flynn, N. Mohan, P. McKiernan et al., "Progress in treatment and outcome for children with neonatal haemochromatosis," *Archives of Disease in Childhood Fetal and Neonatal Edition*, vol. 88, no. 2, pp. F124–F127, 2003.

[3] A. L. Kelly, P. W. Lunt, F. Rodrigues et al., "Classification and genetic features of neonatal haemochromatosis: a study of 27 affected pedigrees and molecular analysis of genes implicated in iron metabolism," *Journal of Medical Genetics*, vol. 38, no. 9, pp. 599–610, 2001.

[4] P. Whitington and J. U. Hibbard, "High-dose immunoglobulin during pregnancy for recurrent neonatal haemochromatosis," *The Lancet*, vol. 364, pp. 1690–1698, 2004.

[5] M. E. Blohm, D. Vesterling-Hörner, G. Calaminus, and U. Göbel, "Alpha 1-fetoprotein (AFP) reference values in infants up to 2 years of age," *Pediatric Hematology and Oncology*, vol. 15, no. 2, pp. 135–142, 1998.

[6] A. Verloes, I. K. Temple, A. Hubert et al., "Recurrence of neonatal haemochromatosis in half sibs born of unaffected mothers," *Journal of Medical Genetics*, vol. 33, no. 6, pp. 444–449, 1996.

[7] A. S. Knisely, G. Mieli-Vergani, and P. Whitington, "Neonatal hemochromatosis," *Gastroenterology Clinics of North America*, vol. 32, no. 3, pp. 877–889, 2003.

[8] P. F. Whitington and P. Malladi, "Neonatal hemochromatosis: is it an alloimmune disease?" *Journal of Pediatric Gastroenterology and Nutrition*, vol. 40, no. 5, pp. 544–549, 2005.

[9] P. Whitington, "Fetal and infantile hemochromatosis," *Hepatology*, vol. 43, no. 4, pp. 654–660, 2006.

[10] E. B. Rand, S. J. Karpen, S. Kelly et al., "Treatment of neonatal hemochromatosis with exchange transfusion and intravenous immunoglobulin," *Journal of Pediatrics*, vol. 155, no. 4, pp. 566–571, 2009.

[11] E. Lopriore, M. L. Mearin, D. Oepkes, R. Devlieger, and P. Whitington, "Neonatal hemochromatosis: management, outcome, and prevention," *Prenatal Diagnosis*, vol. 33, no. 13, pp. 1221–1225, 2013.

[12] F. Babor, B. Hadzik, H. Stannigel, E. Mayatepek, and T. Hoehn, "Successful management of neonatal hemochromatosis by exchange transfusion and immunoglobulin: a case report," *Journal of Perinatology*, vol. 33, no. 1, pp. 83–85, 2013.

2

A Rare Clinical Course of Seronegative Pulmonary-Renal Syndrome

M. Fröhlich-Gildhoff,[1] W. J. Jabs,[2] C. Berhold,[1] M. K. Kuhlmann,[2] U. Ketterer,[1] S. Kische,[1] and H. Ince[1]

[1]*Department of Cardiology and Intensive Care Medicine, Vivantes Klinikum im Friedrichshain, Landsberger Allee 49, 10249 Berlin, Germany*
[2]*Department of Nephrology, Vivantes Klinikum im Friedrichshain, Landsberger Allee 49, 10249 Berlin, Germany*

Correspondence should be addressed to M. Fröhlich-Gildhoff; moritzfg@aol.com

Academic Editor: Zsolt Molnar

Purpose. Pulmonary-renal syndrome (PRS) is characterized by diffuse alveolar hemorrhage and rapidly progressive glomerulonephritis mainly due to autoimmune etiologies. Seronegative PRS is a challenging entity to the clinician, since early diagnosis may be missed leading to delayed appropriate treatment. *Materials and Methods.* We present the clinical course of a 77-year-old patient who was admitted under the suspected diagnosis of pneumogenic sepsis and septic renal failure with fever, dyspnea, and elevated CRP levels. The diagnosis of pulmonary-renal syndrome was initially missed because of the absence of autoantibodies in all serological findings. *Results.* Despite delayed initiation of immunosuppressive therapy and a prolonged period of dialysis and extracorporeal membrane oxygenation the patient recovered well and was released to a rehabilitation center with nearly normalized creatinine levels. The diagnosis of PRS was established by renal biopsy. *Conclusion.* This case illustrates the important differential diagnosis of seronegative pulmonary-renal syndrome in patients with pulmonary and renal impairment.

1. Introduction

Pulmonary-renal syndrome (PRS) is a rare clinical condition defined by rapidly progressive glomerulonephritis (RPGN) and diffuse alveolar hemorrhage (DAH). Its etiology is mainly autoimmune and can be categorized by serological findings (ANCA; anti-GBM antibodies) and renal or pulmonary biopsy. In over 90% of the cases autoantibodies (ANCA, anti-GBM) can be detected, making unclassified PRS a diagnostically challenging entity to the clinician.

We hereby present a case in which the diagnosis of seronegative PRS was established by a pauci-immune RPGN in renal biopsy, in a patient that had undergone immunosuppressive treatment eight months before admission to our hospital due to PRS, positive for both ANCA- and anti-GBM antibodies.

2. Case Report

We report the case of a 77-year-old German woman, who presented to our emergency department due to dyspnea, cough, hemoptysis, and fever.

Initial vital signs were as follows: RR 165/60, heart rate 89 bpm, SpO_2 96%, respiratory rate 28/min, and temperature 38.8°C.

Her past medical history included Goodpasture's syndrome, chronic obstructive pulmonary disease, smoking, high blood pressure, diabetes mellitus type II, and hyperlipidemia.

Eight months before admission the patient had suffered a dialysis-dependent acute kidney failure and an acute respiratory distress syndrome with long-term ventilation, caused by diffuse alveolar hemorrhage. Diagnosis of Goodpasture's syndrome was established by positive serological tests for anti-GBM antibodies and responded well to immunosuppressive therapy with corticoids and cyclophosphamide. Renal biopsy had not been performed, although ANCA also had been tested positive and therefore polyangiitis would have been a likely differential diagnosis. Due to persistent leucopenia and reoccurring infections cyclophosphamide therapy was stopped four months before admission to our hospital and had been replaced by 10 mg prednisolone per day.

On admission to our hospital laboratory results showed an elevation of C-reactive protein level (CRP 94 mg/L) and moderate renal impairment (creatinine 1,3 mg/dL, GFR 38 mL/min) without alterations in white or red blood cell count. Pulmonary radiography showed opacities in the left lower and middle lung zone and antibiotic treatment (Piperacillin/Tazobactam, Ciprofloxacin) was initiated under the suspected diagnosis of pneumonia under immunosuppression.

After progressive worsening of the patient's status with continuous dyspnea even under noninvasive ventilation (FiO_2 1.0), a further increase in CRP (264 mg/L) under escalated antibiotic treatment (vancomycin, Clarithromycin, and Voriconazole), and deteriorated renal function (creatinine 2.7 mg/dL), she was admitted to our intensive care unit on day 6 after hospitalization.

A chest-CT scan showed progressive, diffuse bilateral infiltrates, corresponding to a further decline of the respiratory situation and leading to intubation on day 12 (see Figure 1). Bronchoscopy, performed on day 13, showed signs of pulmonary hemorrhage with microbiological findings of *C. albicans* and no abnormal results in cytological testing.

Laboratory testing for Goodpasture's syndrome (anti-GBM ELISA, Alegria®, Orgentec) on days 5, 26, and 49 as well as vasculitis (MPO-ANCA, PR3-ANCA; ELISA Orgentec and ANAM; immunofluorescence) on days 13, 26, and 49 repeatedly showed negative results. The negative test results hereby differed from the serological testing in the patient's fulminant Goodpasture's syndrome which had occurred eight months earlier.

A further deterioration in pulmonary function with failing oxygenation under highly invasive ventilation protocols resulted in the application of a system of extracorporeal membrane oxygenation (ECMO, CARDIOHELP®, Maquet) on day 16; tracheotomy had been performed on day 26.

Failing kidney function required the initiation of continuous venovenous hemodialysis (CVVHD) from day 25. Urinary testing showed unselective proteinuria of 2300 mg/g creatinine (of which albumin 1462 mg/L) consistent with glomerular damage and mild hematuria (erythrocytes 97/μL) as well as leukocyturia (50/μL). Microscopic exploration showed hyaline cylinders.

In spite of high CRP levels (290 mg/L) we suspected a relapse of a pulmonary-renal syndrome with pulmonary hemorrhage rather than an infection because of low PCT levels and a drop of hemoglobin from 12.6 to 8.1 g/dL within 8 days due to alveolar bleeding. Moreover, the patient showed no clinical improvement under long-lasting broad antibiotic treatment.

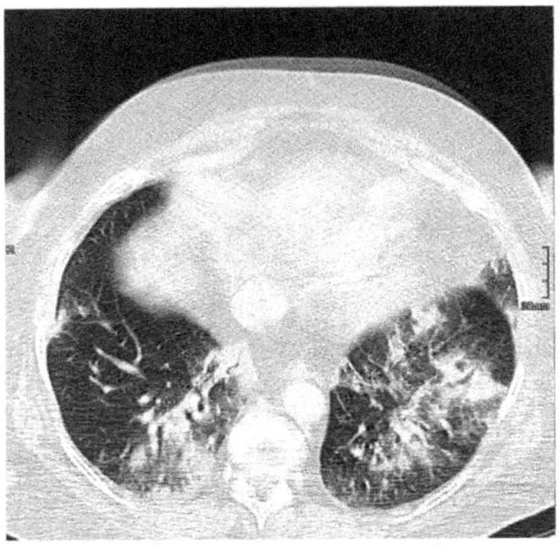

FIGURE 1: Illustrating diffuse bilateral infiltrates of the lung.

Despite repeatedly negative results in laboratory testing for anti-GBM and ANCA a therapy with methylprednisolone (1 g/d) was started on day 26, continued for three days, and followed by a therapy with prednisolone 80 mg per day. It was accompanied by the start of plasma exchange for the duration of 6 days as well as the application of 750 mg of cyclophosphamide on day 31. Under this regime of immunosuppressive therapy the pulmonary and renal function rapidly improved leading to the termination of ECMO therapy and the alternation from CVVHD to intermittent hemodialysis on day 33, which had to be continued until day 50. CRP levels also dropped significantly from 290 to 36 mg/L.

The course of the patient was then complicated by a pneumogenic septic shock with the detection of MRSA in a bronchoalveolar lavage and blood cultures. The situation was stabilized under an escalation of the antibiotic regime to vancomycin and imipenem.

After septic thrombopenia and the impaired hemostatic situation had been improved, renal biopsy was performed on day 44 and revealed scarred intra- and extracapillary glomerulonephritis (crescents) of the pauci-immune type, coherent with rapidly progressive glomerulonephritis and polyangiitis. It also showed diffuse potentially reversible tubular damage and mild benign nephrosclerosis. Despite repetitive dilutions no linear deposition of IgG was observed on the basement membrane by immunofluorescence microscopy.

After the diagnosis of RPGN had histologically been established immunosuppressive therapy was continued with MabThera (Rituximab 1000 mg on days 65 and 79).

Under antibiotic and immunosuppressive therapy the patient's status continually improved. The mobilization of the patient, which initially was complicated by a proximal tetraparesis due to critical illness myopathy (MRI-scan on day 53 showed no signs of myelopathy), eventually showed progress and she could be released to a rehabilitation center on day 104 after admission with a maintenance dosage of prednisolone of 15 mg/d.

Pulmonary function had normalized entirely by the date of discharge. The kidneys showed only moderate impairment (creatinine 1.27 mg/dL; GFR 41 mL/min). The urinalysis showed persistent proteinuria of 888 mg/g creatinine with no further hematuria, probably due to scarred glomeruli.

3. Discussion

Pulmonary-renal syndrome (PRS) is rare and describes the clinical cooccurrence of renal impairment due to glomerulonephritis and a decrease in pulmonary function due to diffuse alveolar hemorrhage. The underlying causes of PRS are heterogeneous and contain a group of autoimmune disorders, which are mainly classified by the detection of antibodies, renal or lung biopsy, or cytological findings in bronchoalveolar lavage. They mainly include ANCA-associated small vessel vasculitis (such as Wegener's granulomatosis, microscopic polyangiitis, and Churg-Strauss vasculitis), Goodpasture's syndrome, systemic lupus erythematosus, Henoch-Schönlein purpura, or cryoglobulinemia. Other rare causes of PRS include drug-induced vasculitis (e.g., propylthiouracil) and subacute endocarditis.

As a particularly deleterious cause for PRS Goodpasture's syndrome is defined by the occurrence of antibodies against the alpha3-NC1-domain of collagen IV in the glomerular or alveolar basement membrane and typical linear deposition of IgG (rarely IgA) observed in part of the basement membrane by immunofluorescence microscopy.

Studies suggest that over 90% of patients with PRS present with one or more antibodies (ANCA, anti-GBM) in the serum, making PRS with no detection of antibodies as in the above-mentioned case very rare [1–3], albeit there have been reports of seronegative relapses in anti-GBM disease after immunosuppressive therapy [4].

In this case two differential diagnoses for the underlying clinical condition seemed possible: a seronegative relapse of anti-GBM disease—which initially had only been diagnosed by circulating antibodies but without renal biopsy—as well as a seronegative ANCA-vasculitis with RPGN and diffuse alveolar hemorrhage.

In the renal biopsy, scarred crescents without linear deposition of IgG along the basement membrane emphasize the possibility of a seronegative ANCA-vasculitis with RPGN. A significant improvement of renal function as in our patient seems to make the diagnosis of an ANCA-associated vasculitis more probable, as anti-GBM diseases like Goodpasture's syndrome usually lead to severe renal impairment and long-term dialysis [5, 6], particularly when treatment is delayed. On the other hand, there have been suggestions that a seronegative anti-GBM disease with predominant pulmonary involvement, as in our case, might be more common than generally suspected and case reports of seroconversion to seronegativity in anti-GBM diseases treated with immunosuppression exist [4]. Additionally, a correlation between cigarette smoking and pulmonary hemorrhage in patients with anti-GBM disease has been demonstrated by Donaghy and Rees [7].

Even though testing by commercially available ELISA-kits, as in our case, is generally considered to be a highly sensitive method for the detection of anti-GBM, the possibility of existing anti-GBM in very low concentrations remains. Furthermore, no tests other than ELISA (e.g., immunoblot, indirect immunofluorescence) have been performed. Importantly, an incidence of 2-3% of seronegative anti-GBM has been estimated by the British reference laboratory for anti-GBM antibodies [8].

The prognosis of PRS derives from simple center experience with low patient numbers. Gallagher et al. observed a 36% early mortality in their single-center study ($n = 14$) with a mean follow-up of four years [9]. Predictors of poor prognosis are crescents in >50% of glomeruli in renal biopsy, serum creatinine levels >5-6 mg/dL, oliguria, or the need for acute dialysis on admission. The early establishment of the correct diagnosis followed by prompt immunosuppressive therapy and plasma exchange are pivotal points in the treatment of PRS.

Diagnosis was missed early in our case due to the complete absence of antibodies, delaying renal biopsy which was performed after immunosuppressive therapy had been started on day 26. The observation of almost complete convalescence of renal and pulmonary function despite delayed disease-specific treatment makes this case very interesting.

Clinical data concerning the course of patients with seronegative PRS is scarce and in most cases the disease leads to end-stage renal failure [1, 10, 11]. As in PRS with a detection of specific antibodies or typical findings in renal or pulmonary biopsy, treatment with corticoids and cyclophosphamide is the basis of any therapy for patients with a suspected seronegative PRS. In some cases plasma exchange has been described to have beneficial effects on patients with seronegative and therefore uncategorizable PRS [12].

4. Conclusion

Seronegative pulmonary-renal syndrome is a rare but potentially life-threatening clinical condition. As the diagnostic process is complicated by the absence of antibodies, end-stage renal disease and even death have been reported as a common consequence of seronegative PRS. This case illustrates the rare instance of renal and pulmonary recovery after therapy with corticosteroids, cyclophosphamide, plasma exchange, and Rituximab, notwithstanding the temporary necessity for renal and pulmonary supportive therapy by dialysis and ECMO.

Consent

Written informed consent was obtained from the patient for the publication of this case report and any accompanying images.

Authors' Contributions

M. Fröhlich-Gildhoff and W. J. Jabs contributed equally.

References

[1] H. Yamaguchi, A. Shirakami, T. Haku et al., "Pulmonary-renal syndrome with negative ANCAs and anti-GBM antibody," *Case Reports in Nephrology*, vol. 2013, Article ID 434531, 6 pages, 2013.

[2] R. Sexena, P. Bygren, B. Arvastson, and J. Wieslander, "Circulating autoantibodies as serological markers in the differential diagnosis of pulmonary renal syndrome," *Journal of Internal Medicine*, vol. 238, no. 2, pp. 143–152, 1995.

[3] J. L. Niles, E. P. Böttinger, G. R. Saurina et al., "The syndrome of lung hemorrhage and nephritis is usually an ANCA-associated condition," *Archives of Internal Medicine*, vol. 156, no. 4, pp. 440–445, 1996.

[4] D. J. Serisier, R. C. W. Wong, and J. G. Armstrong, "Alveolar haemorrhage in anti-glomerular basement membrane disease without detectable antibodies by conventional assays," *Thorax*, vol. 61, no. 7, pp. 636–639, 2006.

[5] F. Madore, J. M. Lazarus, and H. R. Brady, "Therapeutic plasma exchange in renal diseases," *Journal of the American Society of Nephrology*, vol. 7, no. 3, pp. 367–386, 1996.

[6] P. Biesenbach, R. Kain, K. Derfler et al., "Long-term outcome of anti-glomerular basement membrane antibody disease treated with immunoadsorption," *PLoS ONE*, vol. 9, no. 7, article e103568, 2014.

[7] M. Donaghy and A. J. Rees, "Cigarette smoking and lung haemorrhage in glomerulonephritis caused by autoantibodies to glomerular basement membrane," *The Lancet*, vol. 322, no. 8364, pp. 1390–1393, 1983.

[8] A. D. Salama, T. Dougan, J. B. Levy et al., "Goodpasture's disease in the absence of circulating anti-glomerular basement membrane antibodies as detected by standard techniques," *American Journal of Kidney Diseases*, vol. 39, no. 6, pp. 1162–1167, 2002.

[9] H. Gallagher, J. T. C. Kwan, and D. R. W. Jayne, "Pulmonary renal syndrome: a 4-year, single-center experience," *American Journal of Kidney Diseases*, vol. 39, no. 1, pp. 42–47, 2002.

[10] S. C. West, N. Arulkumaran, P. W. Ind, and C. D. Pusey, "Pulmonary-renal syndrome: a life threatening but treatable condition," *Postgraduate Medical Journal*, vol. 89, no. 1051, pp. 274–283, 2013.

[11] Y. Uji, T. Shimizu, T. Yoshioka, H. Yamamoto, Y. Endo, and T. Tani, "A case report of pulmonary-renal syndrome treated with continuous hemodiafiltration and hemodialysis," *Therapeutic Apheresis and Dialysis*, vol. 10, no. 5, pp. 467–471, 2006.

[12] C.-C. Wang, J.-C. Shiang, M.-K. Tsai et al., "Prompt plasmapheresis successfully rescue pulmonary-renal syndrome caused by ANCA-negative microscopic polyangiitis," *Clinical Rheumatology*, vol. 28, no. 12, pp. 1457–1460, 2009.

3

Malignant Catatonia Warrants Early Psychiatric-Critical Care Collaborative Management: Two Cases and Literature Review

Julia Park,[1] Josh Tan,[1] Sylvia Krzeminski,[1] Maryam Hazeghazam,[2] Meghana Bandlamuri,[1] and Richard W. Carlson[1,3,4]

[1] *Department of Medicine, Maricopa Medical Center, Phoenix, AZ, USA*
[2] *Department of Psychiatry, Maricopa Medical Center, Phoenix, AZ, USA*
[3] *College of Medicine, University of Arizona, Phoenix, AZ, USA*
[4] *College of Medicine, Mayo Clinic, Scottsdale, AZ, USA*

Correspondence should be addressed to Julia Park; tojuliapark@gmail.com

Academic Editor: Gil Klinger

Malignant catatonia (MC) is a life-threatening manifestation which can occur in the setting of an underlying neuropsychiatric syndrome or general medical illness and shares clinical and pathophysiological features and medical comorbidities with the Neuroleptic Malignant Syndrome (NMS). The subsequent diagnosis and definitive therapy of MC are typically delayed, which increases morbidity and mortality. We present two cases of MC and review recent literature of MC and NMS, illustrating factors which delay diagnosis and management. When clinical features suggest MC or NMS, we propose early critical care consultation and stabilization with collaborative psychiatric management.

1. Introduction

MC, previously termed "lethal catatonia," is the most severe manifestation within the spectrum of catatonic syndromes. Catatonia is defined as immobility, rigidity, mutism, posturing, excessive motor activity, stupor, negativism, staring, and echolalia. MC represents a life-threatening manifestation that can develop in the context of a neuropsychiatric syndrome or general medical illness and includes behavioral changes, movement disturbances, and autonomic dysregulation [1–5].

Schizophrenia is the most commonly cited inciting condition, although major depression and various toxic-metabolic etiologies have also been implicated. Typical symptoms of MC include catalepsy, stupor, mutism, waxy flexibility, negativism, posturing, autonomic dysfunction, rigidity, fever, and muscle injury [4, 6–10].

Although the potential lethal consequences of MC are well known, diagnosis is often difficult and typically delayed. Due to the fact that both MC and NMS have similar biochemical and neuropharmacologic disturbances, similar clinical features can be seen in both disorders. Current concepts suggest that NMS and malignant catatonia represent a spectrum with biochemical and neuropharmacologic disturbances that involve disturbances of dopamine and GABAergic receptors [11, 12].

The predominant pathophysiology of NMS is central dopamine receptor blockade in the hypothalamus that results in autonomic dysregulation [13]. However, as many patients with either MC or NMS respond to benzodiazepines, it is thought that both share a single biochemical pathway of reduced $GABA_A$ inhibition of the frontal corticostriatal tracts [6, 12].

Standard treatment of MC includes initiation of benzodiazepines and electroconvulsive therapy (ECT). Prior to this approach, the mortality of MC typically exceeded 50%. Recent management strategies which include combined ECT and benzodiazepines result in decreases in morbidity and mortality [14]. Dąbrowski et al. reported full recovery to baseline in up to 80% of patients with this approach [14, 15]. However delay of treatment continues to remain a concerning issue, as recent studies reveal treatment delays are on average 60 days prior to initiation of treatment with benzodiazepines or ECT [16].

We describe two patients with MC that illustrate the problems of misdiagnosis, delayed identifications, and management of critical cardiopulmonary and metabolic disturbances which lead to further delays of definitive therapy. We review clinical features and current management of MC and NMS and propose guidelines for prompt and ongoing collaborative management between psychiatry and critical care services when MC is suspected.

1.1. Case 1. A 55-year-old male with a history of schizophrenia who was noncompliant of medications presented to the hospital with catatonic symptoms and autonomic instability. During the hospital stay, the patient exhibited worsening catatonia, mutism, anorexia, leukocytosis, and autonomic instability. He was treated with rehydration, electrolyte replacement, antibiotics for aspiration pneumonia, and nasoenteral tube feeding. The clinical picture was initially thought to be most consistent with catatonic schizophrenia and the patient was transferred to a psychiatric facility for ECT after fourteen days of medical therapy. During ECT without protection of airway, the patient developed a cardiac arrest with pulseless ventricular tachycardia that was related to dehydration, pneumonia, and sepsis. He was resuscitated, intubated, and admitted to the ICU. The patient had additional complications which included Methicillin Sensitive *Staphylococcus aureus* (MSSA) pneumonia, ischemic colitis, and Vancomycin Resistant Enterococcus (VRE) Urinary Tract Infection (UTI). From the initial presentation to the facility after the cardiac arrest, the diagnosis was delayed by 15 days. Benzodiazepines were initiated at the time of diagnosis and ECT was initiated after medical stabilization that required a total of 26 days from initial presentation. The patient slowly showed signs of clinical improvement in mental status. He was discharged to an extended care inpatient psychiatric facility after nearly 16 months of inpatient psychiatric care.

1.2. Case 2. A 20-year-old male was admitted to inpatient psychiatric care due to acute psychosis. He developed autonomic instability, catatonia, mutism, waxy flexibility, and agitation. He was transferred to a medicine service for treatment of suspected MC. After a poor response to benzodiazepines, institution of ECT was delayed from the time of diagnosis by seventeen days. The delay in treatment was primarily related to exclusion of alternative diagnoses. Critical care was consulted 7 days after admission for MC. The patient was ultimately given a total of 12 sessions of ECT, which resulted in gradual improvement after each dose. During the hospital stay, the patient developed multiple complications including dehydration, urinary tract infection due to *Escherichia coli*, and aspiration pneumonia. The patient's mental status improved. He was discharged home after 4 months of inpatient psychiatric care.

2. Review and Discussion

The cases presented herein illustrate that MC is an emergent and life-threatening illness that is accompanied by multiorgan dysfunction, including cardiopulmonary and metabolic defects requiring concurrent ICU and psychiatric care [1]. Both patients presented in this article suffered severe complications, including cardiopulmonary crisis, infections, dehydration, and prolonged hospital stay. We propose that suspicion of MC should prompt collaborative psychiatric and critical care management with early use of ECT if there is inadequate response to benzodiazepines therapy [7, 17].

We agree with Tuerlings et al. that the high mortality associated with MC is related in part to the failure of rapid and efficient exclusion of alternative diagnoses [18, 19]. The authors reported that delay to first and second treatment was 15 and 60 days, respectively [18]. A decrease in this delay should be a major goal as treatment delay and longer duration of symptoms without treatment have been associated with poorer clinical response [20]. We propose that organic causes be promptly narrowed by psychiatric history, medications changes, overdoses, metabolic derangements, and central nervous system infections. Any suspicion of MC should prompt admission to a critical care unit and stabilization as the diagnostic process proceeds. Currently, no biomarkers exist for MC to assist in diagnosis, although there appears to be an association of elevated d-dimer in the disease [21]. Use of this marker may be helpful in expediting detection of this disease. We further postulate that favorable outcomes may be achieved by collaborative management between critical care and psychiatry, with earlier detection and exclusion of alternative diagnoses, and prompt management of complications associated with MC.

Similarities exist between NMS and MC, thus confounding the picture of a potentially life-threatening disease. Therefore, a comparison of the differences and similarities between the two syndromes is warranted [7, 22–26]. Typically, MC is predominantly manifested by bizarre behavior and mutism, posturing, and catalepsy and with psychiatric disturbances. In contrast, NMS is classically linked to exposure of a neuroleptic agent or atypical antipsychotic, with prominent features of rigidity, autonomic dysfunction, fever, and stupor [4, 11, 26]. Both MC and NMS may lead to muscle injury, aspiration, and metabolic disturbance due to hyperthermia and altered mental status. However, prodromes of MC have psychiatric undertones of psychosis, agitation, stupor, mutism, or anxiety while NMS would present with acute onset of autonomic instability and extrapyramidal side effects after antipsychotic exposure [4, 11, 26]. Therefore, if history excludes exposure to an antipsychotic, the diagnosis of MC would be apparent [3, 4, 22].

Unfortunately, this defining characteristic may be blurred for providers, as the majority of patients with MC have a psychiatric history and therefore have been treated with antipsychotics.

In many instances, the deduction to the diagnosis of NMS or MC requires several days, during which time patients may

Table 1: Complications associated with patient's clinical features.

Clinical features	Potential complications
Autonomic instability	Hypotension, hypertension, arrhythmias, myocardial ischemia, rhabdomyolysis, hemodynamic instability
Decreased movement	Thromboembolic disease, pressure ulcers, rhabdomyolysis
Decreased oral intake	Dehydration, hypovolemia, electrolyte derangements, inability to take oral medications
Catalepsy	Decreased airway clearance, aspiration pneumonia, hypoxemia, pneumonia

already develop medical comorbidities. One of the largest series that reviewed the clinical course of MC was reported by Tuerlings et al. (2010). The mean lag time from first catatonic symptoms to first treatment with benzodiazepines or ECT was 15 days on average. The time lag between the first and second treatment was approximately 27 days. Reported overall improvement with treatment was 76% and complete remission was 58%. Mortality was 9%. Virtually, it is impossible to differentiate NMS from MC on clinical presentation and course. Importantly, both conditions require the same treatment consisting of withdrawal of antipsychotics and initiation of benzodiazepines and ECT as first-line treatments [18].

Whether the diagnosis is MC or NMS, both of the conditions have life-threatening consequences and therefore need ICU and psychiatric collaboration. Alternative diagnoses must be swiftly excluded and benzodiazepines must be utilized within 24 hours as first-line treatment for MC and NMS [18]. Additionally, ECT has been theorized as effective second- if not first-line treatment. ECT should be supplemented after or additionally with benzodiazepines [27–29]. Benzodiazepines are theorized to improve MC and NMS by increasing $GABA_A$ activity. Likewise, the use of ECT may involve GABA activity by inducing a neural storm with increased GABA transmission and clinical improvement [7, 27].

MC typically has a complicated course that involves multiple medical comorbid conditions such as dehydration, aspiration pneumonia, electrolyte disturbances, cardiopulmonary instability, and thromboembolic phenomena. Table 1 lists symptoms and clinical features and associated complications. Psychiatric care including the use of benzodiazepines and ECT is important, but identifying the appropriate level of medical support is crucial [5, 6, 19]. The psychiatric management includes sedative care and ECT treatment for up to 7 days. We suggest that critical care consultation and protection of airway may facilitate safer ECT by close monitoring and prompt care for life-threatening arrhythmias, airway protection, aspiration, hemodynamic instability, ischemia, and fluid and electrolyte balance [17, 30, 31].

3. Conclusion

The previous cases and review describe MC from diagnosis to management and complications. Delays or subtherapeutic treatment with ineffective and less aggressive methods increase morbidity and mortality [16].

No standardized treatment protocols exist for complications of MC, thus causing a delay and hindrance to proper treatment. Prompt identification and institution of life-saving treatments of ECT and pharmacologic therapy with benzodiazepines can be achieved by early critical care consultation for appropriate level of care that is equipped for attention to fluid-electrolyte balance, cardiopulmonary stabilization, and thermoregulation.

References

[1] M. A. Oldham and H. B. Lee, "Catatonia vis-à-vis delirium: the significance of recognizing catatonia in altered mental status," *General Hospital Psychiatry*, vol. 37, no. 6, pp. 554–559, 2015.

[2] P. M. Sadr, M. Hazeghazam, M. Bailon et al., "Management of a severe form of malignant catatonia: useful lessons in diagnosis and management," in *Proceedings of the American Psychiatric Association Annual Meeting*, San Francisco, Calif, USA, March 2013.

[3] V. R. Velamoor, "Neuroleptic malignant syndrome," *Drug Safety*, vol. 19, no. 1, pp. 73–82, 1998.

[4] E. Castillo, R. T. Rubin, and E. Holsboer-Trachsler, "Clinical differentiation between lethal catatonia and neuroleptic malignant syndrome," *The American Journal of Psychiatry*, vol. 146, no. 3, pp. 324–328, 1989.

[5] A. F. Gross, F. A. Smith, and T. A. Stern, "Dread complications of catatonia: a case discussion and review of the literature," *Primary Care Companion to the Journal of Clinical Psychiatry*, vol. 10, no. 2, pp. 153–155, 2008.

[6] G. L. Fricchione, A. F. Gross, J. C. Huffman, G. Bush, and T. A. Stern, "Catatonia, neuroleptic malignant syndrome, and serotonin syndrome," in *Massachusetts General Hospital Handbook of General Hospital Psychiatry*, Elsevier, 2016, https://www clinicalkey.com/#!/content/book/3-s2.0-B9781437719277000212.

[7] M. Fink, "Catatonia: a syndrome appears, disappears, and is rediscovered," *Canadian Journal of Psychiatry*, vol. 54, no. 7, pp. 437–445, 2009.

[8] M. M. Woodbury and M. A. Woodbury, "Neuroleptic-induced catatonia as a stage in the progression toward neuroleptic malignant syndrome," *Journal of the American Academy of Child and Adolescent Psychiatry*, vol. 31, no. 6, pp. 1161–1164, 1992.

[9] W. W. Fleischhacker, B. Unterweger, J. M. Kane, and H. Hinterhuber, "The neuroleptic malignant syndrome and its differentiation from lethal catatonia," *Acta Psychiatrica Scandinavica*, vol. 81, no. 1, pp. 3–5, 1990.

[10] A. Francis, "Catatonia: diagnosis, classification, and treatment," *Current Psychiatry Reports*, vol. 12, no. 3, pp. 180–185, 2010.

[11] F. U. Lang, S. Lang, T. Becker, and M. Jäger, "Neuroleptic malignant syndrome or catatonia? Trying to solve the catatonic dilemma," *Psychopharmacology*, vol. 232, no. 1, pp. 1–5, 2015.

[12] B. T. Carroll, "The universal field hypothesis of catatonia and neuroleptic malignant syndrome," *CNS Spectrums*, vol. 5, no. 7, pp. 26–33, 2000.

[13] G. Northoff, "Catatonia and neuroleptic malignant syndrome: psychopathology and pathophysiology," *Journal of Neural Transmission*, vol. 109, no. 12, pp. 1453–1467, 2002.

[14] M. Dąbrowski and T. Parnowski, "Clinical analysis of safety and effectiveness of electroconvulsive therapy," *Psychiatria Polska*, vol. 46, no. 3, pp. 345–360, 2012.

[15] O. Freudenreich, S. H. Nejad, A. Francis, and G. L. Fricchione, "Psychosis, mania, and catatonia," in *Textbook of Psychosomatic Medicine: Psychiatric Care of the Medically Ill*, J. L. Levenson, Ed., American Psychiatric, Washington, DC, USA, 2011.

[16] J. A. Van Waarde, J. H. A. M. Tuerlings, B. Verwey, and R. C. Van Der Mast, "Electroconvulsive therapy for catatonia: treatment characteristics and outcomes in 27 patients," *The Journal of ECT*, vol. 26, no. 4, pp. 248–252, 2010.

[17] F. Luchini, P. Medda, M. Mariani, M. Mauri, C. Toni, and G. Perugi, "Electroconvulsive therapy in catatonic patients: efficacy and predictors of response," *World Journal of Psychiatry*, vol. 5, no. 2, pp. 182–192, 2015.

[18] J. H. A. M. Tuerlings, J. A. van Waarde, and B. Verwey, "A retrospective study of 34 catatonic patients: analysis of clinical care and treatment," *General Hospital Psychiatry*, vol. 32, no. 6, pp. 631–635, 2010.

[19] B. K. Boyarsky, M. Fuller, and T. Early, "Malignant catatonia-induced respiratory failure with response to ECT," *The Journal of ECT*, vol. 15, no. 3, pp. 232–236, 1999.

[20] J. C. Narayanaswamy, P. Tibrewal, A. Zutshi, R. Srinivasaraju, and S. B. Math, "Clinical predictors of response to treatment in catatonia," *General Hospital Psychiatry*, vol. 34, no. 3, pp. 312–316, 2012.

[21] S. Haouzir, X. Lemoine, M. Petit et al., "The role of coagulation marker fibrin D-dimer in early diagnosis of catatonia," *Psychiatry Research*, vol. 168, no. 1, pp. 78–85, 2009.

[22] J. W. Y. Lee, "Neuroleptic-induced catatonia: clinical presentation, response to benzodiazepines, and relationship to neuroleptic malignant syndrome," *Journal of Clinical Psychopharmacology*, vol. 30, no. 1, pp. 3–10, 2010.

[23] D. A. C. White, "Catatonia and the neuroleptic malignant syndrome—a single entity?" *The British Journal of Psychiatry*, vol. 161, pp. 558–560, 1992.

[24] V. R. Velamoor, "Neuroleptic malignant syndrome," *Drug Safety*, vol. 19, no. 1, pp. 73–82, 1998.

[25] M. Koch, S. Chandragiri, S. Rizvi, G. Petrides, and A. Francis, "Catatonic signs in neuroleptic malignant syndrome," *Comprehensive Psychiatry*, vol. 41, no. 1, pp. 73–75, 2000.

[26] S. Caroff, S. Mann, and P. Keck, "Specific treatment of the neuroleptic malignant syndrome," *Biological Psychiatry*, vol. 44, no. 6, pp. 378–381, 1998.

[27] S. C. Mann, S. N. Caroff, H. R. Bleier, R. E. Antelo, and H. Un, "Electroconvulsive therapy of the lethal catatonia syndrome," *Convulsive Therapy*, vol. 6, no. 3, pp. 239–247, 1990.

[28] J. M. Hawkins, K. J. Archer, S. M. Strakowski, and P. E. Keck Jr., "Somatic treatment of catatonia," *International Journal of Psychiatry in Medicine*, vol. 25, no. 4, pp. 345–369, 1995.

[29] J. M. Davis, P. G. Janicak, P. Sakkas, C. Gilmore, and Z. Wang, "Electroconvulsive therapy in the treatment of the neuroleptic malignant syndrome," *Convulsive Therapy*, vol. 7, no. 2, pp. 111–120, 1991.

[30] W. V. McCall, S. C. Mann, F. E. Shelp, and S. N. Caroff, "Fatal pulmonary embolism in the catatonic syndrome: two case reports and a literature review," *The Journal of Clinical Psychiatry*, vol. 56, no. 1, pp. 21–25, 1995.

[31] W. M. McDonald, T. W. Meeks, W. V. McCall, and C. F. Zorumski, "Electroconvulsive therapy," in *The American Psychiatric Publishing Textbook of Psychopharmacology*, 2009, http://psychiatryonline.org/doi/full/10.1176/appi.books.9781585623860.as44.

4

Euglycemic Diabetic Ketoacidosis in the ICU: 3 Case Reports and Review of Literature

Pablo Lucero [1] **and Sebastián Chapela** [1,2]

[1] *Hospital Británico de Buenos Aires, Intensive Care Services, Argentina*
[2] *Universidad de Buenos Aires, Facultad de Medicina, Departamento de Bioquimica Humana, Argentina*

Correspondence should be addressed to Pablo Lucero; pdlucero@hbritanico.com.ar

Academic Editor: Chiara Lazzeri

Diabetic ketoacidosis (DKA) is an acute complication of diabetes mellitus, both type I and type II, as well as other types with diabetes such gestacional diabetes mellitus. It is characterized by blood glucose levels greater than 250 mg/dL and metabolic acidosis (pH < 7.3 and serum bicarbonate < 15 mEq/dL) with an increased anion gap and the presence of ketone bodies in the blood or urine. Within this pathology, there is a subgroup of pathologies which are characterized by being present with no signs of hyperglycemia, posing a diagnostic challenge due to the absence of the main sign of the pathology and the diversity of their pathophysiology. In this article, we will present 3 clinical cases with 3 different forms of clinical presentation: a case of DKA in pregnancy, a case of DKA associated with the use of sodium-glucose cotransporter 2 (SGLT-2) inhibitors, and a third case related to sepsis, together with a narrative review of the literature on the topic.

1. Introduction

Diabetic ketoacidosis is an acute complication of diabetes. It is diagnosed through laboratory results showing metabolic acidosis with an increased gap and evidence of ketone bodies in the blood or urine. Most of the time, it is present with hyperglycemia. The clinical presentation of this pathology is diverse, going from abdominal pain to sensory deterioration and coma [1].

The pathophysiology of hyperglycemia in diabetic ketoacidosis has 3 cornerstones: an increase in gluconeogenesis, an increase in glycogenolysis and a decrease in peripheral glucose uptake due to a decrease in insulin action in the receptors or a decrease in insulin levels [1]. This prevents glucose from being transported inside the cells and being used as metabolic fuel. On the other hand, there is an increase in lipolysis and fatty acids start being used in the liver, where they are metabolized into ketone bodies, which can be absorbed by most cells [1].

Diabetic ketoacidosis is defined by the presence of blood glucose levels greater than 250 mg/dL, being this the main finding, associated with metabolic acidosis (pH < 7.3 and serum bicarbonate < 15 mEq/dL) with an increased anion gap and the presence of ketone bodies in the blood and/or urine [1]. There are different forms of presentation which differ from the usual presentation described in literature, such as the case of normoglycemic diabetic ketoacidosis. This pathology was first described by Munro in 1973 [2] but, in his work, he studied patients with blood glucose levels under 300mg/dL. Currently, the definition is in line with blood glucose levels under 250mg/dL [1]. 6% of patients show blood glucose levels under 300 mg/dL and around 1% of patients show levels under 180 mg/dL. The most common causes are insulin administration on the way to the hospital and fasting [1]. The diagnosis and treatment of this pathology require a deep pathophysiological knowledge, since it can be triggered by different etiologies. In this review, we will present 3 completely different cases of normoglycemic diabetic ketoacidosis.

2. Clinical Case 1

A 22-year-old woman with a history of diabetes mellitus (diagnosed at 7 years old) is treated with insulin glargine and

Table 1: Patients' laboratory results upon admission to the ICU.

	Na+ (mEq/L)	K+ (mEq/L)	Cl (mEq/L)	pH	HCO2 (mEq/L)	BE (mEq/L)	GAP	Δ CL	Ketonemia	Blood Glucose (mg/dL)
CASE 1	137	4.9	102	7.25	10	-14.9	23	-0.75	+	153
CASE 2	142	3.9	108	7.13	2	-23.7	32	1.5	+	165
CASE 3	140	4.8	109	7.28	7.3	-16.8	23	4	+	132

with good adherence to treatment, with hypothyroidism and 2 previous ICU admissions due to diabetic ketoacidosis in which blood glucose levels were greater than 300 mg/dL.

The patient sought consultation due to vomiting and abdominal pain 12 hours after onset. Upon physical examination, the abdomen was distended with diffuse pain and no signs of peritoneal irritation. Laboratory results showed the following values: pH: 7.25; bicarbonate: 10 mEq/dL; BE: -14.9; blood glucose: 153 mg/dL and positive ketonemia. Admission laboratory results are shown in Table 1. Upon diagnosis of normoglycemic diabetic ketoacidosis, in the context of menstrual cycle alterations and with the aim of studying the trigger, beta subunit of human chorionic gonadotropin levels was requested: 98.928 IU/L. A transvaginal ultrasound was performed and showed a gestational sac with an embryo inside. Reanimation was started with parenteral crystalloids administered at 250 mL/h during 24 hrs. It was interspersed isotonic saline solutions and polyelectrolyte solutions. Total income is 7000 ml / 24 hs. Urinary volume is 2750 ml / 24 hs. Positive balance is 4250 ml/24 hs. Continuous insulin infusion was started, as described in literature (receiving a total of 100 IU in 48 hrs). Progress was shown with improvement of the clinical condition and lab monitoring every 8 hours: pH 7.47; bicarbonate of 22 mEq/dL with blood glucose levels in the normal range (< 200 mg/dl). The usual insulin glargine dose was restored and the patient was discharged.

3. Clinical Case 2

A 50-year-old woman, former smoker, with a history of arterial hypertension, dyslipidemia, left side breast cancer which required chemotherapy, radiation therapy and surgery, hypothyroidism, and diabetes mellitus type II, is treated with 10 mg/day of Dapagliflozin, 1000 mg of Metformin every 12 hours, and NPH insulin at 40 and 60 IU. The patient sought consultation due to abdominal pain, diarrhea and fever. Upon admission, the patient was alert, tachypneic, and being with diffuse abdominal pain with no sign of peritoneal irritation. An abdominal ultrasound was requested and showed the gallbladder with multiple gallstones. The complete laboratory results are shown in Table 1. In the context of leukocytosis, acute kidney failure, and severe metabolic acidosis, the patient was admitted to the ICU with a diagnosis of sepsis. Due to the presence of metabolic acidosis with a gap of 32, a ketonemia test was requested. The result was positive and the patient was diagnosed with euglycemic diabetic ketoacidosis.

After starting treatment with a continuous insulin infusion pump and the administration of water, the patient was discharged from the hospital after 5 days.

4. Clinical Case 3

A 74-year-old male patient with a history of arterial hypertension, noninsulin dependent diabetes mellitus medicated with oral hypoglycemic agents, ischemic cardiopathology with stent placement, nonoliguric chronic kidney failure, and cryptogenic liver cirrhosis required a liver transplant and subsequently suffered portal vein thrombosis requiring anticoagulation. The patient sought consultation after 3 days of passing liquid stools, together with emesis. He denied having fever spikes and, on that date, consulted the emergency ward of this institution, to which he was admitted feeling alert, with AT: 130/64, heart rate: 108 beats per minute, and SO2: 97% on room air. Upon physical examination, the patient was alert, tachypneic, and being with dry mucous membranes. Admission laboratory results are shown in Table 1. A ketonemia test was requested and the result was positive. The clinical presentation was interpreted as dehydration secondary to gastrointestinal losses and euglycemic diabetic ketoacidosis. Reanimation was started with crystalloids, a continuous insulin infusion pump, and the administration of intravenous bicarbonate. After 48 hrs, the patient presented DKA resolution criteria.

5. Discussion

Euglycemic diabetic ketoacidosis is a diagnostic challenge for treating physicians, since there is no hyperglycemia. On the other hand, there are many causes of metabolic acidosis in patients in the intensive care unit, although, when analyzing the gap, high gap metabolic acidosis is less frequent than hyperchloremic acidosis [14]. Therefore, knowing this pathology is key when treating patients with diabetes. Moreover, the triggers are varied and, in this study, we presented 3 cases with two different pathophysiological causes.

This pathology is triggered by multiple causes (Table 2). The following pathophysiological mechanisms are common to all causes: a decrease in insulin action or secretion with a decrease in total glucose uptake at a cellular level, an increase in the production of counterregulatory hormones, and a decrease in glucose production by the liver or an increase in the excretion of glucose in the urine [11, 12].

TABLE 2: Causes of euglycemic diabetic ketoacidosis.

Fasting
Insulin use prior to hospital admission
Pregnancy
Use of SGLT-2
Cocaine abuse
Pancreatitis
Cirrhosis
Use of insulin pump
Sepsis

SGLT-2: type 2 sodium-glucose cotransporter.

The first case deals with a diabetic patient who is pregnant. The reason that normal pregnancy increases blood glucose levels is based on the progressive insulin resistance, which normally occurs. This resistance also explains the worsening of pregestational diabetes during pregnancy. The exogenous insulin loses its effect as the pregnancy progresses. These effects are attributable to the destruction of insulin by the kidney and the action of placental insulinases.

At the beginning of pregnancy, insulin maintains its activity, and its concentration increases due to the hyperplasia of the Beta cells of the pancreatic islets, induced by the high concentrations of placental steroids. As a result of these changes, fasting glycemia decreases. The main effect of insulin in the body is to allow the storage of nutritious substrates to meet energy needs. The provision of food is intermittent while the consumption of energy is constant from where the need for storage arises. The maternal organism stores energies in the form of glucose and fats. In addition, human chorionic gonadotropin causes vomiting, which causes fasting, dehydration, and metabolic acidosis [15].

As pregnancy progresses, the activity of the usual counterregulatory hormones such as human placental lactogen, which is synthesized by the trophoblast and released into the circulation, reduces maternal sensitivity to insulin, increasing postprandial blood glucose levels [10]. Progesterone reduces gastrointestinal motility, increasing glucose uptake [10]. In addition, there is a decrease in insulin sensitivity, particularly in the third trimester, caused by hormonal changes that occur during pregnancy like an increase in estrogen, progestogens, human placental lactogen, and secretion of TNF-α [15]. All these mechanisms induce hyperglycemia in pregnancy. On the other hand, the placenta and the fetus absorb large amounts of glucose, decreasing blood levels when fasting. This leads to an increase in the secretion of maternal fatty acids and their subsequent metabolization in ketone bodies [12].

During late pregnancy, the fetus dramatically increases its glucose-based metabolism and accentuates its anabolic process by growth. On the other hand, the maternal metabolism enters a catabolic process in order to send all the glucose to the fetus through the placenta, using fat as the primary fuel. In the diabetic patient, the decrease in insulin intake profoundly affects the general metabolism, particularly at the level of liver, muscle, and adipose tissue, which are insulin essential action points. The absence of this hormone causes distortion of homeostasis. Plasma levels of glucose, free fatty acids and ketones rise to extreme figures, plasma pH and bicarbonate fall dangerously and there is marked loss of fatty tissue and body mass. If insulin levels are not restored, this case can lead to death.

Finally, the respiratory alkalosis that occurs during pregnancy increases the urinary excretion of bicarbonate, reducing the ability to buffer pH changes caused by the increase in body ketone production [16]. This leads to euglycemic diabetic ketoacidosis in pregnancy.

The incidence rate of diabetic ketoacidosis in all pregnant women with diabetes varies between 0.5 and 3%, being more common in patients with type I diabetes. However, there are more and more cases of patients with type II and gestational diabetes [17, 18]. In a unicentric study in which 223,000 deliveries were analyzed, 14,532 (6.5%) were complicated due to diabetes, just 33 patients presented 40 diabetic ketoacidosis episodes with average blood glucose levels of 380 mg/dL on admission, whereas only 3 cases presented euglycemic diabetic ketoacidosis [18]. The different cases of euglycemic diabetic ketoacidosis in pregnancy, their initial diagnosis, and clinical presentations are analyzed in Table 3. In contrast to most of the cases described in literature, our patient presented with DKA during the first trimester.

The harmful effects of ketoacidosis on the fetus are caused by ketone bodies and glucose passing the placental barrier, dehydration, which leads to decreased placental perfusion and electrolyte imbalance [18]. Fetal acidosis is caused by hyperglycemia, which leads to osmotic diuresis and fetal intravascular volume depletion. Fetal hyperinsulinemia increases oxygen uptake. A decrease in 2,3-DPG increases oxygen affinity for hemoglobin, reducing the amount of oxygen available to the fetus and generating hypoxia [17]. The electrolyte disturbance can not only generate maternal arrhythmias with a subsequent decrease in placental perfusion, but also generate fetal arrhythmias and risk of cardiorespiratory arrest [18]. Although there are no studies that show the long-term consequences for the fetuses born alive, neurodevelopmental alterations were observed. In contrast to other pregnancy complications, a hasty delivery with DKA would be harmful to the fetus. Therefore, it is recommended to stabilize the mother first [19]. Some studies state that fetal mortality in patients with DKA can reach 9% [15] and perinatal mortality is between 9 and 35% [17]. However, there are also authors who argue that ketoacidosis is not associated with a higher mortality rate during the first trimester, nor with a higher rate of malformations [20].

The mainstay of treatment does not differ from the treatment for hyperglycemic ketoacidosis, that is, hydration and insulin. The difference is that, in order to maintain blood glucose levels, the amount of glucose administered must be higher and, in the case of pregnant patients, care should be taken to maintain blood glucose levels suitable for fetal welfare. There is evidence in literature showing that a value of 250 mg/dL (Baha M. 2014) or values between 100 and 150 mg/dL would accomplish this [20].

The second case is associated with the use of sodium-glucose cotransporter 2 (SGLT-2) inhibitors. The incidence

TABLE 3: Cases of euglycemic DKA in pregnancy reported in literature.

Author and Year	Age of the Patient	Gestational Week	Obstetric History	History of Diabetes	Blood Glucose upon Admission	pH upon Admission	Triggering Factor
Darhambulla, 2012 [3]	30 years old	33	Pregnancy: 2 Borns: ?	Recently diagnosed gestational diabetes	95 mg/dL	7.17	Urinary tract infection
Cardonell, 2016 [4]	33 years old	35	Pregnancy: 3 Borns: 2	Diabetes type II	134 mg/dL	7.02	Unknown. During delivery
Chico, 2008 [5]	29 years old	24	Pregnancy: 2 Borns: 1	Diabetes type I	93 mg/dL	7.22	Unknown. During delivery
Franke, 2001 [6]	23 years old	32	Unknown	Recently diagnosed gestational diabetes	127 mg/dL	7.2	Influenza A infection
Kamalakannan, 2003 [7]	28 years old	36	Pregnancy: 5 Borns:?	Diabetes type I	234 mg/dL	7.1	Vomiting and poor treatment adherence
Karpate, 2013 [8]	25 years old	37	Pregnancy: 1 Borns: 0	None	102 mg/dL	N/A	Fasting
Napoli, 2011 [9]	26 years old	34	Pregnancy: 3 Borns: 2	Diabetes type I	211 mg/dL	7.25	Altered food intake
Oliver, 2007 [10]	29 years old	28	N/A	Diabetes type I	205 mg/dL	7.15	Bronchial pneumonia
Rivas, 2016 [11, 12]	39 years old	32	Pregnancy: 2 Borns: 1	None	225 mg/dL	7.15	Emesis
Tarif, 2007 [13]	37 years old	35	Pregnancy: 5 Borns: 4	Gestational diabetes	78 mg/dL	7.32	Emesis and diarrhea

rate of diabetic ketoacidosis in patients treated with SGLT-2 inhibitors varies between 0.16 and 0.76 cases per 1000 patients per year [21, 22]. In a review of literature, 46 cases of diabetic ketoacidosis associated with the use of SGLT-2 were found and, in 70% of the cases, the ketoacidosis was euglycemic [23]. The main mechanism of action is the inhibition of glucose uptake in proximal tubules, increasing glycosuria [24]. In addition, SGLT-2 inhibitors significantly increase plasma glucagon levels through a decrease in paracrine inhibition of insulin and possibly due to the inhibition of glucose transport into pancreatic α cells by SGLT-2 [22]. At the same time, they decrease 3-hydroxybutyrate and acetoacetate elimination at the kidney level [24–28]. Moreover, when blood glucose levels decrease, patients that are being treated with insulin decrease its administration. Therefore, counterregulatory hormone effects predominate, resulting in a lower inhibition of lipolysis and lipogenesis and, thereby, triggering euglycemic ketoacidosis [29–31]. Case reports include the 3 drugs of the gliflozin class: Dapagliflozin [24, 25, 29–35], Canagliflozin [26–28, 31–33, 36, 37], and Empagliflozin [38–40].

The last case deals with a patient with diabetic ketoacidosis associated with dehydration. During fasting, when hepatic glycogen is consumed, there is no source of glucose release into the bloodstream; however, lipolysis and the generation of ketone bodies are increased [41]. Dehydration is also a factor that contributes to the development of euglycemia [42].

Luethi et al. [43] analyzed blood glucose levels, arterial blood gases, and ketonemia and ketonuria in 60 critically ill patients. 63% of the patients developed some degree of ketosis (β-hydroxybutyric levels greater than 0.6 mmol/L). In 12% of the patients, it was severe (greater than 3 mmol/L), and 33 % developed ketonuria (which was only severe in 2% of the patients). The prevalence of ketosis was the same in those who presented glucose peaks greater than 180 mg/dL and those who did not [1]. It is interesting to observe that, in this study [44], only 2 patients out of the 60 developed ketoacidosis based on the criteria set forth by the Joint British Diabetes Society [45] and none of them did, based on the ADA's criteria [11].

Finally, another possible cause of euglycemic ketoacidosis is the administration of insulin before being admitted to the hospital [42]. Other causes are pancreatic lesions developed during pancreatitis due to alcohol consumption, associated with the fasting required by this condition, which would explain the development of euglycemic ketoacidosis [42]. Furthermore, cocaine abuse causes an increase in the secretion of cortisol and noradrenaline by the adrenal gland, in addition to the anorexigenic effects of this drug, which lead to fasting [46].

6. Conclusion

Euglycemic diabetic ketoacidosis is a diagnostic challenge, not only due to the absence of its most important sign, which is hyperglycemia, but also due to its varied triggers. Knowing the different contexts in which it can occur will allow us to suspect euglycemic diabetic ketoacidosis and begin rapid and adequate treatment of the precipitating cause, as well as aggressive hydration, glucose homeostasis through insulin administration, and the adjustment of electrolyte imbalances. A delay results in serious complications both in the fetus (in the case of gestational diabetes) and in the patient, increasing in-hospital morbidity and mortality.

References

[1] A. E. Kitabchi, G. E. Umpierrez, J. M. Miles, and J. N. Fisher, "Hyperglycemic crises in adult patients with diabetes," *Diabetes Care*, vol. 32, no. 7, pp. 1335–1343, 2009.

[2] J. F. Munro, I. W. Campbell, A. C. McCuish, and L. J. Duncan, "Euglycaemic diabetic ketoacidosis," *British Medical Journal*, vol. 2, no. 5866, pp. 578–580, 1973.

[3] B. Franke, D. Carr, and M. H. Hatem, "A case of euglycaemic diabetic ketoacidosis in pregnancy," *Diabetic Medicine*, vol. 18, no. 10, pp. 858-859, 2001.

[4] D. Kamalakannan, V. Baskar, D. M. Barton, and T. A. M. Abdu, "Diabetic ketoacidosis in pregnancy," *Postgraduate Medical Journal*, vol. 79, no. 934, pp. 454–457, 2003.

[5] S. J. Karpate, H. Morsi, M. Shehmar, J. Dale, and C. Patel, "Euglycemic ketoacidosis in pregnancy and its management: case report and review of literature," *European Journal of Obstetrics & Gynecology and Reproductive Biology*, vol. 171, no. 2, pp. 386-387, 2013.

[6] A. Napoli, M. Framarino, A. Colatrella et al., "Eating disorders and diabetic ketoacidosis in a pregnant woman with type 1 diabetes: A case report," *Eating and Weight Disorders*, vol. 16, no. 2, pp. e146–e149, 2011.

[7] R. Oliver, P. Jagadeesan, R. J. Howard, and K. Nikookam, "Euglycaemic diabetic ketoacidosis in pregnancy: An unusual presentation," *Journal of Obstetrics & Gynaecology*, vol. 27, no. 3, p. 308, 2007.

[8] M. Rivas M, P. Belmar Z, P. Durruty A, L. Sanhueza M, and G. López S, "Cetoacidosis diabética normoglicémica en el embarazo: Caso clínico," *Revista Médica de Chile*, vol. 144, no. 10, pp. 1360–1364, 2016.

[9] N. Tarif and W. Al Badr, "Euglycemic diabetic ketoacidosis in pregnancy," *Saudi Journal of Kidney Disease and Transplantation*, vol. 18, no. 4, pp. 590–593, 2007.

[10] B. M. Sibai and O. A. Viteri, "Diabetic ketoacidosis in pregnancy," *Obstetrics & Gynecology*, vol. 123, no. 1, pp. 167–178, 2014.

[11] A. A. Abdin, M. Hamza, M. S. Khan, and A. Ahmed, "ase Report Euglycemic Diabetic Ketoacidosis in a Patient with Cocaine Intoxication," *Case Reports Crit Care*, vol. 2016, 2016.

[12] F. Le Neveu, B. Hywel, and J. N. Harvey, "Euglycaemic ketoacidosis in patients with and without diabetes," *Practical Diabetes*, vol. 30, no. 4, pp. 167–171, 2013.

[13] V. N. Baş, S. Uytun, and Y. A. Torun, "Diabetic euglycemic ketoacidosis in newly diagnosed type 1 diabetes mellitus during Ramadan fasting," *Journal of Pediatric Endocrinology and Metabolism*, vol. 28, no. 3-4, pp. 333–335, 2015.

[14] P. M. Gauthier and H. M. Szerlip, "Metabolic acidosis in the intensive care unit," *Critical Care Clinics*, vol. 18, no. 2, pp. 289–308, 2002.

[15] M. G. Dalfrà, S. Burlina, G. Sartore, and A. Lapolla, "Ketoacidosis in diabetic pregnancy," *The Journal of Maternal-Fetal and Neonatal Medicine*, vol. 29, no. 17, pp. 2889–2895, 2016.

[16] S. N. Bryant, C. L. Herrera, D. B. Nelson, and F. G. Cunningham, "Diabetic ketoacidosis complicating pregnancy," *Journal of Neonatal-Perinatal Medicine*, vol. 10, no. 1, pp. 17–23, 2017.

[17] M. d. Veciana, "Diabetes ketoacidosis in pregnancy," *Seminars in Perinatology*, vol. 37, no. 4, pp. 267–273, 2013.

[18] J. A. Parker and D. L. Conway, "Diabetic Ketoacidosis in Pregnancy," *Obstetrics and Gynecology Clinics of North America*, vol. 34, no. 3, pp. 533–543, 2007.

[19] M. A. Carroll and E. R. Yeomans, "Diabetic ketoacidosis in pregnancy," *Critical Care Medicine*, vol. 33, no. 10, pp. S347–S353, 2005.

[20] R. M. Goldenberg, L. D. Berard, A. Y. Cheng et al., "SGLT2 Inhibitor-associated Diabetic Ketoacidosis: Clinical Review and Recommendations for Prevention and Diagnosis," *Clinical Therapeutics*, vol. 38, no. 12, pp. 2654–2664.el, 2016.

[21] H. Qiu, A. Novikov, and V. Vallon, "Ketosis and diabetic ketoacidosis in response to SGLT2 inhibitors: Basic mechanisms and therapeutic perspectives," *Diabetes/Metabolism Research and Reviews*, vol. 33, no. 5, p. e2886, 2017.

[22] J. A. Levine, S. L. Karam, and G. Aleppo, "SGLT2-I in the Hospital Setting: Diabetic Ketoacidosis and Other Benefits and Concerns," *Current Diabetes Reports*, vol. 17, no. 7, 2017.

[23] J. Rosenstock and E. Ferrannini, "Euglycemic diabetic ketoacidosis: a predictable, detectable, and preventable safety concern with SGLT2 inhibitors," *Diabetes Care*, vol. 38, no. 9, pp. 1638–1642, 2015.

[24] J. Adachi, Y. Inaba, and C. Maki, "Euglycemic diabetic ketoacidosis with persistent diuresis treated with canagliflozin," *Internal Medicine*, vol. 56, no. 2, pp. 187–190, 2017.

[25] D. A. Kelmenson, K. Burr, Y. Azhar, P. Reynolds, C. A. Baker, and N. Rasouli, "Euglycemic Diabetic Ketoacidosis With Prolonged Glucosuria Associated With the Sodium-Glucose Cotransporter-2 Canagliflozin," *Journal of Investigative Medicine High Impact Case Reports*, vol. 5, no. 2, p. 232470961771273, 2017.

[26] M. Jazi and G. Porfiris, "Euglycemic diabetic ketoacidosis in type 2 diabetes treated with a sodium-glucose cotransporter-2 inhibitor," *Canadian Family Physician*, vol. 62, no. 9, pp. 722–e517, 2016.

[27] S. Maraka, A. E. Kearns, N. E. N. Kittah, and D. T. O'Keeffe, "Recurrent euglycemic diabetic ketoacidosis after discontinuation of sodium-glucose cotransporter 2 inhibitor," *Diabetes Research and Clinical Practice*, vol. 118, pp. 77-78, 2016.

[28] S. Ullah, N. Khan, H. Zeb, and H. Tahir, "Metabolic ketoacidosis with normal blood glucose: A rare complication of sodium-glucose cotransporter 2 inhibitors," *SAGE Open Medical Case Reports*, vol. 4, p. 2050313X1667525, 2016.

[29] H. Storgaard, J. I. Bagger, F. K. Knop, T. Vilsbøll, and J. Rungby, "Diabetic Ketoacidosis in a Patient with Type 2 Diabetes After Initiation of Sodium-Glucose Cotransporter 2 Inhibitor Treatment," *Basic & Clinical Pharmacology & Toxicology*, vol. 118, no. 2, pp. 168–170, 2016.

[30] S. Pujara and A. Ioachimescu, "Prolonged Ketosis in a Patient With Euglycemic Diabetic Ketoacidosis Secondary to Dapagliflozin," *Journal of Investigative Medicine High Impact Case Reports*, vol. 5, no. 2, p. 232470961771004, 2017.

[31] F. Brown and T. McColl, "Euglycemic Diabetic Ketoacidosis Secondary to Dapagliflozin Use: A Case Report," *The Journal of Emergency Medicine*, vol. 54, no. 1, pp. 109–111, 2018.

[32] M. Ahmed, M. J. McKenna, and R. K. Crowley, "Diabetic ketoacidosis in patients with type 2 diabetes recently commenced on sglt-2 inhibitors: An ongoing concerN," *Endocrine practice : official journal of the American College of Endocrinology and the American Association of Clinical Endocrinologists*, vol. 23, no. 4, pp. 506–508, 2017.

[33] S. Dizon, E. J. Keely, J. Malcolm, and A. Arnaout, "Insights Into the Recognition and Management of SGLT2-Inhibitor-Associated Ketoacidosis: It's Not Just Euglycemic Diabetic Ketoacidosis," *Canadian Journal of Diabetes*, vol. 41, no. 5, pp. 499–503, 2017.

[34] M. Kim, "Euglycemic diabetic ketoacidosis with SGLT2 inhibitors in lean type 2 diabetes," *Integrative Obesity and Diabetes*, vol. 2, no. 4, 2016.

[35] A. L. Peters, E. O. Buschur, J. B. Buse, P. Cohan, J. C. Diner, and I. B. Hirsch, "Euglycemic diabetic ketoacidosis: a potential complication of treatment with sodium-glucose cotransporter 2 inhibition," *Diabetes Care*, vol. 38, no. 9, pp. 1687–1693, 2015.

[36] J. S. Kum-Nji, A. R. Gosmanov, H. Steinberg, and S. Dagogo-Jack, "Hyperglycemic, high anion-gap metabolic acidosis in patients receiving SGLT-2 inhibitors for diabetes management," *Journal of Diabetes and its Complications*, vol. 31, no. 3, pp. 611–614, 2017.

[37] Alehegn Gelaye, Abdallah Haidar, Christina Kassab, Syed Kazmi, and Prabhat Sinha, "Severe Ketoacidosis Associated with Canagliflozin (Invokana): A Safety Concern," *Case Reports in Critical Care*, vol. 2016, Article ID 1656182, 3 pages, 2016.

[38] N. Candelario and J. Wykretowicz, "The DKA that wasn't: A case of euglycemic diabetic ketoacidosis due to empagliflozin," *Oxford Medical Case Reports*, vol. 2016, no. 7, pp. 144–146, 2016.

[39] P. D. Farjo, K. M. Kidd, and J. L. Reece, "A case of euglycemic diabetic ketoacidosis following long-term empagliflozin therapy," *Diabetes Care*, vol. 39, no. 10, pp. e165–e166, 2016.

[40] W. Ogawa and K. Sakaguchi, "Euglycemic diabetic ketoacidosis induced by SGLT2 inhibitors: Possible mechanism and contributing factors," *Journal of Diabetes Investigation*, vol. 7, no. 2, pp. 135–138, 2016.

[41] J. Prater and J. Chaiban, "Euglycemic diabetic ketoacidosis with acute pancreatitis in a patient not known to have diabetes," *Endocrine Practice*, vol. 1, no. 2, pp. e88–e91, 2015.

[42] N. Luethi, L. Cioccari, M. Crisman, R. Bellomo, G. M. Eastwood, and J. Mårtensson, "Prevalence of ketosis, ketonuria, and ketoacidosis during liberal glycemic control in critically ill patients with diabetes: an observational study," *Critical Care*, vol. 20, no. 1, 2016.

[43] M. W. Savage, K. K. Dhatariya, A. Kilvert et al., "Joint British Diabetes Societies guideline for the management of diabetic ketoacidosis," *Diabetic Medicine*, vol. 28, no. 5, pp. 508–515, 2011.

[44] S. Darbhamulla, N. Shah, and P. Bosio, "Euglycaemic ketoacidosis in a patient with gestational diabetes," *European Journal of Obstetrics & Gynecology and Reproductive Biology*, vol. 163, no. 1, pp. 118-119, 2012.

[45] B. L. Cardonell, B. A. Marks, and M. H. Entrup, "Normoglycemic Diabetic Ketoacidosis in a Pregnant Patient with Type II Diabetes Mellitus Presenting for Emergent Cesarean Delivery," *A & A case reports*, vol. 6, no. 8, pp. 228-229, 2016.

[46] M. Chico, S. N. Levine, and D. F. Lewis, "Normoglycemic diabetic ketoacidosis in pregnancy," *Journal of Perinatology*, vol. 28, no. 4, pp. 310–312, 2008.

Critical Care Management for Novel 2019 SARS-CoV-2 and HCoV-NL63 Coinfection in a Young Immunocompromised Patient: A Chicago Experience

Alejandro Sanchez-Nadales,[1] Miguel Treminio-Quezada,[1] Hasan Abad,[1] Jessica Navarro-Motta,[1] Pamela Contreras-Chavez,[1] Anil Kachru,[2] and Chae Chu[2]

[1]*Department of Medicine, Advocate Illinois Masonic Medical Center, Chicago, IL 60657, USA*
[2]*Department of Pulmonology and Critical Care Medicine, Advocate Illinois Masonic Medical Center, Chicago, IL 60657, USA*

Correspondence should be addressed to Alejandro Sanchez-Nadales; alejandro.sanchez2@advocatehealth.com

Academic Editor: Mehmet Doganay

Background. SARS-CoV-2 is a newly emerged virus that has spread rapidly, exhibiting tremendous morbidity and mortality. Some potential pharmaceutical targets have been identified but are still lacking proper validation. *Case Presentation.* We describe the case of a young, immunosuppressed and critically ill patient with previous Influenza B infection, requiring extracorporeal membrane oxygenation, which was then followed, in the succeeding months, by SARS-CoV-2 infection complicated by severe adult respiratory distress syndrome. Her clinical course exhibited complications, including pulmonary embolism, acute kidney injury, pneumothorax, pneumomediastinum, multiple cardiac arrests, and eventually death. *Conclusion.* Coinfection with other respiratory pathogens and opportunistic infections are possible.

1. Introduction

The Severe Acute Respiratory Syndrome Coronavirus 2 (SARS-CoV-2) is a newly emerged virus that first appeared in December 2019. This pathogen has spread rapidly, exhibiting tremendous morbidity and mortality to such an extent that the World Health Organization (WHO) officially declared the coronavirus disease 2019 (COVID-19) a pandemic on March 11, 2020. Since the first reported death in China on January 11, 2020, over 2.6 million cases and more than 188,000 deaths have been reported worldwide [1]. Dry cough is the most common symptom of COVID-19, with fever occurring in just half of patients [2]. The respiratory, renal, and cardiovascular systems are often affected. Some cases require specialized management in the ICU, with mechanical ventilatory support, with a mortality rate above 50% in those cases, as reported in Europe [3].

Identified risk factors for developing ARDS includes older age, male sex, hypertension, diabetes mellitus (DM), and chronic kidney disease (CKD) [4]. In our patient, type 1 DM, hypertension, and CKD secondary to IgG4 tubulointerstitial nephritis were the associated risk factors. Currently, COVID-19 caused by SARS-CoV-2 remains without definitive therapies. Some potential pharmaceutical targets have been identified but are still lacking proper validation through randomized clinical trials [5]. In this case report, we describe a young, immunosuppressed and critically ill female patient with previous Influenza B infection, which was then followed by SARS-CoV-2 infection in the following months.

2. Case Presentation

We describe the case of a 22-year-old Hispanic female, with a past medical history of biopsy-proven IgG4 tubulointerstitial nephritis on corticosteroids since December 2019, hypertension, and type 1 diabetes mellitus who was admitted twice, since the beginning of 2020, for severe acute hypoxic respiratory failure.

During her first admission in January, she presented with complaints of nonproductive cough and shortness of breath

(SOB) and was diagnosed with multifocal pneumonia, secondary to Influenza B, diagnosed via PCR from a nasopharyngeal swab. She was treated with oseltamivir for 10 days and 3 doses of baloxavir marboxil for double influenza coverage, empiric ceftriaxone-azithromycin for 5 days for superimposed bacterial infection, and continued on sulfamethoxazole/trimethoprim for Pneumocystis prophylaxis. Hospitalization was complicated by hypoxic respiratory failure requiring endotracheal intubation and subsequent venous-venous extracorporeal membrane oxygenation (ECMO) for 5 days, prior to recovery and discharge, after a fourteen-day hospital course.

Two months after initial admission, the patient presented to the emergency department (ED) with one day of SOB, fever, chills, and dry cough. She developed progressive hypoxia requiring endotracheal intubation in the ED despite noninvasive mechanical ventilation. Sequential chest X-ray (CXR) during the first 24 hours did not correlate with the degree of hypoxemia (Figure 1). She was immediately transferred to the ICU, requiring vasopressors and ventilatory support, demanding constant adjustments to the ventilator settings. Early neuromuscular blockade was achieved with rocuronium for management of early severe adult respiratory distress syndrome (ARDS). She was empirically started on meropenem IV 1000 mg Q12H, azithromycin IV 500 mg daily, and hydroxychloroquine 200 mg Q12H, for empiric bacterial and COVID-19 pneumonia treatment, and continued on sulfamethoxazole/trimethoprim 800 mg/160 mg daily for Pneumocystis prophylaxis and prednisone 40 mg daily for IgG nephropathy. Infectious disease and nephrology were consulted. Initial and trended laboratory findings are further elucidated in (Table 1).

On day one of ICU admission, the patient went into pulseless electrical activity (PEA) due to profound hypoxemia and severe acidemia, requiring advanced cardiac life support (ACLS), followed by hypothermic protocol for 24 hours, and initiation of Furosemide drip for volume overload in a setting of acute kidney injury (AKI). ECMO was deemed not appropriate at that time. Additionally, a transthoracic echocardiogram (TTE) performed the same day revealed reduced ejection fraction (EF) estimated at 40-45% and a new free-flowing pericardial effusion (Figure 2). Interestingly, the viral panel evidenced coinfection with the human coronavirus (HCoV) NL63 strain and the novel 2019 coronavirus SARS-CoV-2 via PCR from a nasopharyngeal swab.

As days progressed, she required hemodialysis support and therapeutic anticoagulation for suspected pulmonary embolism (PE). After seven days in the ICU, she spiked fevers along with worsening leukocytosis, and uptrending inflammatory markers, particularly ferritin, D-dimer, and LDH. She was restarted on antibiotics (vancomycin/piperacillin-tazobactam) for possible ventilator-associated pneumonia and received one dose of tocilizumab. Over the next days, her urine output increased and her PEEP and FiO2 requirements were weaned. By day 18, voriconazole was added due to increasing suspicion for superimposed invasive fungal infection, as the sputum cultures grew yeast and β-D-glucan levels were elevated.

Two days later, she was started on inhaled nitric oxide with decreasing doses of corticosteroids. After 25 days in the ICU, she achieved hemodynamically stability, without vasopressors. She improved to the point where she was arousable and able to engage in meaningful social interaction, when off sedation. A follow-up TTE showed recovered EF up to 55-60% and reduction of the pericardial effusion. Chronic hypoxic respiratory failure was attributed to extensive lung fibrosis, with lung transplant as the only definitive management. She underwent tracheostomy. Her urine output was fair while on IV furosemide, but her serum creatinine remained elevated without dialysis, indicating some lack of clearance. She underwent twenty-four-hour urine collection for creatinine clearance which shows markedly decreased kidney function with a creatinine clearance of 6 mL/min. A long-term dialysis catheter (permcath) was placed for continuity of hemodialysis sessions.

After 30 days, a computed tomography (CT) of the chest confirmed a segmental pulmonary embolism, along with a large right pneumothorax, small left pneumomediastinum, and leftward mediastinal shift (Figure 3), which were not observed in daily CXR (Figure 4). A thoracostomy tube was placed. The next day, however, she suffered multiple episodes of arrest with PEA, and despite multiple resuscitations, she perished.

3. Discussion

The SARS-CoV-2 has infected over 2.4 million people across 180 countries in four months, with a huge spectrum of clinical presentations, laboratory results, and imaging [6]. The virus invades cells by binding and crossing the cellular membrane via the angiotensin-converting enzyme 2 (ACE-2) receptor. This protein is found in high concentrations within the lungs and the heart [7, 8]. The most common complications of COVID-19 infection include ARDS, acute kidney injury, electrolyte disturbances, hypoproteinemia, and coagulation disorders. The median time from admission to the development of ARDS was two days in Wuhan, China [4].

Today, seven different coronavirus strains are known to infect humans including the HCoV-229E, HCoV-NL63, and HCoV-HKU1 [9, 10]. By itself, HCoV-NL63 infection has been described mostly in people <30 years [11–13]. This virus may have the ability to evade the human immune system, and thus patients with baseline immunosuppression are susceptible for more severe disease [13]. Coinfection with two different HCoV strains has not been commonly reported, but recently, a study limited to Northern California evidenced that 3.5% infected by SARS-CoV-2 were also positive for other types of coronavirus [14]. Further, superimposed invasive fungal infections have been reported in severe COVID-19, especially on those patients treated with tocilizumab who were concurrently taking immunosuppressive therapy, as it was the case in our patient.

Hospitalized patients with COVID-19 have a high prevalence of kidney disease, and this correlates with greater in-hospital mortality [15]. Decreased kidney function is usually temporal and likely related to profound hypoxia [16]. Avoidance of nephrotoxins to preserve remnant kidney function is indispensable. Furthermore, evidence in patients with DM and SARS-CoV-2 is still limited [17]; however, previous

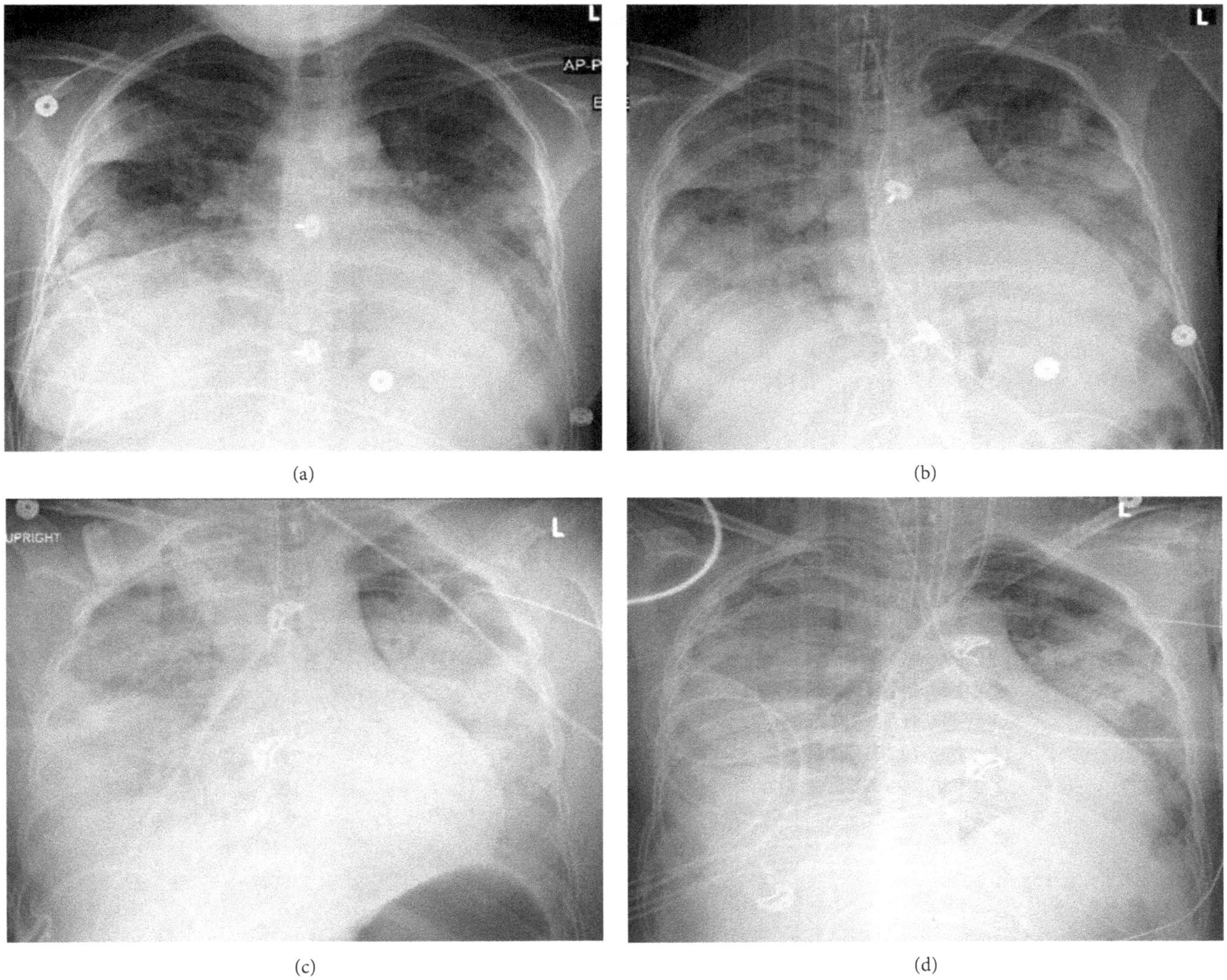

FIGURE 1: CXR with different infiltrates patterns during the initial 24 hours. (a) Initial CXR at the ED revealing bilateral pleural effusions with bibasilar consolidation, increased interstitial markings suggestive of bilateral pulmonary edema, and enlarged cardiac silhouette. (b) After endotracheal intubation with increased confluent airspace opacities throughout the mid-to-lower lungs, findings suggestive of worsening pulmonary edema vs. multifocal infectious process. (c) Findings with the tip of the endotracheal tube overlying the proximal right mainstem bronchus. Otherwise; the bilateral diffuse confluent airspace opacities are not significantly changed. Tube was retracted 2 cm. (d) Ten hours after initial CXR revealing stable cardiomegaly, persistent bilateral fluffy infiltrates and consolidation, and persistent obscuration of the right hemidiaphragm.

studies have described that individuals with diabetes are at risk of severe respiratory disease when infected with respiratory viruses [18].

Abnormal liver function panel, coagulopathies, and elevated D-dimer are common laboratory findings, arising suspicion for disseminated microthrombotic events and collateral pulmonary embolism [19]. Initiating empiric therapeutic anticoagulation is a topic of discussion, without clear criteria. However, recent evidence pointed to the types of patients who will receive the biggest benefits from anticoagulation [20, 21]. It should be started after carefully weighing the risks and benefits as was done in our young patient, who started therapeutic doses of heparin based on elevated D-dimer associated with increasing oxygen demands, prior to PE being confirmed.

Multiple medical interventions have emerged as possible therapeutic targets for SARS-CoV-2, such as corticosteroids, antibiotics, antiparasitics, antiretrovirals, and IL-6 inhibitors. Nevertheless, the safety and efficacy of these agents have not been properly validated through a rigorous randomized clinical trial. Regardless, several retrospective, observational, and open-label studies are now available, although with disparate results. One confusing area has been the use of corticosteroids, which are beneficial in critically ill patients, but their use has been debated in SARS-CoV-2. In our case, the patient was previously on prednisone for tubulointerstitial nephritis, and therapy was continued mostly to avoid adrenal insufficiency [22–24].

Hydroxychloroquine and azithromycin combination shows no clinical benefits in hospitalized patients with severe

Table 1: Laboratory test results.

Laboratory test	Reference values	Day 1	Day 3	Day 6	Day 9	Day 12	Day 15	Day 18	Day 21	Day 24	Day 25
White blood cells ($\times 10^9$/L)	4.2-11	11.9	18.9	12.5	11.1	13.1	15	20.4	22.8	19.8	20.1
Absolute neutrophiles (×103)	1.8-7.7	11.1	18	11.8	9.8	12.2	13.7	19	20.1	17.4	16.8
Absolute lymphocytes ($\times 10^3$)	1.4-4.0	0.5	0.6	0.5	0.9	1	0.6	1	0.7	0.6	0.4
C-reactive protein (mg/dL)	<1		30.1	17.8		10.4	3.4	8.2		1	0.5
Ferritin (ng/mL)	8-252	711	14,188	7,350	4,844	5,127	2,736	2,868	2,927	4,720	5,607
LDH (U/L)	82-240	341	693	862	811	683		715	515		
Procalcitonin (ng/mL)	<0.1	11.32		3.01	3.89	1.22		1.63			
Interleukin-6 (pg/mL)	≤5			16							
Troponin 1 (ng/mL)	<0.05	0.1	0.46	0.07							
NT-proBNP (pg/mL)	<451	30,860		18,041		22,398					
Creatinine (mg/dL)	0.51-0.95	4.87	5.09	5.92	3.73	3.29	4.3	3.04	3.11	2.85	3.01
eGFR (mL/min/1.73 m^3)	>90	12	11	9	16	19	14	21	20	23	21
D-dimer (μg/mL)	<0.57	1.08			14.52	8.23	5.85			3.74	4.42
AST (U/L)	<38	22		59		45	45	82	51	480	264
ALT (U/L)	<64	43		75		17	21	49	72	368	373
Total bilirubin (mg/dL)	0.2-1.0	0.2				0.2	0.2	0.3	0.3	3	4.2
Creatine kinase (U/L)	26-192					43					
Lactate (mmol/L)	0.0-2.0	2.6				1.4					
Triglycerides (mg/dL)	<115			450		315		166	246	672	
pH	7.35-7.45	7.31	7.32	7.36	7.37	7.37	7.33	7.37	7.38	7.38	7.26
PaCO2 (mmHg)	32-45	31	37	33	46	50	47	46	41	34	37
PaO2 (mmHg)	83-108	66	97	72	64	73	60	77	76	63	83
PaO2 to FiO2 ratio	300-500	66	162	120	128	122	86	110	126	157	165
PEEP		12	12	10	12	15	15	18	18	12	10
FiO2 (%)		100	60	60	50	60	70	70	60	40	50
(1,3)-beta-D-glucan (pg/mL)								138(+)			
HCoV-NL63		+									
Novel 2019 SARS-CoV-2		+									

eGFR: estimated glomerular filtration rate; AST: aspartate aminotransferase; ALT: alanine aminotransferase; LDH: lactate dehydrogenase; $PaCO_2$: partial pressure of carbon dioxide; PaO_2: partial pressure of oxygen; FiO_2: fraction of inspired oxygen; O_2 sat: oxygen saturation; PEEP: positive end-expiratory pressure.

COVID-19, despite in vitro antiviral activity [25]. SARS-CoV-2 provokes a hyperinflammatory syndrome with fatal hypercytokinemia (including IL-6) and multiorgan failure [26]. Tocilizumab achieved benefits in isolated cases of SARS-CoV-2 infection, but its overall safety and efficacy are currently being analyzed [27, 28]. Our patient rapidly progressed to ARDS, which precluded a favorable clinical response to antimicrobial therapy. In retrospect, other medications that may have helped our patient include the antiparasitic ivermectin and the antiretroviral remdesivir [29, 30].

A new interesting proposition from Dr. Gattinoni et al. [31, 32] reflects the possibility of different types of lung pathology. Based on his experience in Northern Italy, he stated that only 20 to 30% of patients fulfilled the criteria for severe ARDS. They describe two alternative classifications of ARDS, one referred to as Type L, an unusual form of ARDS, characterized by low elastase, high lung compliance, low ventilation : perfusion ratio, low lung weight without significant edema, and low recruitability and a second referred as Type H, characterized by high elastase, low lung compliance, and significant right-to-left shunt, which is more consistent with standard ARDS criteria. Further, it has been hypothesized that SARS-CoV-2 Type L pneumonia may be related to the loss of regulation of alveoli perfusion and the loss of the hypoxic pulmonary vasoconstriction effect; the reason why it is feasible to think that inhaled nitric oxide may play a pivotal role. In the former guideline, a trial of inhaled pulmonary vasodilator as rescue therapy in patients with severe ARDS and persistent hypoxemia is suggested; however, its routine use is not recommended. In our case, the trial of nitric oxide improved the oxygenation [33].

We provided early neuromuscular blockade as this action provides a higher survival rate in early ARDS [34]. Additionally, strategies such as low TV, high PEEP, and prone position were used. Nevertheless, she developed a large pneumothorax and pneumomediastinum which were never visible on daily CXR, pointing in favor of sustained barotrauma. It is important to be aware of the damage associated with ventilatory support, due to the increased risk of mortality with some strategies [35]. Targeting a driving pressure-limited strategy

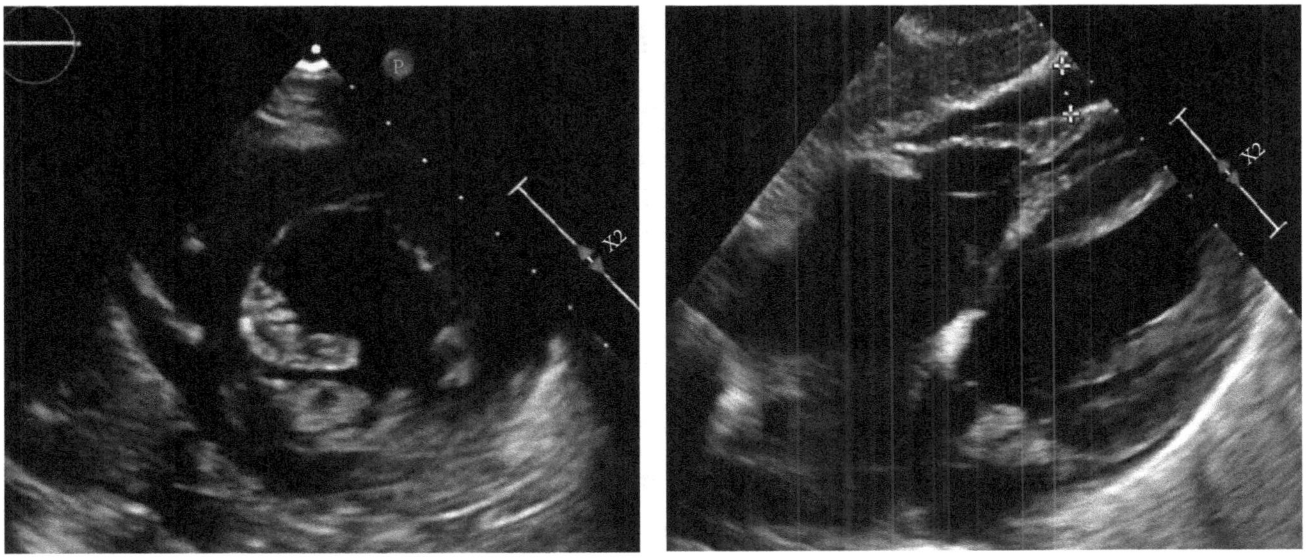

(a) (b)

FIGURE 2: TTE showing a free-flowing pericardial effusion identified circumferentially to the heart. Mild decrease of her left ventricular systolic function, from 50% in January 2020 to 40-45%. (a) Parasternal short axis view. (b) Subxiphoid view.

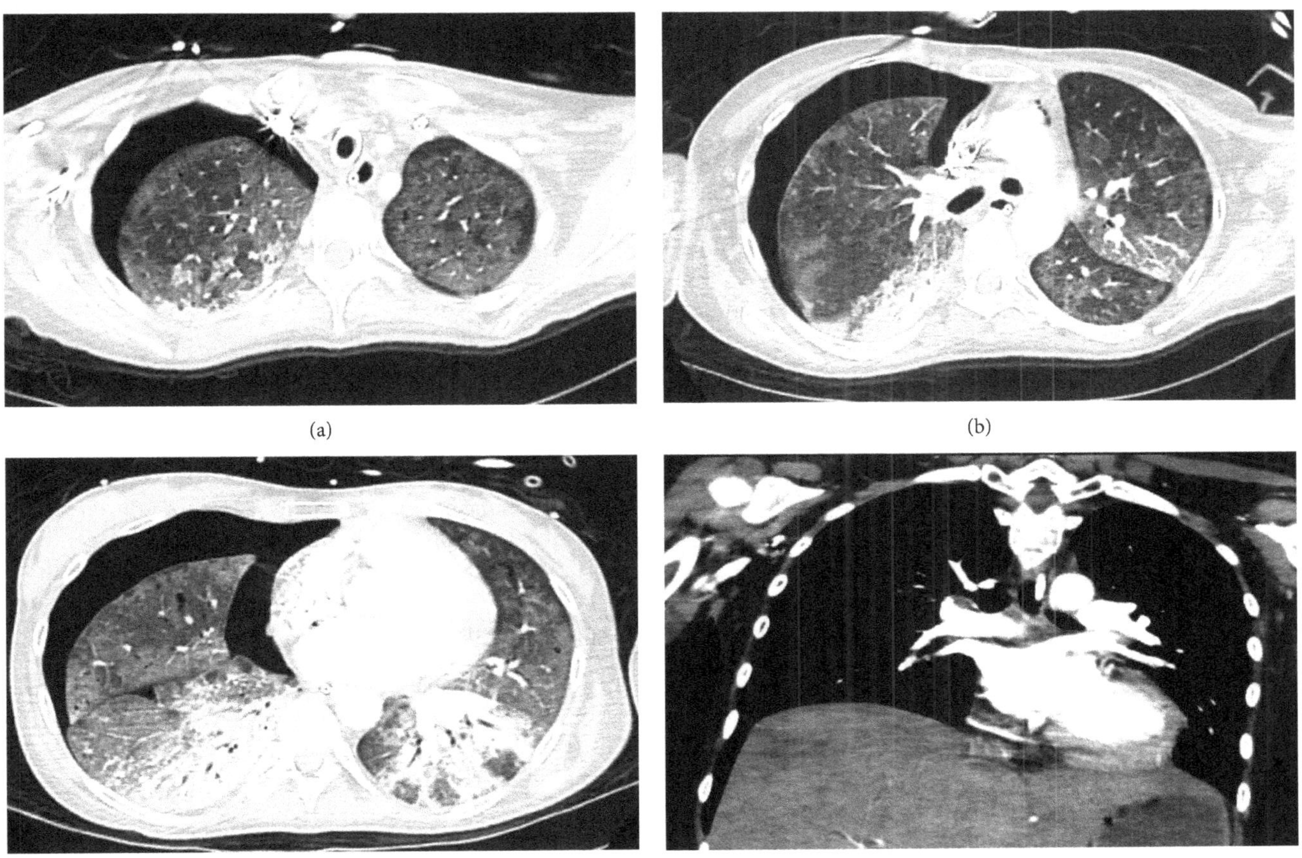

(c) (d)

FIGURE 3: Computed tomography of the Chest. (a–c) Large right pneumothorax with small pneumomediastinum and mediastinal shift compatible with tension pneumothorax (unidentified on daily CXR). Diffuse ground-glass opacities with dense consolidations in both inferior lobes, early fibrosis in the right middle lobe, and multiple pneumatoceles. (d) Acute segmental pulmonary embolism is noted in the posterior segment of the right lower lobe.

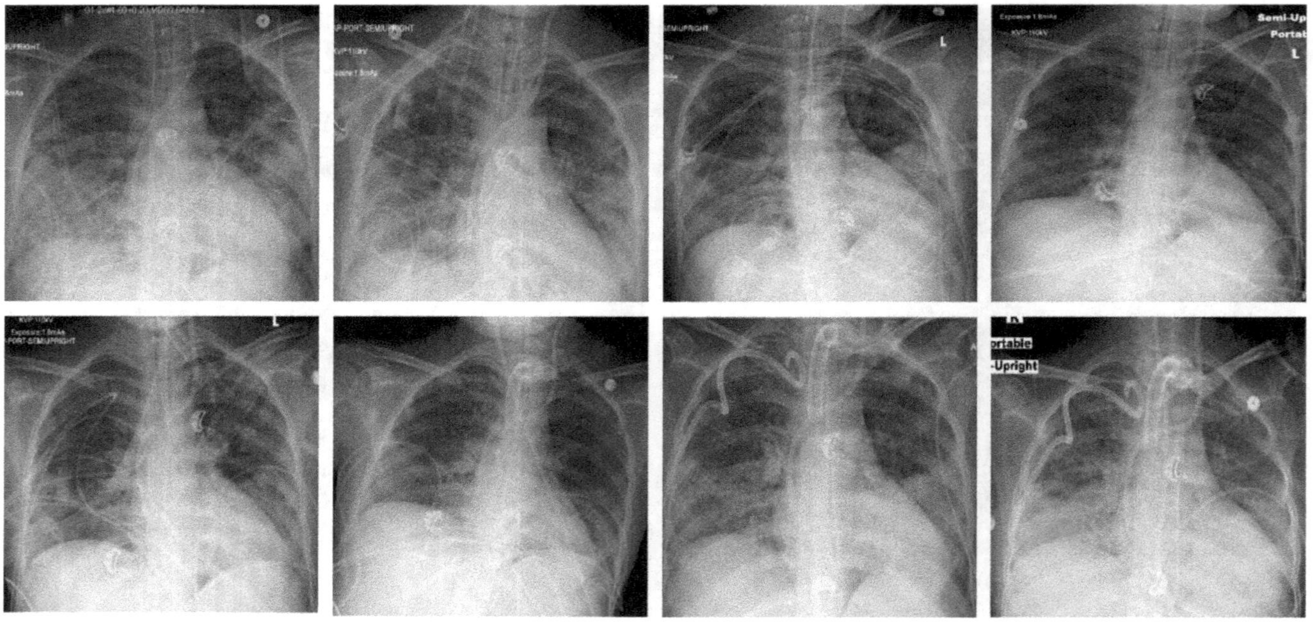

FIGURE 4: CXR progression until tracheostomy and chest tube insertion. Overall images were remarkable for stable appearance of subtle ill-defined hazy opacities throughout both mid to lower lungs. Infiltrates were always most accentuated in the left lung. No evidence of obvious pneumothorax or pneumomediastinum.

provides better outcomes [36]. Physicians should be aware of unrecognizable pneumothorax at CXR as an associated damage for prolonged ventilatory support and barotrauma.

Our patient required ACLS on multiple occasions, with special measures taken, as healthcare workers have the highest risk of contracting SARS-CoV-2. New recommendations include reducing exposure, prioritizing oxygenation strategies with lower aerosolization risk, and considering the appropriateness of resuscitation, based on age, comorbidities, and severity of illness [37].

4. Conclusions

SARS-CoV-2 principally invades pneumocytes via the ACE-2 receptor, generating a significant inflammatory cascade that can render critical illness, associated with high mortality, in the form of ARDS. Coinfection with other respiratory pathogens and opportunistic infections are possible. SARS-CoV-2 infection can elicit different pathophysiological processes which may require multidisciplinary strategies. Of note, inhaled nitric oxide to increase alveolar perfusion should be considered in cases of poor response to "classic" ARDS management.

Abbreviations

ACLS: Advanced cardiac life support
ARDS: Adult respiratory distress syndrome
COVID-19: Coronavirus disease 2019
CXR: Chest X-ray
DM: Diabetes mellitus
ECMO: Extracorporeal membrane oxygenation
NMB: Neuromuscular blockade
ROSC: Return of spontaneous circulation
SARS-CoV-2: Severe acute respiratory syndrome coronavirus 2
SOB: Shortness of breath
TTE: Transthoracic echocardiogram.

Consent

Patient's family consented and gave permission for publication of this data. Informed consent was obtained for this case.

Disclosure

The authors have no relationships relevant to the contents of this paper to disclose..

Authors' Contributions

All authors contributed to manuscript writing and approved the final version. All authors contributed to the conception and design and data analysis and interpretation. ASN contributed to the collection and assembly of data.

References

[1] Worldometers, "Total coronavirus Cases," 2020, https://www.worldometers.info/coronavirus/.

[2] P. K. Bhatraju, B. J. Ghassemieh, M. Nichols et al., "Covid-19 in critically ill patients in the Seattle region—case series," *New England Journal of Medicine*, vol. 382, no. 21, pp. 2012–2022, 2020.

[3] I. Care, N. Audit, and R. Centre, *ICNARC report on COVID-19 in critical care 10*, 2020, https://www.icnarc.org/About/Latest-News/2020/03/27/Report-On-775-Patients-Critically-Ill-With-Covid-19.

[4] C. Wu, X. Chen, Y. Cai et al., "Risk factors associated with acute respiratory distress syndrome and death in patients with coronavirus disease 2019 pneumonia in Wuhan, China," *JAMA internal medicine*, vol. 180, no. 7, p. 934, 2020.

[5] J. M. Sanders, M. L. Monogue, T. Z. Jodlowski, and J. B. Cutrell, "Pharmacologic treatments for coronavirus disease 2019 (COVID-19)," *JAMA*, 2020.

[6] Z. Wu and J. M. McGoogan, "Characteristics of and important lessons from the coronavirus disease 2019 (COVID-19) outbreak in China," *JAMA*, vol. 323, no. 13, p. 1239, 2020.

[7] Y. Yi, P. N. P. Lagniton, S. Ye, E. Li, and R.-H. Xu, "COVID-19: what has been learned and to be learned about the novel coronavirus disease," *International Journal of Biological Sciences*, vol. 16, no. 10, pp. 1753–1766, 2020.

[8] A. H. J. Danser, M. Epstein, and D. Batlle, "Renin-angiotensin system blockers and the COVID-19 pandemic: at present there is no evidence to abandon renin-angiotensin system blockers," *Hypertension*, vol. 75, no. 6, pp. 1382–1385, 2020.

[9] W. Li, R. J. G. Hulswit, S. P. Kenney et al., "Broad receptor engagement of an emerging global coronavirus may potentiate its diverse cross-species transmissibility," in *Proceedings of the National Academy of Sciences*, vol. 115no. 22, pp. E5135–E5143, 2018.

[10] L. van der Hoek, K. Pyrc, M. F. Jebbink et al., "Identification of a new human coronavirus," *Nature medicine*, vol. 10, no. 4, pp. 368–373, 2004.

[11] P. K. Kiyuka, C. N. Agoti, P. K. Munywoki et al., "Human coronavirus NL63 molecular epidemiology and evolutionary patterns in rural coastal Kenya," *The Journal of Infectious Diseases*, vol. 217, no. 11, pp. 1728–1739, 2018.

[12] S.-H. Huang, M.-C. Su, N. Tien et al., "Epidemiology of human coronavirus NL63 infection among hospitalized patients with pneumonia in Taiwan," *Journal of Microbiology, Immunology and Infection*, vol. 50, no. 6, pp. 763–770, 2017.

[13] A. Vabret, T. Mourez, J. Dina et al., "Human coronavirus NL63, France," *Emerging Infectious Diseases*, vol. 11, no. 8, pp. 1225–1229, 2005.

[14] D. Kim, J. Quinn, B. Pinsky, N. H. Shah, and I. Brown, "Rates of co-infection between SARS-CoV-2 and other respiratory pathogens," *JAMA*, vol. 323, no. 20, p. 2085, 2020.

[15] Y. Cheng, R. Luo, K. Wang et al., "Kidney disease is associated with in-hospital death of patients with COVID-19," *Kidney International*, vol. 97, no. 5, pp. 829–838, 2020.

[16] T. Chen, D. Wu, H. Chen et al., "Clinical characteristics of 113 deceased patients with coronavirus disease 2019: retrospective study," *BMJ*, vol. 368, 2020.

[17] J. S. Hirsch, J. H. Ng, D. W. Ross et al., "Acute kidney injury in patients hospitalized with COVID-19," *Kidney International*, vol. 98, no. 1, pp. 209–218, 2020.

[18] R. Gupta, A. Ghosh, A. K. Singh, and A. Misra, "Clinical considerations for patients with diabetes in times of COVID-19 epidemic," *Diabetes & Metabolic Syndrome*, vol. 14, no. 3, pp. 211-212, 2020.

[19] P. Xu, Q. Zhou, and J. Xu, "Mechanism of thrombocytopenia in COVID-19 patients," *Annals of Hematology*, vol. 99, no. 6, pp. 1205–1208, 2020.

[20] S. Cui, S. Chen, X. Li, S. Liu, and F. Wang, "Prevalence of venous thromboembolism in patients with severe novel coronavirus pneumonia," *Journal of Thrombosis and Haemostasis*, vol. 18, no. 6, pp. 1421–1424, 2020.

[21] N. Tang, H. Bai, X. Chen, J. Gong, D. Li, and Z. Sun, "Anticoagulant treatment is associated with decreased mortality in severe coronavirus disease 2019 patients with coagulopathy," *Journal of Thrombosis and Haemostasis*, vol. 18, no. 5, pp. 1094–1099, 2020

[22] A. Bhimraj, R. L. Morgan, A. H. Shumaker et al., "Infectious Diseases Society of America Guidelines on the Treatment and Management of Patients with COVID-19," *Clinical Infectious Diseases*https://www.idsociety.org/practice-guideline/covid-19-guideline-treatment-and-management/.

[23] M. S. Baek, Y. Lee, S.-B. Hong, C.-M. Lim, Y. Koh, and J. W. Huh, "Effect of corticosteroid therapy in the early phase of acute respiratory distress syndrome: a propensity-matched cohort study," *The Korean Journal of Internal Medicine*, 2020.

[24] D. Annane, S. M. Pastores, W. Arlt et al., "Critical illness-related corticosteroid insufficiency (CIRCI): a narrative review from a Multispecialty Task Force of the Society of Critical Care Medicine (SCCM) and the European Society of Intensive Care Medicine (ESICM)," *Intensive care medicine*, vol. 43, no. 12, pp. 1781–1792, 2017.

[25] J. M. Molina, C. Delaugerre, J. L. Goff et al., "No evidence of rapid antiviral clearance or clinical benefit with the combination of hydroxychloroquine and azithromycin in patients with severe COVID-19 infection," *Médecine et Maladies Infectieuses*, pp. 30085–30088, 2020.

[26] C. Huang, Y. Wang, X. Li et al., "Clinical features of patients infected with 2019 novel coronavirus in Wuhan, China," *The Lancet*, vol. 395, no. 10223, pp. 497–506, 2020.

[27] ClinicalTrialsgov, "Tocilizumab in COVID-19 pneumonia (TOCIVID-19)," Identifier: NCT04317092.

[28] ClinicalTrialsgov, "Tocilizumab for SARS-CoV2 severe pneumonitis," Identifier: NCT04315480.

[29] L. Caly, J. D. Druce, M. G. Catton, D. A. Jans, and K. M. Wagstaff, "The FDA-approved drug ivermectin inhibits the replication of SARS-CoV-2 _in vitro_," *Antiviral Research*, vol. 178, p. 104787, 2020.

[30] J. Grein, N. Ohmagari, D. Shin et al., "Compassionate use of remdesivir for patients with severe Covid-19," *New England Journal of Medicine*, vol. 382, no. 24, pp. 2327–2336, 2020.

[31] L. Gattinoni, D. Chiumello, P. Caironi et al., "COVID-19 pneumonia: different respiratory treatments for different phenotypes?," *Intensive Care Medicine*, vol. 46, no. 6, pp. 1099–1102, 2020.

[32] L. Gattinoni, S. Coppola, M. Cressoni, M. Busana, S. Rossi, and D. Chiumello, "COVID-19 Does Not Lead to a "Typical" Acute Respiratory Distress Syndrome," *American Journal of Respiratory and Critical Care Medicine*, vol. 201, no. 10, pp. 1299-1300, 2020.

[33] W. Alhazzani, M. H. Møller, Y. M. Arabi et al., "Surviving Sepsis campaign: guidelines on the management of critically ill adults with coronavirus disease 2019 (COVID-19)," *Intensive Care Medicine*, vol. 46, no. 5, pp. 854–887, 2020.

[34] L. Papazian, J. M. Forel, A. Gacouin et al., "Neuromuscular Blockers in Early Acute Respiratory Distress Syndrome," *New England Journal of Medicine*, vol. 363, no. 12, pp. 1107–1116, 2010.

[35] M. B. P. Amato, M. O. Meade, A. S. Slutsky et al., "Driving pressure and survival in the acute respiratory distress syndrome," *New England Journal of Medicine*, vol. 372, no. 8, pp. 747–755, 2015.

[36] G. Bellani, A. Grassi, S. Sosio et al., "Driving Pressure Is Associated with Outcome during Assisted Ventilation in Acute Respiratory Distress Syndrome," *Anesthesiology*, vol. 131, no. 3, pp. 594–604, 2019.

[37] D. P. Edelson, C. Sasson, P. S. Chan et al., "Interim Guidance for Basic and Advanced Life Support in Adults, Children, and Neonates With Suspected or Confirmed COVID-19," *Circulation*, vol. 141, no. 25, pp. e933–e943, 2020.

6

Gastric Emphysema in a Critically Ill Patient Successfully Treated without Surgery

Hiromi Ihoriya,[1] Tetsuya Yumoto,[1] Masaya Iwamuro,[2] Noritomo Fujisaki,[1] Takaaki Osako,[1] Hiromichi Naito,[1] and Atsunori Nakao[1]

[1]*Advanced Emergency and Critical Care Medical Center, Okayama University Hospital, Japan*
[2]*Department of Gastroenterology and Hepatology, Okayama University Graduate School of Medicine, Dentistry, and Pharmaceutical Sciences, Japan*

Correspondence should be addressed to Tetsuya Yumoto; tyumoto@cc.okayama-u.ac.jp

Academic Editor: Kenneth S. Waxman

Gastric emphysema is a relatively rare clinical entity caused by injury to the gastric mucosa. A 62-year-old Japanese male with a history of heavy alcohol consumption and smoking was admitted to the emergency intensive care unit due to severe hypercapnic respiratory acidosis. His body mass index was only 12.6. Ten days after initiation of enteral feeding, he complained of abdominal pain. Computed tomography revealed intraluminal air in the distended gastric wall. Esophagogastroduodenoscopy showed diffuse edema, redness, and erosion throughout the stomach. Based on the findings of narrow angle and short distance of the aorta-superior mesenteric artery, the patient was diagnosed with gastric emphysema associated with superior mesenteric artery syndrome. He was successfully managed nonoperatively with treatments including intravenous antibiotics, gastric decompression, and bowel rest. Physicians should be aware of this unusual condition in such critically ill patients complaining of abdominal pain and needing close monitoring and observation to exclude gastric necrosis or perforation.

1. Introduction

Gastric emphysema, which is characterized by the accumulation of gas within the wall of the stomach with or without concomitant portal venous gas, is a relatively rare clinical entity. It can develop secondary to mechanical injury of the gastric surface resulting from elevation of intraluminal pressure such as malignant obstruction of the stomach outlet, superior mesenteric artery syndrome (SMAS), or excessive vomiting [1–5]. Although gastric emphysema is usually self-limiting and resolves spontaneously, it can be challenging to differentiate from emphysematous gastritis and mortality from the condition remains high [6]. To our knowledge, gastric emphysema has never been reported in a critically ill patient. Herein, we describe a rare case of gastric emphysema that might have been induced by SMAS in a patient with malnutrition and alcoholism. This paper should help raise physician awareness of this potentially critical condition.

2. Case Presentation

A 62-year-old Japanese male with a history of heavy alcohol consumption and smoking was brought to the emergency department due to altered mental status. He was confused and disoriented, with a Glasgow Coma Scale score of 8 (E2V2M4). His vital signs were as follows: respiratory rate: 36 breaths/min; pulse rate: 124 beats/min, blood pressure: 122/84 mmHg; and temperature: 35.9°C. Physical examination was unremarkable except for gross emaciation (height: 160 cm; weight: 32.2 kg; body mass index: 12.6). Also, no obvious abnormal neurological findings including paralysis or ocular movement disorder were observed. Arterial blood gas analysis revealed severe respiratory acidosis with pH: 7.187; $PaCO_2$: 110.3 mmHg; PaO_2: 145.9 mmHg; $HCO3^-$: 30.6 mmol/L; base excess: 6.8 mmol/L; lactate: 4.0 mmol/L; glucose: 104 mg/dl on 10 L/min of oxygen. Laboratory data showed hyponatremia of 117 mEq/L without any other abnormal findings. The patient was intubated and mechanically

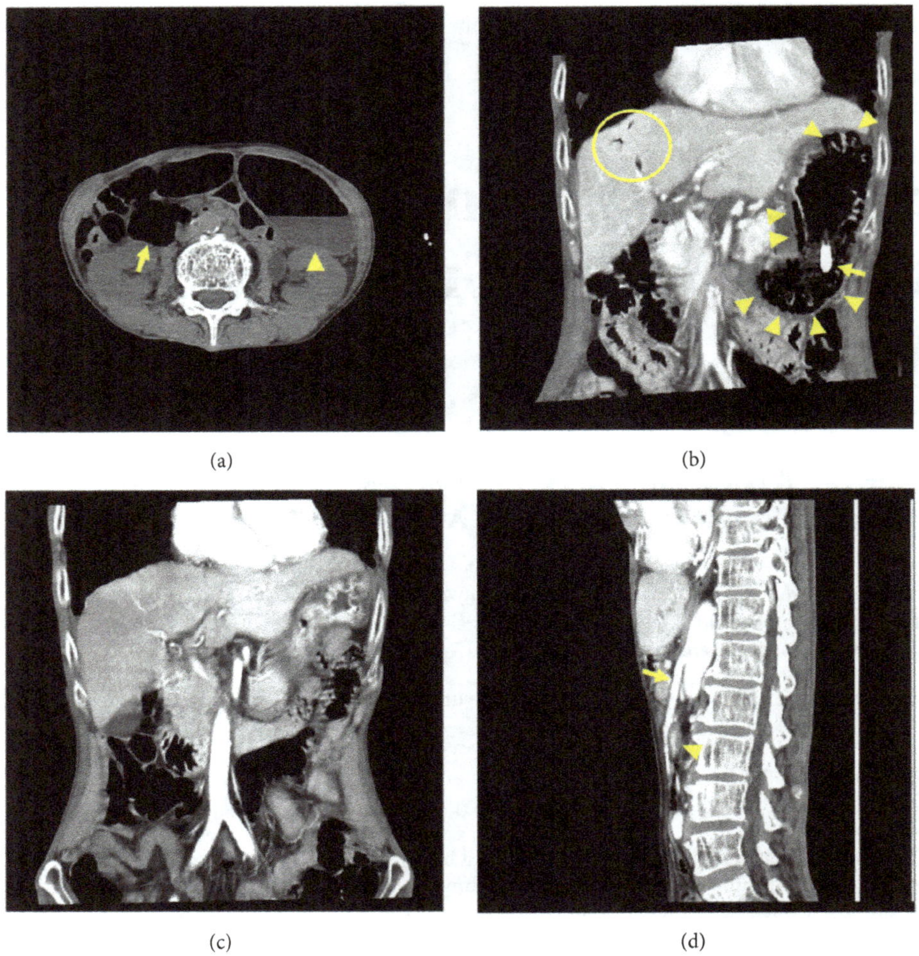

FIGURE 1: Plain abdominal CT scan on admission showing dilatation of the stomach (arrowhead) and second portion of the duodenum (arrow) (a). Contrast-enhanced CT scan on hospital day 11 showing gas within the wall of a distended stomach (arrowheads) and portal vein (circled region). An arrow demonstrating the tip of the feeding tube (b). Follow-up CT scan showing improvement of gas in the stomach and portal vein (c). Sagittal view showing an acute angle of the aorto-superior mesenteric artery (arrow) and a collapsed duodenum (arrowhead) (d).

ventilated due to his altered level of consciousness resulting from severe hypercapnic respiratory failure. While computed tomography (CT) examination of the head revealed no abnormalities, abdominal CT showed dilatation of the stomach and second portion of duodenum (Figure 1(a)). He was admitted to the emergency intensive care unit for further management.

The patient received intravenous omeprazole for stress ulcer prophylaxis and ampicillin/sulbactam for suspected aspiration pneumonia from day 1. When his estimated original $PaCO_2$ level was restored (around 60 mmHg), his neurological state improved. On the second day, an enteral feeding was initiated through a nasogastric tube at 10 mL/h and advanced by 5 mL/day every 48 hours, as no gastric contents had been drained. Tracheostomy was performed on day 5 because prolonged ventilatory support had been expected.

On day 11, he complained of epigastric and left upper quadrant tenderness without guarding or rebound tenderness. In addition, a total of 500 cc of gastric fluid mixed with a material resembling coffee-grounds was drained through the nasogastric tube. His white blood cell count rose to 22,130 /μL with neutrophils 95.8%. Persistent abdominal pain and detection of ascites by ultrasound led us to perform contrast-enhanced CT, which revealed intraluminal air in the distended gastric wall with hepatic portal venous gas (Figure 1(b)). Esophagogastroduodenoscopy (EGD) demonstrated edema, redness, and erosion, with a white coating throughout the stomach without evidence of active bleeding or obvious necrotic lesions (Figure 2(a)).

As the patient had been hemodynamically stable with benign abdominal findings and without elevation of lactate levels, he was successfully managed with nonoperative treatments including intravenous vancomycin and meropenem, bowel rest, and nasogastric tube decompression. Blood cultures obtained on day 11 showed no growth. Follow-up abdominal CT scan on day 19 showed improvement of the

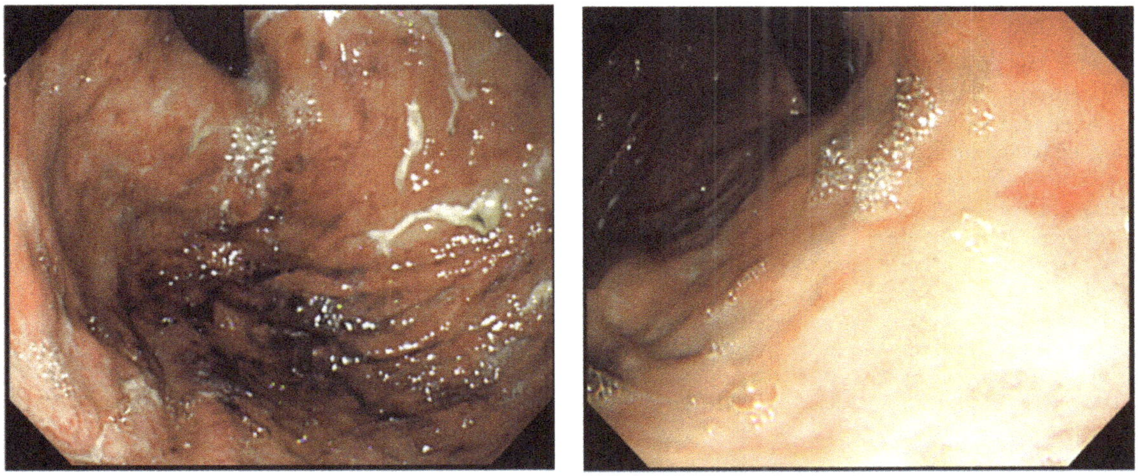

(a) (b)

FIGURE 2: Esophagogastroduodenoscopy demonstrating diffuse mucosal edema, redness, and erosive lesions with white coating throughout the stomach (a), which was resolved (b).

gas in the stomach and portal vein (Figure 1(c)). The aorta-superior mesenteric artery (SMA) angle and distance were 17 degrees and 4 mm, respectively (Figure 1(d)), suggesting SMAS as an underlying condition. Complete resolution of the erosive lesions was confirmed on repeat EGD on the same day (Figure 2(b)). Enteral nutrition was resumed uneventfully. Thereafter, the patient was transferred to another hospital for rehabilitation.

3. Discussion

Our case highlights the need to consider gastric emphysema, which might have been caused by SMAS, in a critically ill and malnourished patient complaining of abdominal pain. Conservative treatment was effective in treating gastric emphysema in patients with stable hemodynamic status without evidence of gastric necrosis or perforation.

Gastric emphysema is considered a relatively benign condition characterized by intraluminal gas in the stomach resulting from mucosal trauma. It is important to differentiate between gastric emphysema and emphysematous gastritis, both of which exhibit similar radiological findings of gas in the stomach wall with or without portal venous gas [6, 7]. Emphysematous gastritis is a distinct clinical entity related to infection of the gastric wall by gas-forming organisms [8]. The proposed predisposing factors for gastric emphysema resulting from mucosal trauma include gastrointestinal malignancy, gastric volvulus, SMAS, repetitive vomiting, or even nasogastric tube placement [1–7, 9], while immunosuppression, diabetes mellitus, ingestion of corrosives, alcoholism, or nonsteroidal anti-inflammatory drugs have been reported as common underlying conditions in a patient with emphysematous gastritis [6, 8, 10]. Surgical intervention may be warranted in patients with emphysematous gastritis due to development of necrosis or perforation of the stomach [8, 11]. In addition to proper hemodynamic monitoring and management and intravenous antibiotics, EGD should be performed to exclude ischemic stomach [6]. In the present case, benign abdominal findings with hemodynamic stability as well as without evidence of obvious necrotic lesions based on CT examination allowed us to treat the patient with conservative methods including broad-spectrum antibiotics, gastric decompression, and bowel rest.

SMAS is an unusual digestive condition characterized by compression of the third portion of the duodenum due to narrowing of the aorta-SMA angle as a result of extreme weight loss [12]. This clinical entity may cause gastric emphysema, which would be attributed to the elevation of intragastric pressure resulting from intestinal obstruction. To date, only a few cases of gastric emphysema associated with SMAS have been reported [3, 13–15]. Our patient was compatible with SMAS based on the findings of aorta-SMA angle and distance of below 25 degrees and 8 mm, respectively [16]. In addition to SMAS, underlying malnutrition and/or nonocclusive mesenteric ischemia might have contributed to the development of gastric emphysema in the present case [17–19].

As such, this was the first report of gastric emphysema that might have been caused by SMAS in a critically ill and malnourished patient admitted to the intensive care unit due to severe hypercapnic respiratory failure. Critical care physicians should be aware of this clinical entity in such severely ill patients complaining of abdominal pain. Careful hemodynamic monitoring and repetitive physical examination are necessary to exclude gastric necrosis or perforation, which need surgical intervention. Early diagnosis and proper management allow for successful nonoperative management in patients with gastric emphysema.

References

[1] S. Lee and JN. Rutledge, "Gastric emphysema," *The American Journal of Gastroenterology*, vol. 79, no. 11, pp. 899–904, 1984.

[2] M.-S. Soon, H.-H. Yen, A. Soon, and O. S. Lin, "Endoscopic ultrasonographic appearance of gastric emphysema," *World Journal of Gastroenterology*, vol. 11, no. 11, pp. 1719–1721, 2005.

[3] J. E. Lim, G. L. Duke, and S. R. Eachempati, "Superior mesenteric artery syndrome presenting with acute massive gastric dilatation, gastric wall pneumatosis, and portal venous gas," *Surgery*, vol. 134, no. 5, pp. 840–843, 2003.

[4] M. P. Parikh, M. Sherid, V. Ganipisetti, V. Gopalakrishnan, M. Habib, and M. Tripathi, "Vomiting-induced gastric emphysema and hepatoportal venous gas: A case report and review of the literature," *Case Reports in Medicine*, vol. 2015, Article ID 413230, 4 pages, 2015.

[5] P. Sharma and E. G. Akl, "A combination of intramural stomach and portal venous air: conservative treatment," *Journal of Community Hospital Internal Medicine Perspectives (JCHIMP)*, vol. 6, no. 1, p. 30519, 2016.

[6] K. Matsushima, E. J. Won, M. R. Tangel, L. M. Enomoto, D. M. Avella, and D. I. Soybel, "Emphysematous gastritis and gastric emphysema: similar radiographic findings, distinct clinical entities," *World Journal of Surgery*, vol. 39, no. 4, pp. 1008–1017, 2015.

[7] Z. G. Naqvi, N. Shahzad, A. R. Alvi, and S. Effendi, "Intramural gas in stomach along with acute calculus cholecystitis: an unusual association," *BMJ Case Reports*, vol. 2013, 2013.

[8] B. A. Wormer and G. Mostafa, "Emphysematous gastritis with delayed gastric perforation," *Journal of Gastrointestinal Surgery*, vol. 17, no. 7, pp. 1336–1338, 2013.

[9] N. A. Zenooz, M. R. Robbin, and V. Perez, "Gastric pneumatosis following nasogastric tube placement: a case report with literature review," *Emergency Radiology*, vol. 13, no. 4, pp. 205–207, 2007.

[10] J. Iannuzzi, T. J. Watson, and V. R. Litle, "Emphysematous gastritis: a young diabetic's recovery," *International Journal of Surgery Case Reports*, vol. 3, no. 4, pp. 125–127, 2012.

[11] P. A. Ferrada, "Successful surgical treatment of emphysematous gastritis on a patient with poor cardiac function," *The American Surgeon*, vol. 78, no. 2, pp. E66–E67, 2012.

[12] L. B. Cohen, S. P. Field, and D. B. Sachar, "The superior mesenteric artery syndrome. The disease that isn't, or is it?" *Journal of Clinical Gastroenterology*, vol. 7, no. 2, pp. 113–116, 1985.

[13] T. Ichikawa, H. Yamamuro, J. Koizumi et al., "Duodenal emphysema complicated with superior mesenteric artery syndrome in a patient with cerebral paralysis: a case report," *The Tokai Journal of Experimental and Clinical Medicine*, vol. 40, no. 2, pp. 40–43, 2015.

[14] Y. Sakamoto, K. Mashiko, H. Matsumoto, Y. Hara, N. Kutsukata, and Y. Yamamoto, "Gastric pneumatosis and portal venous gas in superior mesenteric artery syndrome," *Indian Journal of Gastroenterology*, vol. 25, no. 5, pp. 265-266, 2006.

[15] A. Martínez-Pérez, R. Trullenque-Juan, S. Santarrufina-Martínez, and E. Armañanzas-Villena, "Massive gastrointestinal pneumatosis in a patient with celiac disease and superior mesenteric artery syndrome," *Revista Española de Enfermedades Digestivas*, vol. 107, no. 11, pp. 709-710, 2015.

[16] S. Neri, S. S. Signorelli, E. Mondati et al., "Ultrasound imaging in diagnosis of superior mesenteric artery syndrome," *Journal of Internal Medicine*, vol. 257, no. 4, pp. 346–351, 2005.

[17] R. Udassin, I. Aviad, I. Vinograd, and S. Nissan, "Isolated emphysematous gastritis in an infant," *Gastrointestinal Radiology*, vol. 9, no. 1, pp. 9–12, 1984.

[18] T. Kim, H. U. Kim, and H. J. Song, "A case of gastric emphysema in anorexia nervosa presenting as acute gastric distension," *The Korean Journal of Gastroenterology*, vol. 60, no. 5, pp. 315–319, 2012.

[19] S. Bourcier, A. Oudjit, G. Goudard et al., "Diagnosis of non-occlusive acute mesenteric ischemia in the intensive care unit," *Annals of Intensive Care*, vol. 6, no. 1, p. 112, 2016.

7

A Critically Ill Child with Gangrenous Appendicitis Masquerading as Hollow Viscous Perforation

Ashish Lal Shrestha,[1] Santosh Maharjan,[2] Anil Dev Pant,[3] and Pankaj Bahadur Nepali[3]

[1]*Department of Pediatric Surgery, Grande International Hospital, Tokha Road, Kathmandu, Nepal*
[2]*Department of Radiodiagnosis, Grande International Hospital, Tokha Road, Kathmandu, Nepal*
[3]*Department of Pathology, Grande International Hospital, Tokha Road, Kathmandu, Nepal*

Correspondence should be addressed to Ashish Lal Shrestha; butchgrunty@yahoo.com

Academic Editor: Kenneth S. Waxman

Background. Severe complications of acute appendicitis (AA) hitherto well described are less common in clinical practice nowadays. When a septic child is encountered with a short history of abdominal symptoms and disproportionate signs of peritonitis further complicated by radiological findings causing a diagnostic conundrum, management becomes exceedingly demanding. *Case Presentation.* A 10-year-old previously healthy boy presented to the emergency room with generalized abdominal pain associated with fever and jaundice for a day. Blood workup revealed leucopenia, hyperbilirubinemia, hyponatremia, and elevated CRP. Initial radiological evaluation suggested hollow viscous perforation. He was diagnosed to have hollow viscous perforation peritonitis in severe sepsis. At laparotomy, generalized peritoneal contamination was found, the source of which could be traced down to the gangrenous perforated appendix. *Conclusion.* Complicated appendicitis, in children, can present with baffling findings. Timely identification of an ill child, adequate workup, prompt resuscitation, and source control are imperative for a successful outcome.

1. Introduction

Appendicitis can present with complications like gangrene, perforation, and peritonitis with the incidence of perforation being reported ~30% in children [1]. While the risks are more for younger children due to inexpressibility and language coherence, amongst the older ones, the delayed presentation seems to be accountable [1].

The incidence of adult appendicular perforation presenting with pneumoperitoneum is estimated to be 0-7% while no similar data seems to exist in children [2].

In 70% of adults with peritonitis, pneumoperitoneum is an expected finding that can be linked with perforated peptic ulcer in most, perforated sigmoid diverticulitis in a few, and an anastomotic leak in postoperative patients in the rest, thereby tending to overlook an appendicular etiology [2, 3].

Confounded by limitations in history taking and nonspecific examination findings, it becomes even a bigger diagnostic challenge in children We present an interesting case of a boy presenting with generalized peritonitis in severe sepsis with pneumoperitoneum initially thought to have peptic ulcer perforation and on further evaluation found to have a gangrenous perforated appendicitis.

2. Case Report

A 10-year-old Nepalese boy presented to the emergency room (ER) for sudden periumbilical pain that became generalized over the day associated with fever, bilious vomiting, abdominal distension, and obstipation. General examination revealed fever (101 degrees F), tachycardia (120 beats per minute), and tachypnea (40 breaths per minute). His blood pressure was 90/60 mmHg, and capillary refill time was 3 seconds. He looked dehydrated with a dry and coated tongue and seemed to be in notable distress. Abdominal examination revealed generalized distension with tenderness, guarding, and absent bowel sounds on auscultation.

His hemogram showed leucopenia (total leukocyte count (TLC): 2550 cells/Cu.mm and differential leukocyte count: polymorphs: 58%, lymphocytes: 14%, eosinophils: 1%, monocytes: 26%, and basophils: 1%) and elevated C-reactive protein (CRP): 90 mg/l.

Biochemical tests showed moderate hyponatremia (Na+: 128 mmol/l) and normal liver panel except for mild hyperbilirubinemia (2.6 mg/dl). Urinalysis was normal.

Abdominal radiograph revealed free air under the diaphragm as shown in Figure 1. Ultrasound abdomen showed distended gassy bowel.

He was diagnosed to have hollow viscous perforation peritonitis with a source probably in the proximal gastrointestinal tract. Nasogastric decompression was initiated along with aggressive fluid resuscitation, first dose intravenous broad-spectrum antibiotics (piperacillin-tazobactam, amikacin, and metronidazole), and analgesics.

He underwent an emergency exploratory midline laparotomy under general anesthesia. Intraoperatively generalized peritonitis was found with putrid pus and fibrinous flakes in the subdiaphragmatic regions, Morrison's pouch, both paracolic gutters, and pelvis. The appendix was found to be gangrenous and perforated at its base as shown in Figure 2. Appendectomy and thorough peritoneal irrigation with normal saline was performed. Although the base was perforated, the adjoining caecum was healthy along with a portion of appendicular stump that allowed transfixing sutures done doubly with 3-0 Vicryl. A 20Fr ADK drain was left to drain the pelvis.

The fascia was repaired with interrupted 1 Vicryl without tension and skin with staplers.

Postoperatively, he was monitored in PICU (Pediatric Intensive Care Unit) with continuation of supportive care. While in PICU, his vital signs remained stable with the maintenance of intake-output balance and correction of metabolic acidosis.

On postoperative day (POD) 3, his TLC improved to 7210 cells/Cu.mm, CRP remained >90 mg/l, total bilirubin was 2.2 mg/dl, and serum sodium levels normalized (Na +:136 m mol/l).

On postoperative day 5, TLC was 6650 cells/Cu.mm, CRP was 23 mg/l, and total bilirubin was 0.9 mg/dl. Peritoneal pus had grown Pseudomonas aeruginosa that was sensitive to the antibiotics that he was receiving. Since the drain output was insignificant, it was removed.

He had an uneventful postoperative course, and after a total of 7 days, intravenous antibiotics were discontinued and he was subsequently discharged.

The histopathology showed appendicular mucosa with suppuration, ulceration, and full-thickness inflammation along with myonecrosis. The lumen contained fecal material. The findings were suggestive of gangrenous appendicitis with periappendiceal inflammation as shown in Figure 3.

At follow-up a week later, he had recovered well. At the same visit, skin staplers were removed as shown in Figure 4.

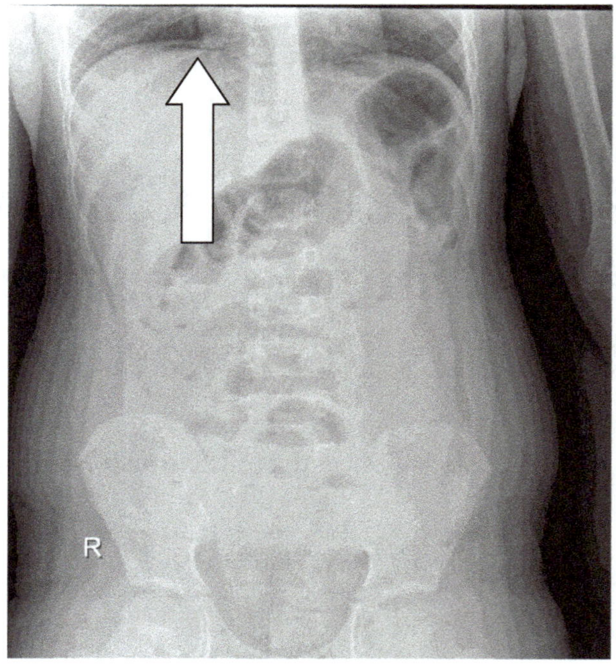

Figure 1: Plain abdominal erect radiograph showing subdiaphragmatic free air.

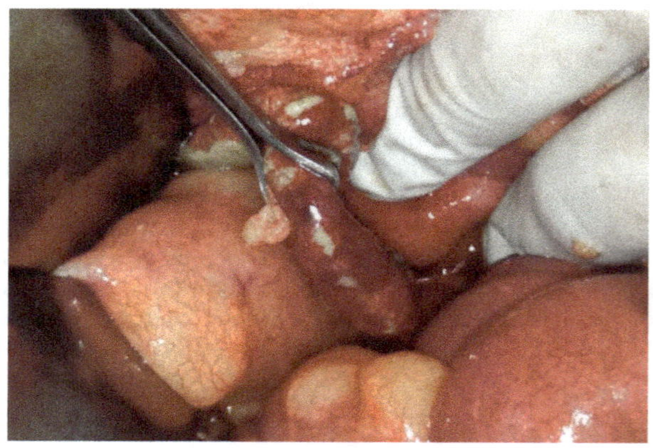

Figure 2: Intraoperative appearance of a gangrenous perforated appendix.

3. Discussion

Peritonitis in children is a well-established entity, and appendicular perforation as a cause is also widely known [4, 5]. The temporal profile in the natural history of appendicitis results in various stages of inflammation including complications like gangrene and perforation, the prediction of which is not easy [1].

Generally, the intraluminal lymphoid hyperplasia is the pathogenic mechanism causing AA. But any process that could occlude its lumen causing an increase in luminal pressure could induce inflammation. This would allow bacterial translocation, transmural suppuration, and eventual necrosis with perforation [2]. However, pneumoperitoneum remains an uncommon finding with appendicular perforation owing to the lumen that is already obstructed [2].

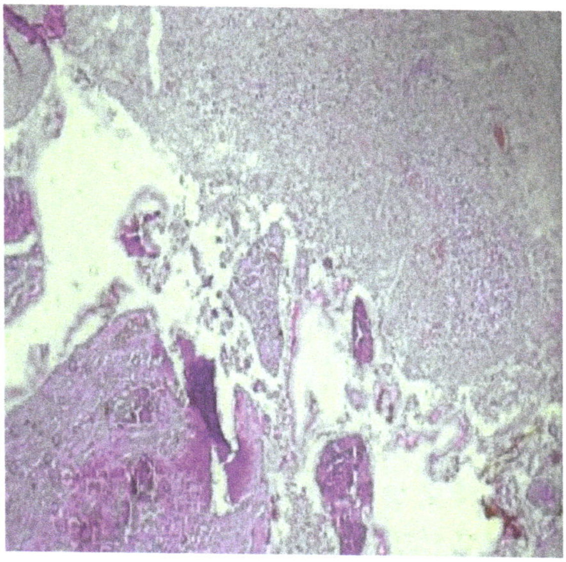

(a)

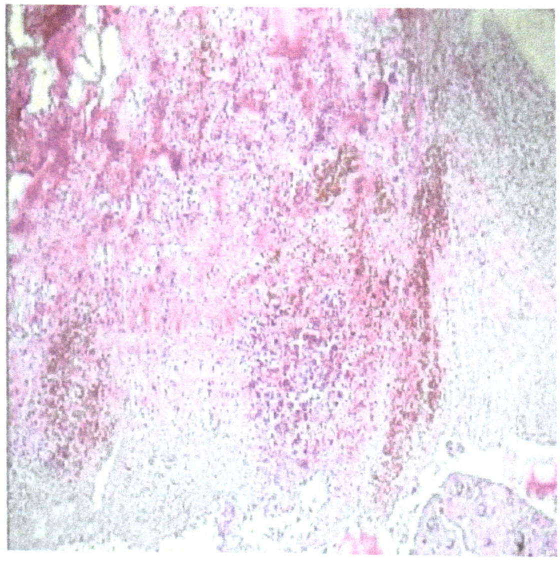

(b)

FIGURE 3: Histopathological appearance of the appendix at 40x magnifications showing (a) fecalith and mucosal ulceration and (b) full-thickness inflammation and myonecrosis.

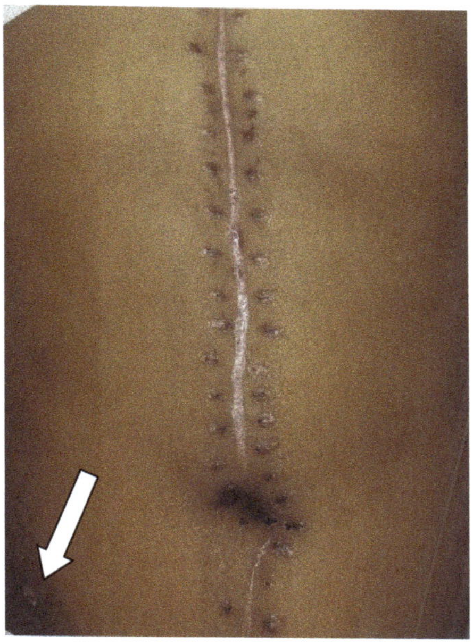

FIGURE 4: Midline laparotomy scar with drain insertion site, after surgical clip removal at 1-week follow-up.

In few patients, the intestinal free air may overcome the obstruction, escape into the peritoneal cavity, and manifest as free air in plain abdominal erect films. In others, the bacteria involved in periappendicular abscess could be responsible for gas formation [2]. Though minimal (3 ml) air is sufficient to manifest pneumoperitoneum on a plain and erect abdominal radiograph, the finding coexisting with a perforated appendix is rather rare even in adult patients [6]. The fact that no large studies are reported in children could mean that it is even more exceedingly rare in children [7].

Whatever the cause of pneumoperitoneum or peritonitis, the initial workup and resuscitation always take precedence over the diagnostic confirmation. When presented with a critically ill child with such findings, the first and foremost step is to attain hemodynamic stability, with a prompt and adequate resuscitation meanwhile continuing further evaluation to plan a definite management [8]. Pain control with appropriate analgesics and first dose antibiotics need not be delayed till the definitive diagnosis is made.

If a plain radiograph at ER suggests pneumoperitoneum with background findings of peritonitis in sepsis, the next definitive step is source control. As with our patient, we decided to proceed with a midline laparotomy and complete exploration in order to clear pus from the deeper peritoneal recesses and to avoid abscesses in the postoperative period apart from trying to avoid missing an upper gastrointestinal pathology. A formal exploration in this case was unavoidable in view of (1) unknown focus of infection and free air and (2) general peritoneal contamination.

4. Conclusion

Appendicular perforation peritonitis presenting with sepsis and free peritoneal air on a plain radiograph is a rare phenomenon or rather an uncommon presentation of a much common disease process. The finding may present with dilemma in diagnosis and surgical approach. However, with generalized peritoneal contamination, complete abdominal exploration is imperative to avoid missing findings and to attain adequate source control. Regardless of surgical findings, the initial steps of resuscitation and workup are paramount.

Abbreviations

AA: Acute appendicitis
PICU: Pediatric intensive care unit
TLC: Total leukocyte count
CRP: C-reactive protein.

Consent

Written informed consent was obtained from the patient for publication of this case report and accompanying images.

Authors' Contributions

Ashish Lal Shrestha participated in the surgical and perioperative management of the patient and conception and design of the report and wrote the paper. Santosh Maharjan reported the radiological findings. Anil Dev Pant and Pankaj Bahadur Nepali performed the histopathological analysis of the report. All have been involved in the diagnosis and patient care. All the authors read and approved the final paper.

Acknowledgments

We would like to thank the ward staff of PICU and the Pediatric Ward of Grande International Hospital for helping with the management of our patient.

References

[1] E. C. Howell, E. D. Dubina, and S. L. Lee, "Perforation risk in pediatric appendicitis: assessment and management," *Pediatric Health, Medicine and Therapeutics*, vol. 9, pp. 135–145, 2018.

[2] C. W. Y. Wong, P. H. Y. Chung, L. C. L. Lan, and K. K. Y. Wong, "Acute appendicitis presenting as pneumoperitoneum in a teenage boy undergoing chemotherapy: Figure 1," *BML Case Reports*, vol. 2015, article bcr2015210347, 2015.

[3] S. ŞSahin, T. ÇCavusolu, M. Kubat, and H. ÇCalisş, "A rare cause of pneumoperitoneum: perforated appendicitis," *Journal of Ayub Medical College Abbottabad*, vol. 28, no. 2, pp. 415-416, 2016.

[4] E. Mutabazi, A. Bonane, A. J. Ndibanje, and J. Rickard, "Epidemiological study of peritonitis among children and factors predicting mortality at a tertiary referral hospital in Rwanda," *East and Central African Journal of Surgery*, vol. 22, no. 3, p. 21, 2018.

[5] O. D. Osifo and S. O. Ogiemwonyi, "Peritonitis in children: our experience in Benin City, Nigeria," *Surgical Infections*, vol. 12, no. 2, pp. 127–130, 2011.

[6] K. K. Chan, "Acute appendicitis with pneumoperitoneum," *Singapore Medical Journal*, vol. 3, 1962.

[7] L. Duman, "Pneumoperitoneum," *Annals of Pediatric Surgery*, vol. 10, no. 1, pp. 20-21, 2014.

[8] B. Tan, J. J.-M. Wong, R. Sultana et al., "Global case-fatality rates in pediatric severe sepsis and septic shock: a systematic review and meta-analysis," *JAMA Pediatrics*, vol. 173, no. 4, pp. 352–362, 2019.

8

Gastric Emphysema in a Critically Ill Patient Successfully Treated without Surgery

Hiromi Ihoriya,[1] Tetsuya Yumoto ,[1] Masaya Iwamuro ,[2] Noritomo Fujisaki,[1] Takaaki Osako,[1] Hiromichi Naito ,[1] and Atsunori Nakao[1]

[1] *Advanced Emergency and Critical Care Medical Center, Okayama University Hospital, Japan*
[2] *Department of Gastroenterology and Hepatology, Okayama University Graduate School of Medicine, Dentistry, and Pharmaceutical Sciences, Japan*

Correspondence should be addressed to Tetsuya Yumoto; tyumoto@cc.okayama-u.ac.jp

Academic Editor: Kenneth S. Waxman

Gastric emphysema is a relatively rare clinical entity caused by injury to the gastric mucosa. A 62-year-old Japanese male with a history of heavy alcohol consumption and smoking was admitted to the emergency intensive care unit due to severe hypercapnic respiratory acidosis. His body mass index was only 12.6. Ten days after initiation of enteral feeding, he complained of abdominal pain. Computed tomography revealed intraluminal air in the distended gastric wall. Esophagogastroduodenoscopy showed diffuse edema, redness, and erosion throughout the stomach. Based on the findings of narrow angle and short distance of the aorta-superior mesenteric artery, the patient was diagnosed with gastric emphysema associated with superior mesenteric artery syndrome. He was successfully managed nonoperatively with treatments including intravenous antibiotics, gastric decompression, and bowel rest. Physicians should be aware of this unusual condition in such critically ill patients complaining of abdominal pain and needing close monitoring and observation to exclude gastric necrosis or perforation.

1. Introduction

Gastric emphysema, which is characterized by the accumulation of gas within the wall of the stomach with or without concomitant portal venous gas, is a relatively rare clinical entity. It can develop secondary to mechanical injury of the gastric surface resulting from elevation of intraluminal pressure such as malignant obstruction of the stomach outlet, superior mesenteric artery syndrome (SMAS), or excessive vomiting [1–5]. Although gastric emphysema is usually self-limiting and resolves spontaneously, it can be challenging to differentiate from emphysematous gastritis and mortality from the condition remains high [6]. To our knowledge, gastric emphysema has never been reported in a critically ill patient. Herein, we describe a rare case of gastric emphysema that might have been induced by SMAS in a patient with malnutrition and alcoholism. This paper should help raise physician awareness of this potentially critical condition.

2. Case Presentation

A 62-year-old Japanese male with a history of heavy alcohol consumption and smoking was brought to the emergency department due to altered mental status. He was confused and disoriented, with a Glasgow Coma Scale score of 8 (E2V2M4). His vital signs were as follows: respiratory rate: 36 breaths/min; pulse rate: 124 beats/min, blood pressure: 122/84 mmHg; and temperature: 35.9°C. Physical examination was unremarkable except for gross emaciation (height: 160 cm; weight: 32.2 kg; body mass index: 12.6). Also, no obvious abnormal neurological findings including paralysis or ocular movement disorder were observed. Arterial blood gas analysis revealed severe respiratory acidosis with pH: 7.187; $PaCO_2$: 110.3 mmHg; PaO_2: 145.9 mmHg; $HCO3^-$: 30.6 mmol/L; base excess: 6.8 mmol/L; lactate: 4.0 mmol/L; glucose: 104 mg/dl on 10 L/min of oxygen. Laboratory data showed hyponatremia of 117 mEq/L without any other abnormal findings. The patient was intubated and mechanically

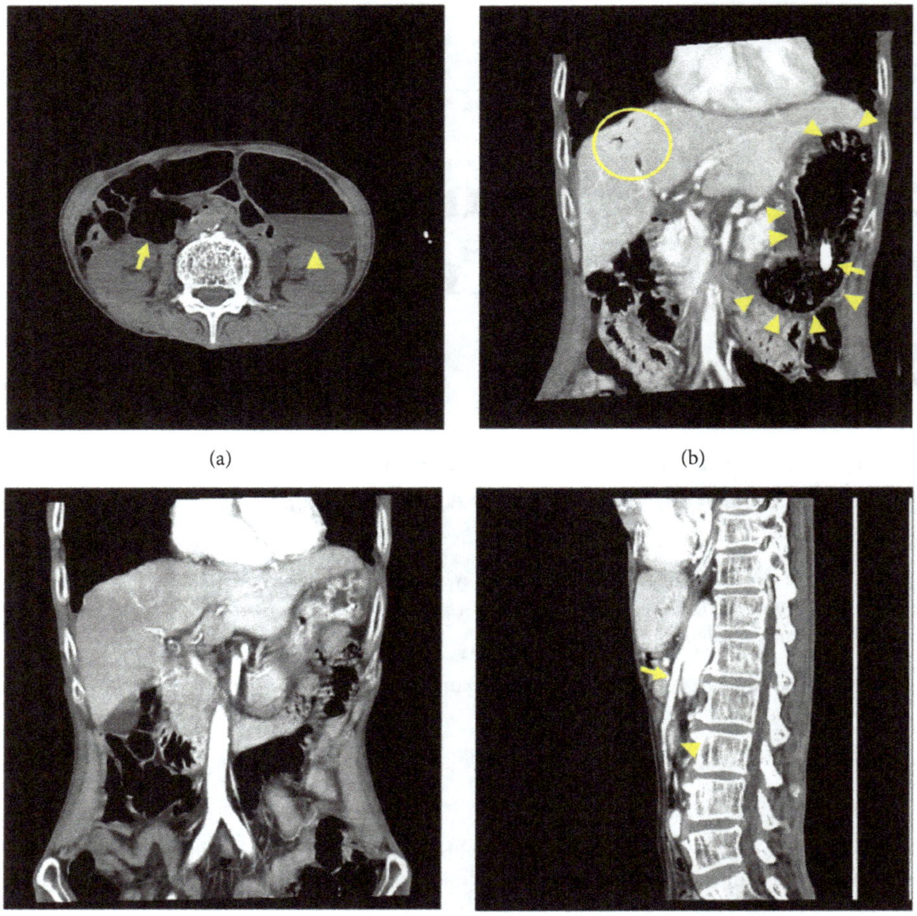

(a) (b) (c) (d)

Figure 1: Plain abdominal CT scan on admission showing dilatation of the stomach (arrowhead) and second portion of the duodenum (arrow) (a). Contrast-enhanced CT scan on hospital day 11 showing gas within the wall of a distended stomach (arrowheads) and portal vein (circled region). An arrow demonstrating the tip of the feeding tube (b). Follow-up CT scan showing improvement of gas in the stomach and portal vein (c). Sagittal view showing an acute angle of the aorto-superior mesenteric artery (arrow) and a collapsed duodenum (arrowhead) (d).

ventilated due to his altered level of consciousness resulting from severe hypercapnic respiratory failure. While computed tomography (CT) examination of the head revealed no abnormalities, abdominal CT showed dilatation of the stomach and second portion of duodenum (Figure 1(a)). He was admitted to the emergency intensive care unit for further management.

The patient received intravenous omeprazole for stress ulcer prophylaxis and ampicillin/sulbactam for suspected aspiration pneumonia from day 1. When his estimated original $PaCO_2$ level was restored (around 60 mmHg), his neurological state improved. On the second day, an enteral feeding was initiated through a nasogastric tube at 10 mL/h and advanced by 5 mL/day every 48 hours, as no gastric contents had been drained. Tracheostomy was performed on day 5 because prolonged ventilatory support had been expected.

On day 11, he complained of epigastric and left upper quadrant tenderness without guarding or rebound tenderness. In addition, a total of 500 cc of gastric fluid mixed with a material resembling coffee-grounds was drained through the nasogastric tube. His white blood cell count rose to 22,130 /μL with neutrophils 95.8%. Persistent abdominal pain and detection of ascites by ultrasound led us to perform contrast-enhanced CT, which revealed intraluminal air in the distended gastric wall with hepatic portal venous gas (Figure 1(b)). Esophagogastroduodenoscopy (EGD) demonstrated edema, redness, and erosion, with a white coating throughout the stomach without evidence of active bleeding or obvious necrotic lesions (Figure 2(a)).

As the patient had been hemodynamically stable with benign abdominal findings and without elevation of lactate levels, he was successfully managed with nonoperative treatments including intravenous vancomycin and meropenem, bowel rest, and nasogastric tube decompression. Blood cultures obtained on day 11 showed no growth. Follow-up abdominal CT scan on day 19 showed improvement of the

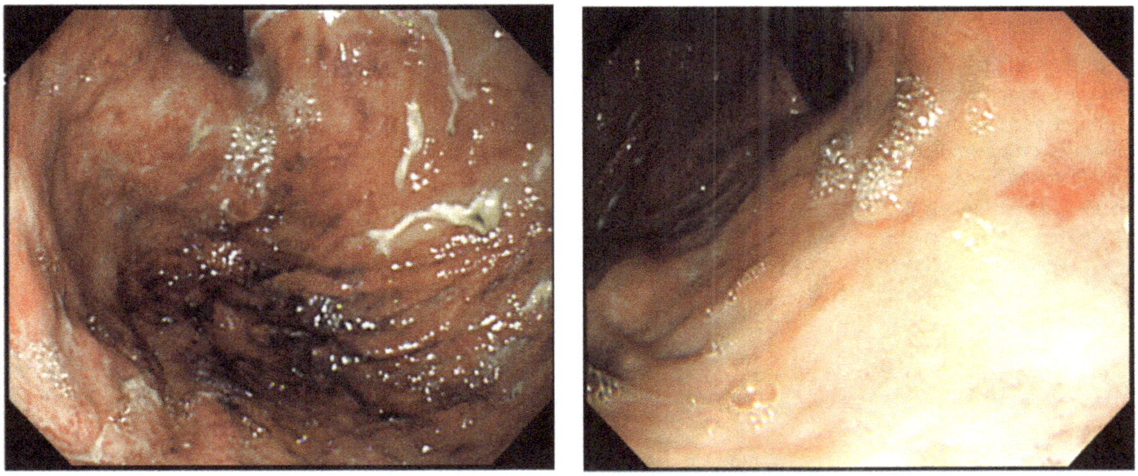

(a) (b)

FIGURE 2: Esophagogastroduodenoscopy demonstrating diffuse mucosal edema, redness, and erosive lesions with white coating throughout the stomach (a), which was resolved (b).

gas in the stomach and portal vein (Figure 1(c)). The aorta-superior mesenteric artery (SMA) angle and distance were 17 degrees and 4 mm, respectively (Figure 1(d)), suggesting SMAS as an underlying condition. Complete resolution of the erosive lesions was confirmed on repeat EGD on the same day (Figure 2(b)). Enteral nutrition was resumed uneventfully. Thereafter, the patient was transferred to another hospital for rehabilitation.

3. Discussion

Our case highlights the need to consider gastric emphysema, which might have been caused by SMAS, in a critically ill and malnourished patient complaining of abdominal pain. Conservative treatment was effective in treating gastric emphysema in patients with stable hemodynamic status without evidence of gastric necrosis or perforation.

Gastric emphysema is considered a relatively benign condition characterized by intraluminal gas in the stomach resulting from mucosal trauma. It is important to differentiate between gastric emphysema and emphysematous gastritis, both of which exhibit similar radiological findings of gas in the stomach wall with or without portal venous gas [6, 7]. Emphysematous gastritis is a distinct clinical entity related to infection of the gastric wall by gas-forming organisms [8]. The proposed predisposing factors for gastric emphysema resulting from mucosal trauma include gastrointestinal malignancy, gastric volvulus, SMAS, repetitive vomiting, or even nasogastric tube placement [1–7, 9], while immunosuppression, diabetes mellitus, ingestion of corrosives, alcoholism, or nonsteroidal anti-inflammatory drugs have been reported as common underlying conditions in a patient with emphysematous gastritis [6, 8, 10]. Surgical intervention may be warranted in patients with emphysematous gastritis due to development of necrosis or perforation of the stomach [8, 11]. In addition to proper hemodynamic monitoring and management and intravenous antibiotics, EGD should be performed to exclude ischemic stomach [6]. In the present case, benign abdominal findings with hemodynamic stability as well as without evidence of obvious necrotic lesions based on CT examination allowed us to treat the patient with conservative methods including broad-spectrum antibiotics, gastric decompression, and bowel rest.

SMAS is an unusual digestive condition characterized by compression of the third portion of the duodenum due to narrowing of the aorta-SMA angle as a result of extreme weight loss [12]. This clinical entity may cause gastric emphysema, which would be attributed to the elevation of intragastric pressure resulting from intestinal obstruction. To date, only a few cases of gastric emphysema associated with SMAS have been reported [3, 13–15]. Our patient was compatible with SMAS based on the findings of aorta-SMA angle and distance of below 25 degrees and 8 mm, respectively [16]. In addition to SMAS, underlying malnutrition and/or nonocclusive mesenteric ischemia might have contributed to the development of gastric emphysema in the present case [17–19].

As such, this was the first report of gastric emphysema that might have been caused by SMAS in a critically ill and malnourished patient admitted to the intensive care unit due to severe hypercapnic respiratory failure. Critical care physicians should be aware of this clinical entity in such severely ill patients complaining of abdominal pain. Careful hemodynamic monitoring and repetitive physical examination are necessary to exclude gastric necrosis or perforation, which need surgical intervention. Early diagnosis and proper management allow for successful nonoperative management in patients with gastric emphysema.

References

[1] S. Lee and JN. Rutledge, "Gastric emphysema," *The American Journal of Gastroenterology*, vol. 79, no. 11, pp. 899–904, 1984.

[2] M.-S. Soon, H.-H. Yen, A. Soon, and O. S. Lin, "Endoscopic ultrasonographic appearance of gastric emphysema," *World Journal of Gastroenterology*, vol. 11, no. 11, pp. 1719–1721, 2005.

[3] J. E. Lim, G. L. Duke, and S. R. Eachempati, "Superior mesenteric artery syndrome presenting with acute massive gastric dilatation, gastric wall pneumatosis, and portal venous gas," *Surgery*, vol. 134, no. 5, pp. 840–843, 2003.

[4] M. P. Parikh, M. Sherid, V. Ganipisetti, V. Gopalakrishnan, M. Habib, and M. Tripathi, "Vomiting-induced gastric emphysema and hepatoportal venous gas: A case report and review of the literature," *Case Reports in Medicine*, vol. 2015, Article ID 413230, 4 pages, 2015.

[5] P. Sharma and E. G. Akl, "A combination of intramural stomach and portal venous air: conservative treatment," *Journal of Community Hospital Internal Medicine Perspectives (JCHIMP)*, vol. 6, no. 1, p. 30519, 2016.

[6] K. Matsushima, E. J. Won, M. R. Tangel, L. M. Enomoto, D. M. Avella, and D. I. Soybel, "Emphysematous gastritis and gastric emphysema: similar radiographic findings, distinct clinical entities," *World Journal of Surgery*, vol. 39, no. 4, pp. 1008–1017, 2015.

[7] Z. G. Naqvi, N. Shahzad, A. R. Alvi, and S. Effendi, "Intramural gas in stomach along with acute calculus cholecystitis: an unusual association," *BMJ Case Reports*, vol. 2013, 2013.

[8] B. A. Wormer and G. Mostafa, "Emphysematous gastritis with delayed gastric perforation," *Journal of Gastrointestinal Surgery*, vol. 17, no. 7, pp. 1336–1338, 2013.

[9] N. A. Zenooz, M. R. Robbin, and V. Perez, "Gastric pneumatosis following nasogastric tube placement: a case report with literature review," *Emergency Radiology*, vol. 13, no. 4, pp. 205–207, 2007.

[10] J. Iannuzzi, T. J. Watson, and V. R. Litle, "Emphysematous gastritis: a young diabetic's recovery," *International Journal of Surgery Case Reports*, vol. 3, no. 4, pp. 125–127, 2012.

[11] P. A. Ferrada, "Successful surgical treatment of emphysematous gastritis on a patient with poor cardiac function," *The American Surgeon*, vol. 78, no. 2, pp. E66–E67, 2012.

[12] L. B. Cohen, S. P. Field, and D. B. Sachar, "The superior mesenteric artery syndrome. The disease that isn't, or is it?" *Journal of Clinical Gastroenterology*, vol. 7, no. 2, pp. 113–116, 1985.

[13] T. Ichikawa, H. Yamamuro, J. Koizumi et al., "Duodenal emphysema complicated with superior mesenteric artery syndrome in a patient with cerebral paralysis: a case report," *The Tokai Journal of Experimental and Clinical Medicine*, vol. 40, no. 2, pp. 40–43, 2015.

[14] Y. Sakamoto, K. Mashiko, H. Matsumoto, Y. Hara, N. Kutsukata, and Y. Yamamoto, "Gastric pneumatosis and portal venous gas in superior mesenteric artery syndrome," *Indian Journal of Gastroenterology*, vol. 25, no. 5, pp. 265-266, 2006.

[15] A. Martínez-Pérez, R. Trullenque-Juan, S. Santarrufina-Martínez, and E. Armañanzas-Villena, "Massive gastrointestinal pneumatosis in a patient with celiac disease and superior mesenteric artery syndrome," *Revista Española de Enfermedades Digestivas*, vol. 107, no. 11, pp. 709-710, 2015.

[16] S. Neri, S. S. Signorelli, E. Mondati et al., "Ultrasound imaging in diagnosis of superior mesenteric artery syndrome," *Journal of Internal Medicine*, vol. 257, no. 4, pp. 346–351, 2005.

[17] R. Udassin, I. Aviad, I. Vinograd, and S. Nissan, "Isolated emphysematous gastritis in an infant," *Gastrointestinal Radiology*, vol. 9, no. 1, pp. 9–12, 1984.

[18] T. Kim, H. U. Kim, and H. J. Song, "A case of gastric emphysema in anorexia nervosa presenting as acute gastric distension," *The Korean Journal of Gastroenterology*, vol. 60, no. 5, pp. 315–319, 2012.

[19] S. Bourcier, A. Oudjit, G. Goudard et al., "Diagnosis of non-occlusive acute mesenteric ischemia in the intensive care unit," *Annals of Intensive Care*, vol. 6, no. 1, p. 112, 2016.

9

Complete Heart Block as a Clinical Feature in Critically Ill Coronavirus Disease 2019 (COVID-19) Patients: A Case Series of Three Cases

Farook Ahmad,[1,2] Priti Gandre,[1] Julien Nguekam,[1] Alanna Wall,[1] ShiYu Ong,[1] Abdul N. Karuppamakkantakath,[1] Konstantinos Tasopoulos,[1] Muhammad Athar Sadiq,[3] Sazzli Kasim,[2] and Jeronimo M. Cuesta[1]

[1]*Critical Care Unit, North Middlesex University, Hospital NHS Trust, Sterling Way, London N18 1QX, UK*
[2]*Cardiology Unit, Medical Department of Universiti Teknologi MARA (UiTM) Sungai Buloh, Malaysia*
[3]*Cardiology Unit, Department of Medicine, Sultan Qaboos University, Muscat 123, Oman*

Correspondence should be addressed to Farook Ahmad; farook.ahmad@nhs.net

Academic Editor: Mehmet Doganay

Background. Novel coronavirus-19 disease (COVID-19) is associated with significant cardiovascular morbidity and mortality. However, there have been very few reports on complete heart block (CHB) associated with COVID-19. This case series describes clinical characteristics, potential mechanisms, and short-term outcomes of critically ill COVID-19 patients complicated by CHB. *Case Summary.* We present three cases of new-onset CHB in critically ill COVID-19 patients. Patient 1 is a 41-year-old male with well-documented history of Familial Mediterranean Fever (FMF) who required mechanical ventilator support for acute hypoxic respiratory failure from severe COVID-19 pneumonia. He developed new-onset CHB without a hemodynamic derangement but subsequently had acute coronary syndrome complicated by cardiogenic shock. Patient 2 is a 77-year-old male with no past medical history who required intubation for severe COVID-19 pneumonia acute hypoxic respiratory failure. He developed CHB with sinus pause requiring temporary pacing but subsequently developed multiorgan failure. Patient 3 is 36-year-old lady 38 + 2 weeks pregnant, gravida 2 para 1 with no other medical history, who had an emergency Lower Section Caesarean Section (LSCS) as she required intubation for acute hypoxic respiratory failure. She exhibited new-onset CHB without hemodynamic compromise. The CHB resolved spontaneously after 24 hours. *Discussion.* COVID-19-associated CHB is a very rare clinical manifestation. The potential mechanisms for CHB in patients with COVID-19 include myocardial inflammation or direct viral infiltration as well as other causes such as metabolic derangements or use of sedatives. Patients diagnosed with COVID-19 should be monitored closely for the development of bradyarrhythmia and hemodynamic instability.

1. Introduction

In January 2020, the World Health Organization declared the outbreak of novel coronavirus, SARS-CoV-2 (COVID-19) a Public Health Emergency of International Concern [1, 2]. The primary clinical manifestation of COVID-19 is the respiratory system, but involvement of other systems has been reported, especially the cardiovascular system [1–3]. Cardiovascular complications of COVID-19 include myocardial infarction, myocarditis, heart failure, cardiogenic shock, and cardiac arrhythmias [3]. However, CHB is a very rare cardiovascular complication of COVID-19 disease. We present a case series of 3 patients with no prior cardiovascular history and otherwise normal cardiac structure and function who were admitted to the Intensive Care Unit with COVID-19 and developed CHB during their clinical course. We believe that this is a rare yet fatal cardiovascular complication of COVID-19 disease. Thus, it is important for clinicians to be aware of this severe manifestation of the disease.

2. Case 1

Patient 1 was a 41-year-old businessman, with history of Familial Mediterranean Fever (FMF) on long-term colchicine, who presented to our institution with 1 week of fever associated with pleuritic chest pain and breathlessness. On arrival, he was noted to be hypotensive with elevated jugular venous pressure as well as severe respiratory distress requiring mechanical ventilator support. A nasopharyngeal swab test for SARS-CoV-2 by polymerase chain reaction was positive, and he was treated with Tocilizumab and Dexamethasone as per institutional practice. He was further managed in the Intensive Care Unit (ICU) for COVID-19 pneumonitis. Initial laboratory investigations showed lymphopenia (688 cells/mm^3) and raised inflammatory markers (CRP 110 mg/L, fibrinogen 888 mg/dL, and D-dimer 11000 ng/mL Fibrinogen Equivalent Units (FEU)). His renal markers, electrolytes, and troponin T on admission were all within normal limits (Table 1, Supplementary Data). Electrocardiogram (ECG) on presentation showed normal sinus rhythm at a rate of 82 beats per minute (bpm), normal intervals, normal axis, and no ST-T wave changes. There was no previous ECG for comparison.

He was proned immediately after endotracheal intubation. On day 5 of ICU admission, the patient was noted to be in complete heart block on cardiac telemetry monitoring. Figure 1(a) shows that a 12-lead electrocardiogram performed confirmed the diagnosis of CHB with a ventricular rate of approximately 50 bpm. Immediate laboratory investigations including thyroid function, cardiac biomarkers, and electrolytes were unremarkable. Echocardiogram revealed a normal left ventricular ejection fraction with no regional wall motion abnormalities or valvular pathology. The ongoing medication list was checked and found to be unremarkable for precipitating atrioventricular (AV) block. The complete heart block continued with a spontaneous and stable ventricular rate of 40-45 beats per minute with stable hemodynamics for a further three days. It was managed conservatively under vigilant monitoring with invasive cardiac output monitoring. On day 8 of ICU admission, he acutely deteriorated and had cardiogenic shock requiring noradrenaline and adrenaline. ECG showed ST elevation in AVR with global ST depression (Figure 1(b)). Cardiac troponins were significantly raised, and a repeat 2-D echocardiogram showed global hypokinesia with severely reduced ejection fraction of 20%. Shortly after, the patient deteriorated further and developed ventricular tachycardia (Figure 1(c)) and passed away later that day following a failed cardiopulmonary resuscitation (CPR). A timeline event for this patient is provided in Table 2, Supplementary data.

3. Case 2

Patient 2 is a 77-year-old Italian man with no significant past medical history who was brought in by ambulance to the emergency department with acute onset of shortness of breath for 3-day duration. He was noted to be severely hypoxic with $SpO_2 < 50\%$ upon arrival of paramedics at his residential home. He was intubated and proned immediately upon arrival from the emergency department. A nasopharyngeal swab was positive for SARS-CoV-2 by polymerase chain reaction and was treated with Tocilizumab and Dexamethasone as per institutional practice. Initial laboratory workup showed lymphopenia (628 cells/mm^3) and elevated inflammatory markers (CRP 128 mg/L, fibrinogen 818 mg/dL, and D-dimer 17000 ng/mL FEU). His other laboratory workup was within normal limits, including a normal troponin T (Table 1, Supplementary Data). His initial ECG showed a normal sinus rhythm with heart rate of 94 bpm, but no other abnormalities were found. There was no previous ECG for comparison. Chest radiography revealed bilateral ground-glass opacities and computed tomography pulmonary angiogram (CTPA) showed extensive patchy peripheral ground-glass opacification throughout the thorax but no evidence of pulmonary embolism. Echocardiogram revealed a normal left ventricular ejection fraction with no regional wall motion abnormalities or valvular pathology.

The clinical course in ICU was complicated by shock on day 7 of admission which progressed into multiorgan failure and support requiring continuous renal replacement therapy and hepatic failure as well as elevated troponin level (peak troponin T level was 5003 ng/L). He was also noted to have bradycardia with cardiac telemetry monitoring which revealed a CHB with occasional sinus pause, and the 12-lead ECG showed a CHB (Figure 2). These episodes of AV block alternating with CHB continued with increasing inotropic support. Laboratory investigations for electrolytes and thyroid function were all within normal limits. A balloon flotation temporary pacing wire was inserted successfully using bedside echocardiogram guidance, and he was scheduled for permanent pacemaker implantation. Unfortunately, he developed refractory hypoxic respiratory failure and was deemed not a suitable candidate for Extracorporeal Membrane Oxygenation (ECMO). Successive family conferences resulted in family shifting the focus of care to comfort measures. He passed away on day 10 of admission. A timeline event for this patient is provided in Table 2, Supplementary data.

4. Case 3

Patient 3 is a 36-year-old pregnant female, gravida 2 para 1 (G2P1) with previous Lower Segment Caesarean Section (LSCS) and currently at 38 + 2 weeks pregnant presented with acute onset of shortness of breath for 4-day duration associated with fever, myalgias, and diarrhea for 4-day duration. On arrival to the emergency department, the patient was noted to be febrile with a temperature of 38.8°C, tachycardic with a heart rate of 105 bpm, respiratory rate of 32 breaths per minute, and severely hypoxic with an oxygen saturation of 82% on room air. Her nasopharyngeal swab tested positive for SARS-CoV-2 by polymerase chain reaction and was treated with Tocilizumab and Dexamethasone as per institutional practice. Chest radiography revealed bilateral infiltrates. Initial lab workup revealed mildly elevated white blood cell count with lymphopenia (700 cells/mm^3), elevated procalcitonin (6.4 ng/mL), LDH (610 U/L), D-dimer

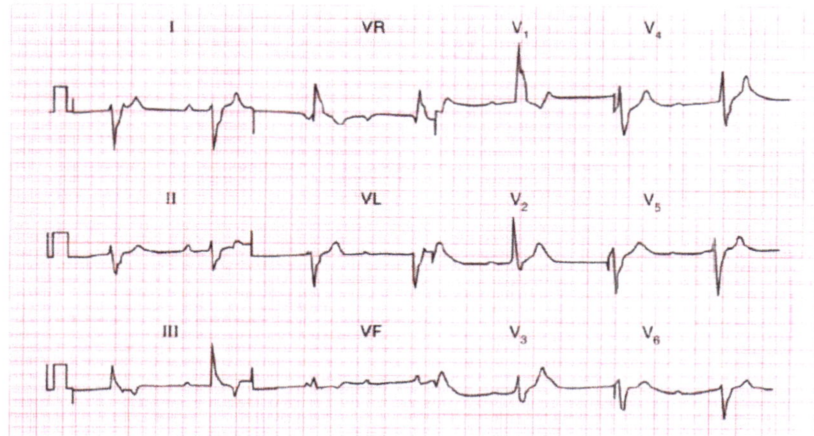

(a)

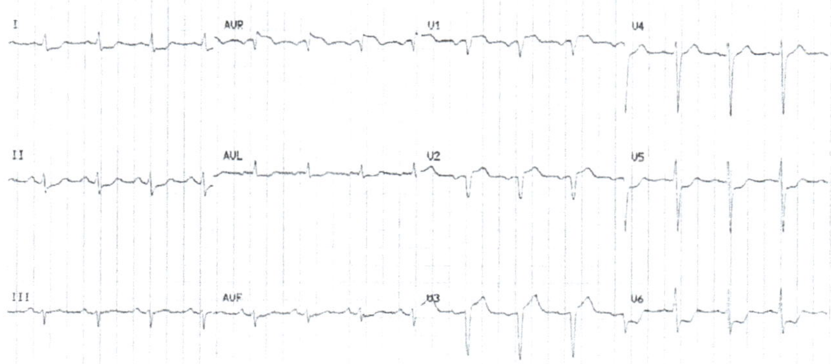

(b)

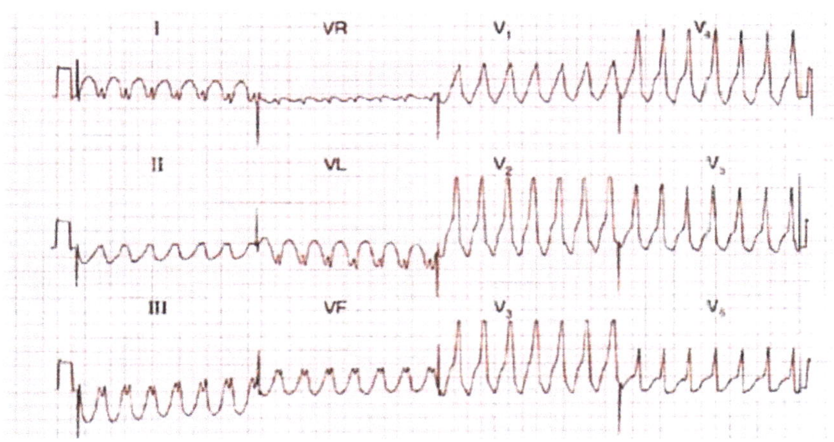

(c)

FIGURE 1: (a) ECG of patient 1 on day 5 ICU admission showing CHB with ventricular escape rhythm rate approximately 50 bpm. (b) ECG of patient 1 on day 8 admission showing ST elevation in lead AVR and ST depression at leads 1, AVL, II, AVF, V5, and V. (c) ECG of patient 1 on day 8 admission showing ventricular tachycardia and subsequently pulseless electrical activity (not recorded).

14000 ng/mL FEU, but normal troponin T < 0.01 ng/mL (Table 1, Supplementary data). ECG on admission (Figure 3(a)) showed sinus tachycardia at 167 bpm, normal intervals, normal axis, and absence of ischemic findings. She was commenced on noninvasive ventilation and had CTPA that showed severe extensive bilateral patchy ground-glass opacification throughout but no evidence of pulmonary embolism. She was intubated for worsening hypoxic respiratory failure and underwent a LSCS with no further complication and was subsequently admitted to ICU.

Her course of admission was complicated by progressive hypoxemia requiring prone ventilation. On day 3, the patient was noted to be in shock requiring inotropic support. Her ECG showed sinus tachycardia with diffuse T wave inversion. Echocardiogram showed global hypokinesia with depressed ejection fraction of 30% but normal septal thickness of

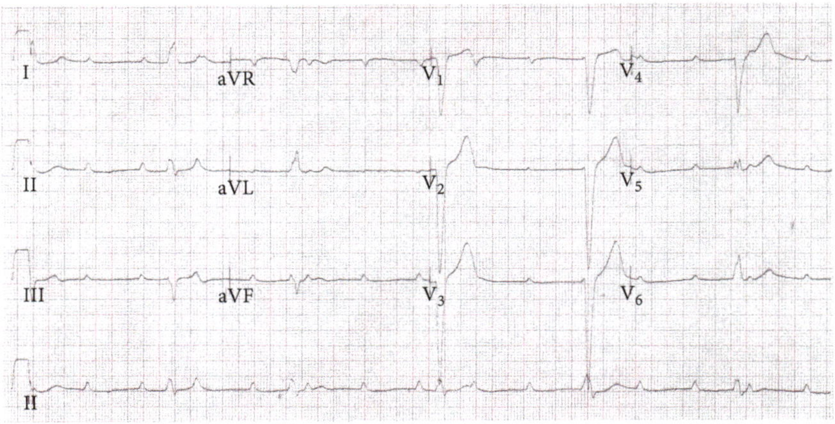

FIGURE 2: ECG for patient 2 on day 7 of admission showing CHB with ventricular rate approximately 35 bpm.

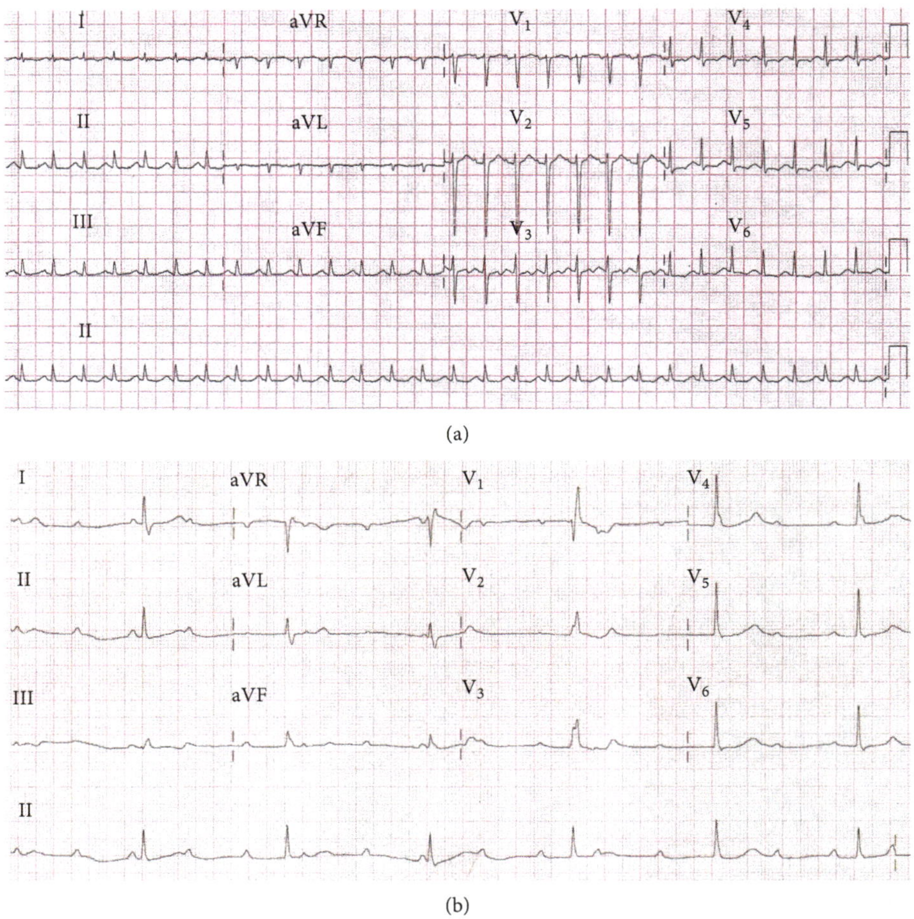

FIGURE 3: (a) ECG on admission for patient 3 showing sinus tachycardia. (b) ECG for patient 3 on day 5 admission showing complete heart block CHB with narrow QRS, suggesting distal AV node focus as origin of escape rhythm.

1.2 cm. Her serum CK was elevated at 600 U/L. A diagnosis of myocarditis was made [4], and she was continued on supportive care.

On day 5 of admission to ICU, intermittent complete heart block was seen on telemetry for less than 24 hours and 12-lead ECG showed a CHB with narrow QRS, suggesting distal AV node focus as origin of escape rhythm (Figure 3(b)). However, she was managed conservatively with vigilant monitoring as she was receiving prone ventilation for refractory hypoxia at the time and she was stable on single, nonescalating inotropic support. Her laboratory investigations for electrolytes and thyroid function were all within normal range. The CHB resolved gradually with improvement in hypoxemia. She was deemed not a suitable candidate for ECMO as the pAO_2/FiO_2 ratio improved with proning maneuvers. A repeat echocardiography shows improved ejection fraction to 50%. The patient was subsequently discharged to another critical care facility for continuation in management and was stable at the time of writing this report. She was also planned for repeat echocardiography as outpatient cardiology clinic follow-up. A timeline event for this patient is provided in Table 2, Supplementary data.

5. Discussion

The SARS-CoV-2 virus has caused a worldwide pandemic infecting millions of people, targeting primarily the respiratory system [1–3]. Cardiovascular complications have been reported with varying incidences as one of the manifestations that confer a worse prognosis [4]. Possible etiologies for cardiovascular complications include hypoxemia, electrolyte and metabolic abnormalities, microthrombi, and/or cardiomyopathy from direct invasion to the cardiomyocytes. Cardiac arrhythmias affecting the atrioventricular (AV) node have been reported in association with cardiac injury in critically ill COVID-19 patients [4, 5].

In our case series, initial and subsequent troponin levels were normal for all the patients. In addition, echocardiography results were not suggestive of underlying cardiomyopathy. This indicates a new onset AV node disease, from either direct infiltration of the AV node, i.e., focused involvement of the AV node, or the AV block being secondary to the critical illness itself. Possible etiologies for new-onset AV node disease include coronary artery disease (CAD); functional, structural, or valvular heart diseases; thyroid disease; medications; and infections [6–8]. Thus, the escape rhythm tended to be narrow, similar to the sinus in morphology, and of adequate rate to support normal hemodynamics without requiring temporary pacing as seen in patient no. 3. The hemodynamic instability requiring temporary pacing in patient 2 is probably contributed by multiple underlying causes rather than the complete heart block alone. Patient 1, meanwhile, has well-documented history of FMF. It has been previously reported that FMF patients are prone to develop CAD, mostly due to increased inflammatory activity and endothelial dysfunction [9]. Several studies and case reports have described the pericardial involvement in FMF patients including acute and recurrent pericarditis, constrictive pericarditis, pericardial effusion, and cardiac tamponade [10]. However, there is no report to suggest a direct correlation between COVID-19 and FMF with cardiac arrhythmia especially CHB and/or acute coronary syndrome.

The implication of the development of AV block in critically ill COVID-19 patients remains undetermined. In this case series, we have had mixed outcomes from the new onset of AV node disease. The resolution of AV block in patient 3 without further intervention suggests that a temporary or even permanent pacemaker is not required, while patient 2 required immediate temporary pacing wire insertion. Often the prone positioning and clinical status of these exceptional diagnoses make insertion of pacemaker very difficult, which otherwise would be the primary option to treat complete heart block.

While in the midst of the pandemic, we have also noted that sinus bradycardia is a very common finding in critically ill COVID-19 patients. However, these cases were not reported due to the fact that sinus bradycardia commonly occurs in patients with mechanical ventilator support and concurrently on high doses of sedatives and NMBA agent.

Previous publications on cardiovascular manifestation of critically ill COVID-19 mostly focus on acute coronary syndrome and/or myocarditis. To our knowledge, atrioventricular block is a very rare clinical manifestation of COVID-19 patients. Thus, it is important for clinicians to be aware of such a possible severe manifestation with undesirable outcome. We hope that this series will lead to future investigations of the pathophysiology of COVID-19 on the cardiovascular conduction system.

6. Conclusion

CHB can be a clinical manifestation of critically ill COVID-19 patients. Vigilant monitoring and due clinical suspicion are necessary to detect this in a timely manner. The prognosis of the AV node involvement remains unknown and will need future investigations as well as long-term follow-up.

Consent

Written and informed consent for publication was obtained from the next of kin of the 3 patients described in this case series.

References

[1] Z. Xu, L. Shi, Y. Wang et al., "Pathological findings of COVID-19 associated with acute respiratory distress syndrome," *The Lancet Respiratory Medicine*, vol. 8, no. 4, pp. 420–422, 2020.

[2] D. Wang, B. Hu, C. Hu et al., "Clinical characteristics of 138 hospitalized patients with 2019 novel coronavirus-infected pneumonia in Wuhan, China," *JAMA*, vol. 323, no. 11, pp. 1061–1069, 2020.

[3] C. L. Huang, Y. M. Wang, W. X. Li et al., "Clinical features of patients infected with 2019 novel coronavirus in Wuhan, China," *The Lancet*, vol. 395, no. 10223, pp. 497–506, 2020.

[4] S. Babapoor-Farrokhran, D. Gill, J. Walker, R. T. Rasekhi, B. Bozorgnia, and A. Amanullah, "Myocardial injury and COVID-19: possible mechanisms," *Life Sciences*, vol. 1, p. 253, 2020.

[5] T. Eneizat Mahdawi, H. Y. Wang, F. I. Haddadin, D. al-Qaysi, and J. V. Wylie, "Heart block in patients with coronavirus disease 2019: a case series of 3 patients infected with SARS-CoV-2," *HeartRhythm Case Reports*, vol. 6, no. 9, pp. 652–656, 2020.

[6] R. Gopinathannair, F. M. Merchant, D. R. Lakkireddy et al., "COVID-19 and cardiac arrhythmias: a global perspective on arrhythmia characteristics and management strategies," *Journal of Interventional Cardiac Electrophysiology*, vol. 59, no. 2, pp. 329–336, 2020.

[7] M. Zoob and K. S. Smith, "Aetiology of complete heart-block," *British Medical Journal*, vol. 2, no. 5366, pp. 1149–1154, 1963.

[8] M. Lev, "Anatomic basis for atrioventricular block," *The American Journal of Medicine*, vol. 37, no. 5, pp. 742–748, 1964.

[9] M. P. Grimaldi, G. Candore, S. Vasto et al., "Role of the pyrin M694V (A2080G) allele in acute myocardial infarction and longevity: a study in the Sicilian population," *Journal of Leukocyte Biology*, vol. 79, no. 3, pp. 611–615, 2006.

[10] A. Dabestani, L. M. Noble, J. S. Child, J. Krivokapich, and A. D. Schwabe, "Pericardial disease in familial Mediterranean fever: an echocardiographic study," *Chest*, vol. 81, no. 5, pp. 592–595, 1982.

Massive Pulmonary Embolism Complicating Coronavirus Disease 2019 (COVID-19) Pneumonia

Shruti Hegde,[1] Gemini Yesodharan,[1] John Tedrow,[2] and Alena Goldman[1]

[1]*Division of Cardiovascular Medicine, Department of Medicine, St. Elizabeth's Medical Center, Tufts University School of Medicine, USA*
[2]*Division of Pulmonary and Critical Care Medicine, Department of Medicine, St. Elizabeth's Medical Center, Tufts University School of Medicine, USA*

Correspondence should be addressed to Shruti Hegde; shruti.hegde1587@gmail.com

Academic Editor: Ricardo Jorge Dinis-Oliveira

Background. Patients with severe COVID-19 pneumonia are hypercoagulable and are at risk for acute pulmonary embolism. Timely diagnosis is imperative for their prognosis and recovery. This case describes an otherwise healthy 55-year-old man with respiratory failure requiring mechanical ventilatory support secondary to COVID-19 pneumonia. Massive acute pulmonary embolism with right heart failure complicated his course. *Case.* A healthy 55-year-old man presented to our emergency department (ED) with a sore throat, cough, and myalgia. A nasopharyngeal swab was obtained, and he was discharged for home quarantine. His swab turned positive for SARS-CoV-2 infection on real-time reverse transcriptase-polymerase chain reaction assay (RT-PCR) on day 2 of his ED visit. A week later, he represented with worsening shortness of breath, requiring intubation for hypoxic respiratory failure due to COVID-19 pneumonia. Initially, he was easy to oxygenate, had no hemodynamic compromise, and was afebrile. On day 3, he became febrile and developed significant hemodynamic instability requiring maximum vasopressor support and oxygenation difficulty. His ECG revealed sinus tachycardia with S1Q3T3 pattern. On bedside TTE, there was evidence of right heart strain and elevated pulmonary artery systolic pressure of 45 mmHg. All data was indicative of a massive APE as the etiology for his hemodynamic collapse. A decision was made to forgo computed tomography pulmonary angiography (CTPA), given his clinical instability, and systemic thrombolytic therapy was administered. Within the next 12-24 hours, his hemodynamic status significantly improved. *Conclusions.* This case highlights the importance of considering massive APE in COVID-19 patients as a cause of the sudden and rapid hemodynamic decline. Furthermore, timely diagnosis can be made to aid in appropriate management with the help of bedside TTE and ECG in cases where CTPA is not feasible secondary to the patient's hemodynamic instability.

1. Introduction

After its initial outbreak in Wuhan, China, in December 2019, SARS-CoV-2 has rapidly spread worldwide with 5,405,029 cases as of May 24th, 2020 [1, 2].

Our understanding of the etiology of multiorgan failure of severe COVID-19 infection is still incomplete. In critically ill patients with severe COVID-19 pneumonia, there is a correlation between elevated inflammatory markers and markers of hypercoagulability and adverse clinical outcome [3]. High D-dimer levels are commonly associated with venous thromboembolism and acute pulmonary embolism but are difficult to interpret in the setting of severe clinical illness. CTPA is typically done to confirm the diagnosis of APE. However, in cases of rapid clinical deterioration with hemodynamic instability, bedside echocardiogram and electrocardiogram in conjunction with a clinical pretest probability of acute venous thromboembolism can serve as vital diagnostic tools and aids in timely treatment. We describe a case of a previously healthy 55-year old with COVID-19 pneumonia complicated by APE.

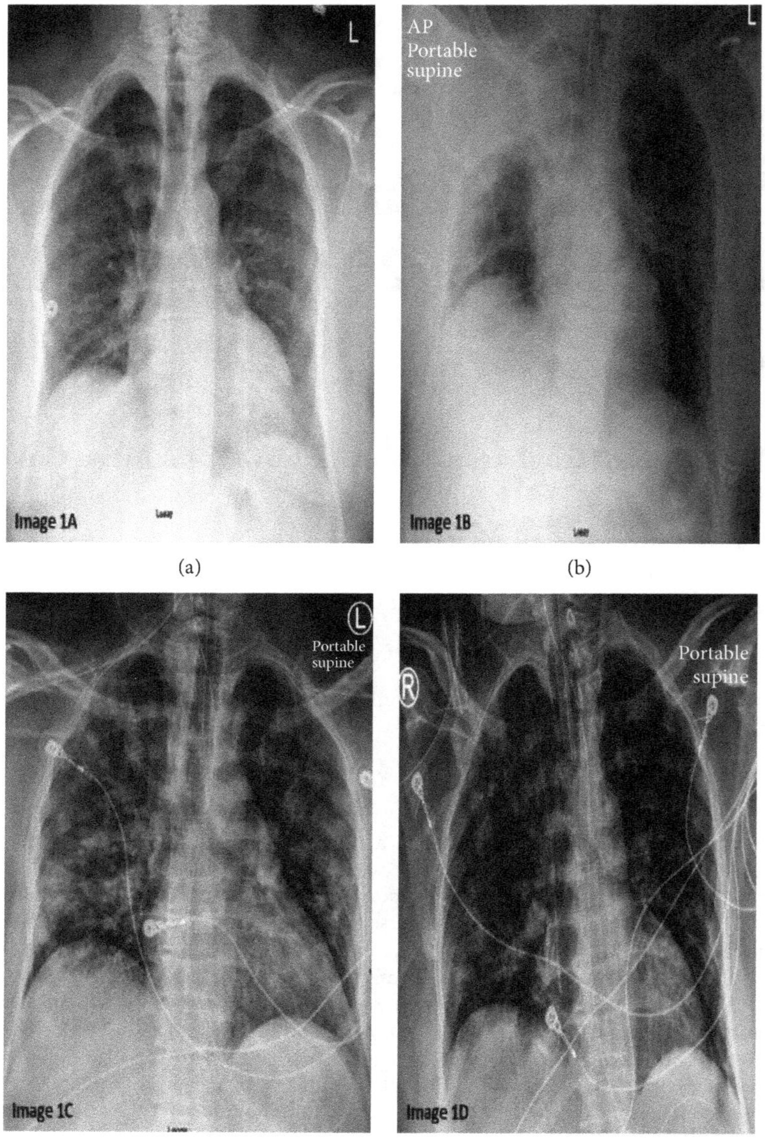

(a) (b)

(c) (d)

Figure 1: (a) Chest X-ray, PA view on initial presentation to emergency room showing increased interstitial markings bilaterally. (b) Chest X-ray, AP view done on patient's second emergency room visit showing bilateral patchy consolidations and worse in right lung fields. (c) Chest X-ray, PA view on hospital day 3 showing persistent bilateral patchy consolidations improved from hospital day 1. (d) Chest X-ray, PA view on hospital day 7 showing improved bilateral consolidations.

2. Case Presentation

A 55-year-old male without prior medical history presented to the emergency department (ED) with dry cough, sore throat, mouth sores, and myalgias for a week. He was afebrile with stable vitals. Physical examination revealed vesicular lesions on the buccal mucosa and the sublingual area, with posterior pharyngeal erythema, but no edema or midline shift. The lungs were clear. He worked as a taxi driver but denied obvious sick contacts. Chest X-ray (CXR) revealed increased vascular markings, especially at the left base (Figure 1(a)). 12 lead ECG showed sinus rhythm with normal axis, right bundle branch block, and inverted anterior T waves without other changes. Nasal swabs for coronavirus and influenza were obtained, and he was discharged home with instructions for self-quarantine for 14 days. Nasopharyngeal swab turned positive for SARS-CoV-2 on RT-PCR assay in two days.

The patient returned to the ED a week later, with worsening shortness of breath over 24 hours. He was afebrile, with a blood pressure of 143/80 mmHg and a resting heart rate of 88 beats per minute, respiratory rate of 38 per minute, and with oxygen saturation of 88% on 4 liters by nasal cannula. CXR revealed bilateral patchy infiltrates consistent with multifocal pneumonia, right greater than left lung field, and he was intubated with the diagnosis of COVID-19 pneumonia (Figure 1(b)). Laboratory data revealed an unremarkable

TABLE 1: Blood work of patient at the time of admission, on the day of event, and on day 8 of admission.

Laboratory measure	Reference range	Day 1	Day 3 (at the time of APE)	Day 5	Day 8
White blood cell ($x10^3/\mu L$)	4.5-11	7.0	21.7	43.1*	37*
Red blood cell ($x10^6/\mu L$)	4.0-5.5	4.99	3.82	3.42	3.78
Hemoglobin (g/dL)	12-17	14.5	11.2	10.4	11.2
Hematocrit (%)	35-50	43.8	37.9	31.5	37.9
Platelet count ($x10^3/\mu L$)	150-400	179	131	158	130
ESR (mm/hr)	0-20	90	NA	NA	NA
Sodium (mmol/L)	137-146	137	141	136	135
Potassium (mmol/L)	3.5-5.3	4.0	5.3	4.2	3.9
Chloride (mmol/L)	98-107	99	94	95	98
Bicarbonate (mmol/L)	23-32	26	14	20	24
Blood urea nitrogen (mg/dL)	5-25	10	38	25	42
Creatinine (mg/dL)	0.6-1.4	1.0	1.8	2.4**	3.0***
Ferritin (ng/mL)	30-400	1181	47646	NA	NA
Aspartate amino transferase (AST) (U/L)	15-41	216	>7000	2985	295
Alanine aminotransferase (ALT) (U/L)	14-63	159	4828	3168	975
Troponin T (ng/mL)	≤0.03	<0.01	<0.01	0.77	0.66
NT-pro-B-type natriuretic peptide (NT-pro-BNP) (pg/mL)	0-900	90	8244	3601	2801
Total creatine kinase (U/L)	49-397	133	NA	NA	NA
Creatine kinase MB (CKMB) (ng/mL)	0-6.0	NA	25.3	4.6	2.5
C-reactive protein (CRP) (mg/dL)	<0.5	22.91	31.57	NA	4.93*
C-reactive protein high sensitivity (mg/L)	1.0-3.0	162.7	NA	NA	NA
D-dimer, quantitative (μg/mLFEU)	<0.5	2.74	>20.0	NA	NA
Fibrinogen (mg/dL)	171-459	736	NA	NA	NA
PTT (sec)	23.3-35.9	28	38	75.4#	78.2#
Arterial blood gas (ABG)	Reference range	VC, FiO_2 40%, PEEP 12, TV 400	VC, FiO_2 100%, PEEP 14, TV 600	VC, FiO_2 40% PEEP 10, TV 400	Spontaneous/CPAP FiO_2 40%, PEEP 5
ABG (pH)	7.35-7.45	7.4	7.04	7.41	7.45
ABG partial pressure CO_2 (mmHg)	35-45	46	63.5	35.1	38.2
ABG partial pressure O_2 (mmHg)	80-100	215	70.6	139	113
ABG measured O_2 saturation (%)	94-98	99	90	99.8	99

*On hydrocortisone sodium succinate 50 mg intravenous every 8 hours. ** On continuous veno-venous hemodialysis. *** On intermittent hemodialysis. #On therapeutic heparin drip at 15.5 mls/hr (100 units/mL). DVT/PE anticoagulation protocol with heparin 25000 units/250 mL. Bolus dose of 80 units/kg. Initial infusion 18 units/kg/hr. Infusion adjusted to maintain target at PTT of 65-104 seconds. VC: volume control ventilation mode; FiO_2: fraction of inspired oxygen in percent; PEEP: positive end expiratory pressure in cmH_2O; TV: tidal volume in milliliter.

complete blood count and basic metabolic panel, AST, and ALT of 216 U/L and 159 U/L, respectively. He was stabilized on assist control (AC) ventilation with tidal volume (TV) of 400 mL, positive end expiratory pressure (PEEP) of 12 mmHg, and FiO_2 of 40%. On these settings, his arterial PaO_2 was 99%. He was maintained on midazolam drip for sedation. Azithromycin 250 mg once daily and hydroxychloroquine 200 mg Q12 hours were started.

The next day, he became febrile to 102F, and broad-spectrum antibiotics were added to cover for possible bacterial superinfection. Laboratory values were notable for leukocytosis of 14000/μL, creatinine of 1.8 mg/dL, ferritin of 1181 ng/mL, CRP of 163 mg/L, ESR of 90 mm/hr, fibrinogen of 736 mg/dL, and D-dimer of 2.74 μg/mLFEU. His LFTs and ventilator requirements remained stable on hospital day 2.

On hospital day 3, he became progressively hypotensive, tachycardiac, and hypoxic. He quickly escalated to requiring maximum doses of norepinephrine, epinephrine, vasopressin, and phenylephrine. Despite increased ventilator support with FiO_2 of 100%, PEEP of 14 mmHg, and TV 500 mL, his arterial blood gas (ABG) was notable for a pH of 6.86, pCO_2 of 84 mmHg, PaO_2 of 63%, and bicarbonate of 17 mg/dL. His peak inspiratory airway pressure was 25 cmH_2O and plateau pressure of 24 cmH_2O. Laboratory data showed worsening leukocytosis to 22,000/μL, creatinine of 3.1 mg/dL, AST of >7000 U/L, ALT 4828 U/L, troponin T < 0.01, CKMB 25.3 ng/mL, NT-pro-BNP of 8244 pg/dL, CRP of 31.6 mg/dL, ferritin 47,646 ng/mL, and D-dimer of >20 μg/mL/FEU (Table 1). Repeat CXR showed persistent bilateral patchy opacities (Figure 1(c)). Bedside 12 lead

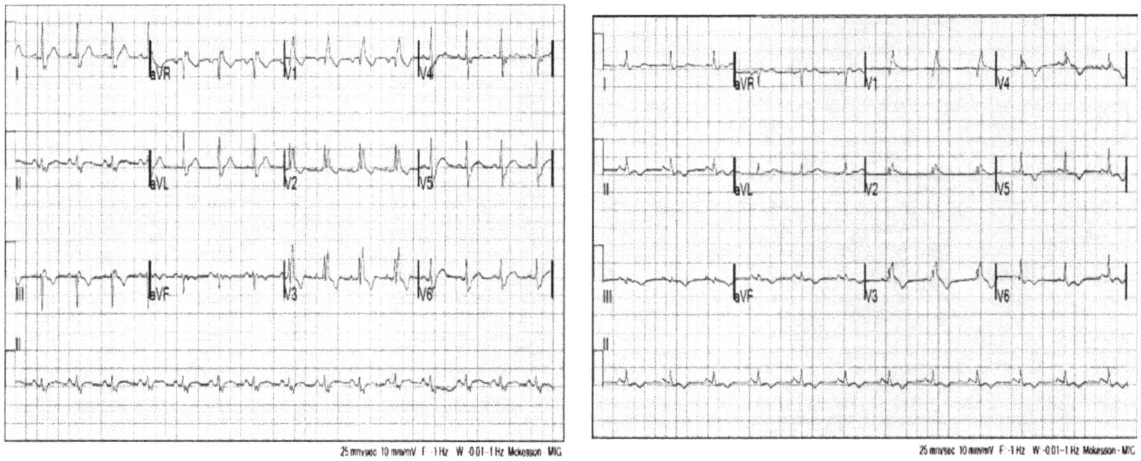

(a) (b)

FIGURE 2: (a) 12 lead EKG on the day of acute pulmonary embolism diagnosis showing sinus rhythm, heart rate of 90 bpm, PR interval of 145 ms, QRS duration of 145 ms, QTc of 420 ms, and QRS axis of 35 degrees. S1Q3T3 RV strain pattern with right bundle branch block (RBBB). (b) 12 lead EKG on day 5 of ICU admission: sinus rhythm, heart rate of 70 bpm, PR interval of 130 ms, QRS duration of 150 ms, QTc of 430 ms, QRS axis of 17 degrees, and RBBB. Diffuse T wave changes.

ECG revealed evidence of RV strain (Figure 2(a)). Bedside echocardiogram revealed severe right ventricular dilation, moderate tricuspid regurgitation, and severely reduced right ventricular function with global hypokinesis ventricle apical sparing, a.k.a. McConnell's sign (94% specificity for the diagnosis of APE) [4] (Movie 1-4). Given hemodynamic instability, a decision was made to proceed directly with systemic thrombolytic therapy in the form of tissue plasminogen activator (alteplase) (TPA) 100 mls at 50 mL/hr. He was then initiated on a heparin infusion as per standard DVT/PE protocol. Over the next day, there was a steady improvement in his hemodynamics. He unfortunately suffered acute oliguric kidney injury and required CVVHD.

By day 5, the patient was weaned off vasopressors. By day 10, he was extubated to nasal cannula. By day 14, at the time of submission, he was discharged to acute rehabilitation facility on room air and apixaban 2.5 mg twice daily given hemodialysis requirement. Repeat CXR and ECG are shown in Figures 1(d) and 2(b), respectively.

3. Discussion

We describe a patient with COVID-19 pneumonia complicated by APE, which was diagnosed by bedside tests and successfully treated with thrombolysis.

From the available data from our Chinese colleagues, some of the severe COVID-19 complications correlate with the host inflammatory process and cytokine storm induced by the virus [5, 6]. In our patient, the hypercoagulable state was evident by increased D-dimer and fibrinogen levels, which is not uncommon for the degree of illness. Critically elevated levels of CRP and ESR were observed around the time of APE diagnosis. A heightened inflammatory response resulting in prothrombotic milieu could be one of the possible causes of APE in our patient. Younger patients with a robust immune system may be more susceptible to these complications, and early initiation of immunomodulating therapy is under investigation in this patient subgroup.

Critically ill COVID-19 pneumonia patients fulfill three criteria of Virchow's triad: prolonged immobilization, inflammatory state, and the possibility of endothelial cell damage. A recent study by Obi et al. done on critically ill patients with influenza A H1N1 ARDS, empirical systemic heparin anticoagulation significantly reduced the incidence of pulmonary embolism without increased hemorrhagic complications [7]. A study from Wuhan, China, on 183 consecutive patients with COVID-19 showed that nonsurvivors had markedly elevated levels of D-dimer and fibrin degradation product compared to survivors indicating a higher prothrombotic risk [8]. Empiric therapeutic anticoagulation was used in some severe COVID-19 patients in Wuhan [9]. Initiating empiric anticoagulation, particularly in higher-risk groups of patients, needs more data at this time.

In a recently published study in Lancet [10], retrospective analysis of 25 patients with COVID-19 pneumonia who underwent CTPA due to suspected APE and other clinical concerns found APE in ten patients (40%) of the cohort. Emboli were predominantly located in small branches of the pulmonary artery. The thrombus was partly or entirely resorbed after initiation of systemic anticoagulation therapy for three patients who underwent a follow-up CTPA [10]. In our patient, timely treatment of APE aborted progressive obstructive shock that would have undoubtedly resulted in the patient's demise.

4. Conclusion

Our case is one of the few descriptions of a massive APE in a patient with severe SARS-CoV2 pneumonia, promptly diagnosed, and successfully treated with systemic thrombolysis. A bedside echocardiogram and a 12 lead ECG aided in the timely diagnosis of APE as a cause of the sudden hemodynamic collapse and rapid change in oxygenation and ventilation status of our patient. Bedside diagnosis was crucial for both fast therapeutics and avoiding transportation of a critically ill COVID-19 positive patient for an urgent CTPA, thus avoiding cross-contamination and conserving PPE. Further research is required to determine the cause and effect relationship between overactive inflammatory response and risk of development of venous thromboembolic complications in this critically ill patient cohort, as well as to elucidate safety and best anticoagulation choices. Likewise, studies are needed to establish an effect of direct antiviral and immunomodulating therapy on decreasing thromboembolic complications.

5. Limitations

The inability to confirm APE with CTPA is a limitation of our case. However, clinical indicators, bedside tests, and clinical response to therapy were sufficient for diagnosis of a massive APE complicating COVID-19 pneumonia.

Additional Points

Learning Objectives. (1) Patients with severe coronavirus disease 2019 (COVID-19) pneumonia are hypercoagulable and are at risk for acute pulmonary embolism (APE). (2) Massive acute pulmonary embolism should always be considered in the differential diagnosis for sudden and rapid hemodynamic decline in patients with COVID-19. (3) Critical care bedside echocardiography along with other clinical indicators helps in timely diagnosis and thus treatment of APE in patients with COVID-19 pneumonia, which is lifesaving.

Consent

No written consent has been obtained from the patient as there is no patient identifiable data included in the current case report.

Acknowledgments

The authors thank the faculty involved in the Division of Cardiovascular Medicine and critical care faculty at St. Elizabeth's Medical Center, Tufts University School of Medicine.

Supplementary Materials

Movie 1A-: transthoracic echocardiography (TEE) parasternal long axis view shows enlarged right ventricle (RV) and a small under filled hyperdynamic left ventricular (LV) cavity. Movie 1B: TTE parasternal short axis view at the level of mitral valve showing enlarged right ventricular (RV) cavity with flattened "D-shaped" interventricular septum (IVS). Movie 1C: TTE apical four-chamber view shows enlarged right ventricle (RV) with severely reduced right ventricular function and global hypokinesis of the right ventricle sparing the apex (McConnell's sign encircled). Also, note the flattening and shift of IVS towards left ventricle (LV). Movie 1D: TTE apical four-chamber view with color Doppler across tricuspid valve (TV) shows moderate tricuspid regurgitation (arrow). Also, seen is the enlarged right ventricle (RV) with severely reduced right ventricular function and McConnell's sign. *(Supplementary Materials)*

References

[1] P. Zhou, X. L. Yang, X. G. Wang et al., "A pneumonia outbreak associated with a new coronavirus of probable bat origin," *Nature*, vol. 579, no. 7798, pp. 270–273, 2020.

[2] "Coronavirus COVID-19 Global Cases by Center for Systems Science and Engineering at Johns Hopkins University," May 2020, https://coronavirus.jhu.edu/map.html.

[3] H. Wang, S. Luo, Y. Shen et al., "Multiple enzyme release, inflammation storm and hypercoagulability Are Prominent Indicators For disease Progression In COVID-19: a multi-centered, Correlation Study with CT imaging score," *The Lancet*, 2020.

[4] M. V. McConnell, S. D. Solomon, M. E. Rayan, P. C. Come, S. Z. Goldhaber, and R. T. Lee, "Regional right ventricular dysfunction detected by echocardiography in acute pulmonary embolism," *The American Journal of Cardiology*, vol. 78, no. 4, pp. 469–473, 1996.

[5] W. J. Guan, Z. Y. Ni, Y. Hu et al., "Clinical characteristics of coronavirus disease 2019 in China," *New England Journal of Medicine*, vol. 382, no. 18, pp. 1708–1720, 2020.

[6] X. Yang, Y. Yu, J. Xu et al., "Clinical course and outcomes of critically ill patients with SARS-CoV-2 pneumonia in Wuhan, China: a single-centered, retrospective, observational study," *The Lancet Respiratory Medicine*, vol. 8, no. 5, pp. 475–481, 2020.

[7] A. T. Obi, C. J. Tignanelli, B. N. Jacobs et al., "Empirical systemic anticoagulation is associated with decreased venous thromboembolism in critically ill influenza A H1N1 acute respiratory distress syndrome patients," *Journal of Vascular Surgery. Venous and Lymphatic Disorders*, vol. 7, no. 3, pp. 317–324, 2019.

[8] N. Tang, D. Li, X. Wang, and Z. Sun, "Abnormal coagulation parameters are associated with poor prognosis in patients with novel coronavirus pneumonia," *Journal of Thrombosis and Haemostasis*, vol. 18, no. 4, pp. 844–847, 2020.

[9] Y. Zhang, W. Cao, M. Xiao et al., "Clinical and coagulation characteristics of 7 patients with critical COVID-2019 pneumonia and acro-ischemia," *Zhonghua Xue Ye Xue Za Zhi*, vol. 41, 2020.

[10] J. Chen, X. Wang, S. Zhang et al., "Findings of acute pulmonary embolism in COVID-19 patients," *SSRN Electronic Journal*, 2020.

11

Acute Pancreatitis Induced by Diabetic Ketoacidosis with Major Hypertriglyceridemia: Report of Four Cases

Karama Bouchaala, Mabrouk Bahloul, Sabrine Bradii, Hela Kallel, Kamilia Chtara, and Mounir Bouaziz

Department of Intensive Care, HabibBourguiba University Hospital, Sfax, Tunisia

Correspondence should be addressed to Mabrouk Bahloul; bahloulmab@yahoo.fr

Academic Editor: Kenneth S. Waxman

Acute pancreatitis (AP) is a real clinical challenge. Acute pancreatitis remains a common cause of emergency department consultations and a major cause for hospitalization. Gallstones and drinking a lot of alcohol are the most frequent causes of AP. Moreover, AP can be induced by diabetic ketoacidosis (DKA) complicated by hypertriglyceridemia. We report 4 cases of DKA with hypertriglyceridemia complicated by AP in previously undiagnosed diabetes patients. All of our patients presented to the emergency ward with abdominal pain. Their physical exam showed epigastric tenderness. An abdominal CT scan was performed for each patient, showing an AP grade E. Laboratory samples showed high serum glucose levels. They had metabolic acidosis with elevated anion gap. They had high lipasemia and amylasemia. Their lipid panel was disturbed with a high level of cholesterol (from 12.8 mmol/l to 33 mmol/l) and triglyceridemia (from 53 to 133 mmol/l). Our patients were admitted into our ICU where they received fluid resuscitation and intravenous insulin, and their triglycerides rates decreased gradually. Two patients recovered to a good health state, and the two others developed septic shock, requiring the use of large-spectrum antibiotics, and acute kidney injury (AKI) with refractory metabolic acidosis, requiring hemodialysis. Despite the intensive treatment, they developed an unrecoverable multiorgan failure. Through our case series, we aim to highlight the importance of making an early diagnosis, which can be difficult in some situations due to overlapping signs; however, it is crucial for a good recovery. A good understanding of the pathway of hypoinsulinemic states causing hypertriglyceridemia then AP is important because it is the key to best management.

1. Introduction

Acute pancreatitis (AP) is a real clinical challenge. Nowadays, acute pancreatitis represents a common cause of emergency department consultations and a major cause for hospitalization. Gallstones and drinking a lot of alcohol are the most frequent causes of AP [1]. Moreover, AP can be induced by diabetic ketoacidosis (DKA), complicated by hypertriglyceridemia [2]. However, and to the best of our knowledge, the association of this triad of pancreatitis, hypertriglyceridemia, and diabetic ketoacidosis and its treatment has not been widely discussed in the literature in both adults and children [3]. Rapid diagnosis is difficult due to overlapping signs, but it is crucial for adequate management. We report 4 cases of DKA with hypertriglyceridemia complicated by AP in previously undiagnosed diabetes patients.

2. Case Reports

2.1. Case 1. A previously healthy 12-year-old girl, with a 10-day history of nausea, polyuria, and polydipsia, was brought to the emergency department for abdominal pain and vomiting. The patient did not have any history of alcohol consumption or medical health problems besides this presenting complaint. She was admitted in the pediatric unit. On admission to the ICU, the physical exam

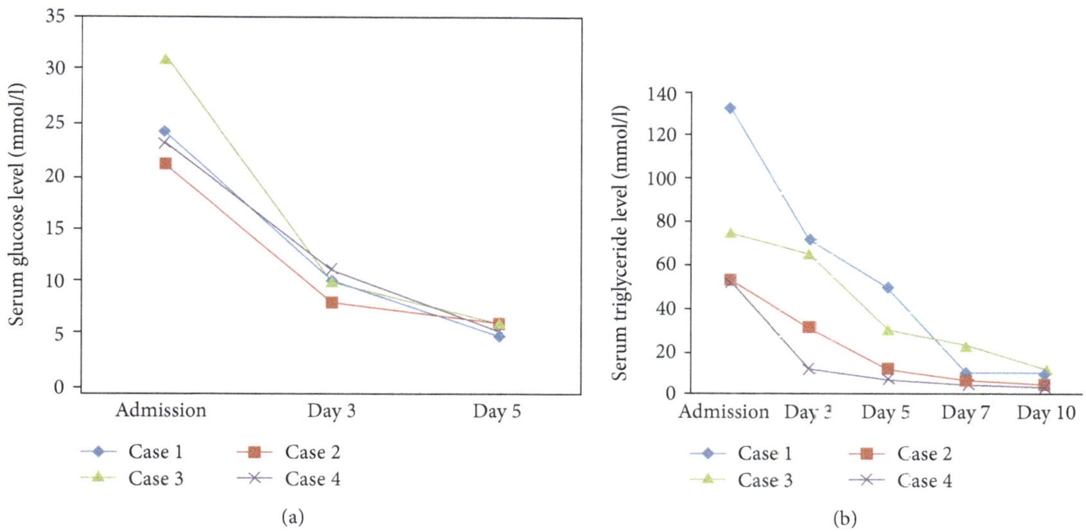

Figure 1: Evolution of serum glucose (a) and serum triglyceride (b) and level under treatment in all patients.

showed diffuse abdominal pain. She had sunken eyes with a clear acetone-smelling breath.

Her blood pressure was at 80/40 mmHg, pulse at 140 beats/min, respiration rate at 35/min, pulse oxygen saturation (SpO_2) under air room at 96%, and body temperature at 38°C. Laboratory samples showed serum glucose level at 24 mmol/l, pH at 7.19, bicarbonate at 10 mmol/l, anion gap at 26, lipase at 260 U/l, amylase at 244 U/l, cholesterol at 33 mmol/l, and serum triglyceride = 133 mmol/l. WBC count was at 14650/mm^3 and glycated hemoglobin was at 11.0%. Aspartate aminotransferase (AST), alanine aminotransferase (ALT), alkaline phosphatase, and bilirubin values were normal.

The abdominal ultrasound exam was normal. An abdominal CT scan was performed showing an AP grade E with three fluid collections and the presence of retroperitoneal air. The diagnosis of AP induced by DKA with concurrent hypertriglyceridemia was obtained, and the patient was transferred to our ICU for an adequate management. Continuous insulin infusion and fluid administration were initiated. The patient's health state improved. Her triglyceride rate decreased gradually (Figure 1). Continuous insulin was switched to subcutaneous insulin, and the patient was discharged after five days.

2.2. Case 2. A 12-year-old female child with no medical history and no history of prior biliary colic or alcohol consumption was admitted in the pediatric unit for abdominal pain and fever. Questioning the parents' revealed that, for 4 weeks, she had been suffering from polyuria and polydipsia associated with a significant loss of weight. The patient's health status deteriorated gradually, with abdominal pain and fever. The physical exam showed diffuse abdominal tenderness with an important decrease of bowel sounds. Her blood pressure was at 60/30 mmHg, pulse at 160 beats/min, temperature at 39°C, and respiratory rate at 30/min. The laboratory exams showed serum glucose level at 21 mmol/l, hemoglobin A1c at 16.5%, pH = 7.24, bicarbonate at 5 mmol/l, anion gap at 36, serum sodium = 142 mmol/l, serum potassium = 2.7 mmol/l, lipase = 411 U/l, amylase = 361 U/l, cholesterol = 12.8 mmol/l, and serum triglyceride = 53 mmol/l with apparent lipema in the lab test tubes. The other biochemical values were at the normal range, particularly the aspartate aminotransferase (AST), alanine aminotransferase (ALT), alkaline phosphatase, and bilirubin values.

Computed tomography (CT) scan revealed gastric distension, changes in the interstitium of the pancreas, and intrahepatic bile duct dilatation. The imaging did not show any other anomaly causing acute pancreatitis, in particular, a gallstone disease or extrahepatic duct dilatation. The patient developed respiratory distress needing the use of mechanical ventilation, then she was transferred to the intensive care unit. In ICU, she underwent fluid infusion, catecholamine prescription, and insulin infusion. During her ICU stay, she developed septic shock, requiring large-spectrum antibiotics, and acute kidney injury (AKI) with refractory metabolic acidosis, requiring hemodialysis. Despite the intensive treatment, the patient developed a multiorgan failure. She died 12 days after ICU admission.

2.3. Case 3. A 37-year-old male presenting with 2 weeks of polyuria, polydipsia, and epigastric pain and vomiting was admitted in an intensive care unit for consciousness alteration. Taking his medical history by interrogating his parents did not reveal any alcohol abuse or a prior history of biliary colic.

On admission, the initial assessment showed a Glasgow Coma Scale Score at 8/15, body temperature at 38.3°C, heart rate at 120 beats/min, blood pressure at 80/45 mmHg, respiratory rate at 30 breaths/min, and an oxygen saturation of 93% under room air. He needed intubation and mechanical ventilation.

The laboratory tests showed serum glucose at 32 mmol/l, pH = 7.31, bicarbonate = 10.7 mmol/l, serum sodium = 132 mmol/l, serum potassium = 3.9 mmol/l, lipase = 511 U/l, cholesterol = 12.8 mmol/l, serum triglyceride = 75 mmol/l,

WBC count = 3900/mm^3, platelet count = 101000/mm^3, and CRP at 496 mg/l. Aspartate aminotransferase, alanine aminotransferase, alkaline phosphatase, and bilirubin values were at the normal range.

An abdominal CT scan with contrast was obtained showing an acute pancreatitis grade E with two fluid collections in the pancreas. There was no evidence for gallstones. He was aggressively hydrated and received IV insulin.

A repeat abdomen CT scan, performed 7 days later, showed a necrotic fluid collection which was infected. An endoscopic drainage was performed. The patient's neurological status deteriorated with no sign of waking up and multiple episodes of seizures. A brain CT scan was performed, showing cortical and subcortical hypodense lesion in the right frontal area.

During his ICU stay, the patient developed septic shock with multiorgan failure. He died 45 days after ICU admission.

2.4. Case 4. A 42-year-old man with no significant medical history, presented after 10 days of polyuria and polydipsia, was admitted into the emergency department for vomiting and abdominal pain. No history of alcohol consumption was found.

The physical exam showed a diffuse abdominal tenderness. His blood pressure was at 100/70 mmHg, pulse at 130 beats/min, temperature at 37°C, and respiratory rate at 32 beats/min.

The laboratory tests showed serum glucose level at 23 mmol/l, hemoglobin A1c at 16.5%, pH = 7.26, bicarbonate = 7 mmol/l, anion gap = 36, serum sodium = 143 mmol/l, serum potassium = 2.9 mmol/l, lipase = 441 U/l, amylase = 361 U/l, cholesterol = 12.8 mmol/l, and triglyceridemia = 53 mmol/l with apparent lipema in the lab test tubes. WBC count was at 9200/mm^3, platelet count at 153000/mm^3, CRP at 330 mg/l, AST = 35 IU/l, ALT = 28 IU/l, bilirubin = 26 mmol/l, and the alkaline phosphatase=120 IU/l.

Computed tomography (CT) scan revealed an acute pancreatitis grade E with two fluid collections in the pancreas associated with peritoneal effusion. Fluid bolus and continuous insulin infusion were initiated. The patient's health state improved, and he was discharged after seven days.

All patient characteristics and laboratory results on admission are summarized in Tables 1 and 2, respectively. Figure 1 shows the evolution of triglyceride and blood glucose levels under treatment in all studied patients.

3. Discussion

Our cases confirm that AP can be induced by diabetic ketoacidosis (DKA) complicated by hypertriglyceridemia apart from any biliary cause or gallstone disease.

The literature analysis showed that the association between diabetic ketoacidosis, hypertriglyceridemia, and acute pancreatitis has rarely been reported. In fact, the triad of DKA with hypertriglyceridemia-induced acute pancreatitis occurs in 4% of cases [2]. It can affect both adults and children, as in our cases.

Table 1: Patients' characteristics.

	Case 1	Case 2	Case 3	Case 4
Age (years)	12	12	37	42
SAPSII in admission (points)	39	45	75	68
SOFA in admission (points)	16	20	18	16
ICU stay (days)	5	12	45	7
Mechanical ventilation (days)	0	12	45	0

Table 2: Laboratory results on ICU admission.

	Case 1	Case 2	Case 3	Case 4
Glucose serum (mmol/l)	24	21	32	42
Triglyceride (mmol/l)	133	53	75	53
Lipase (IU/l)	260	411	511	441
WBC/mm^3	14650	21500	3900	9200
Platelet/mm^3	88940	65000	101000	153000
pH	7.19	7.24	7.31	7.26
HCO_3^- (mmol/l)	10	5	20.7	7
PaO_2 (mmHg)	65	75	79	62
$PaCO_2$ (mmHg)	12	14	45	20
PaO_2/FiO_2 (%)	309	150	131	88
Serum sodium (mmol/l)	135	142	132	143
Serum potassium (mmol/l)	2.5	2.7	3.9	2.9
Chloride (mmol/l)	98	88	99	87
CRP (mg/l)	350	214	496	330

As far as the physiological side is concerned, there is a bidirectional relationship between dysglycemia and pancreatitis [4]. Acute pancreatitis could induce a beta cell dysfunction and transient insulin deficiency, and it could also increase insulin resistance due to systemic inflammation [5].

In this case, glycemic control can be achieved after remission of systemic inflammatory response and insulin infusion.

On the other hand, diabetes increases the risk of hypertriglyceridemia (HTG) which can induce acute pancreatitis. The mechanism by which HTG causes AP is still not completely understood. Many animal models have yielded some theories [6–8]. The first theory postulates that pancreatic lipase hydrolyses excess TG with the accumulation of free fatty acids in the pancreas. Free fatty acids then cause acinar cell and pancreatic capillary injury. The resultant ischemia creates an acidic environment, which further enhances free fatty acid toxicity [6].

The second hypothesis suggests that the hyperviscosity which is due to elevated levels of chylomicrons in these pancreatic capillaries leads to ischemia. HTG has also been shown to contribute to and accelerate the inflammatory cascade in animal models of AP [6].

The triad of acute pancreatitis (AP) coexisting with diabetes ketoacidosis (DKA) and hypertriglyceridemia (HTG) has a worse prognosis than a simple AP. In fact, this triad has the potential for devastating consequences with multiorgan failure. Many studies seek to evaluate AP outcomes in patients with and without DKA. According to Tsuang et al.'s analysis [6], the DKA group had significantly higher inpatient mortality compared to non-DKA-patients. DKA patients had almost 5 times higher odds of having AKI than those without DKA. Moreover, DKA subjects have a higher risk of ileus, shock, ARDS/mechanical ventilation, and/or SIRS [6]. They also need more parenteral nutrition, higher hospital charges, and longer in-hospital stay [2]. Other studies confirmed that the development of organ dysfunction and necrosis was present, more often observed in the hypertriglyceridemia-induced acute pancreatitis group than in the non-hypertriglyceridemia-induced acute pancreatitis group [2]. Making an early diagnosis is difficult due to overlapping signs, but it is important for a good recovery. In our study, all 4 patients were managed with fluid repletion and intravenous insulin infusion. Lipid-lowering treatments were started to decrease serum triglycerides. In our cases, 2 patients recovered relatively quickly, while 2 others died because they had severe pancreatitis and multiorgan failure, sepsis, and acute respiratory distress syndrome.

In our third case, the patient developed severe neurological signs with seizures. Pancreatic encephalopathy (PE) is very plausible. PE is a serious complication of severe acute pancreatitis, and it is considered a poor prognosis sign. The pathogenesis is not well elucidated. Many factors can be included: pancreatin activation, excessive release of cytokines and oxygen free radicals, microcirculation abnormalities of hemodynamic disturbance, ET-1/NO ratio, hypoxemia, bacterial infection, water and electrolyte imbalance, and vitamin B1 deficiency [7]. Understanding these factors is very important because it is the key to the prevention and best management of PE.

4. Conclusion

HTG-AP is associated with more complications and poor outcomes. The published studies concerning the mechanism of HTG-AP are in slow progress worldwide. Prospective ones enrolling a larger number of patients are still warranted to have more knowledge about HTG-AP and to promote the development of its therapeutic strategies.

Authors' Contributions

All authors contributed in drafting the manuscript. All authors read and approved the final manuscript.

References

[1] S. E. Roberts, S. Morrison-Rees, A. John, J. G. Williams, T. H. Brown, and D. G. Samuel, "The incidence and aetiology of acute pancreatitis across Europe," *Pancreatology*, vol. 17, no. 2, pp. 155–165, 2017.

[2] Y. Wang, B. M. Attar, K. Hinami et al., "Concurrent diabetic ketoacidosis in hypertriglyceridemia-induced pancreatitis: how does it affect the clinical course and severity scores," *Pancreas*, vol. 46, no. 10, pp. 1336–1340, 2017.

[3] P. K. Sharma, M. Kumar, and D. K. Yadav, "Severe hypertriglyceridemia causing pancreatitis in a child with new-onset type-I diabetes mellitus presenting with diabetic ketoacidosis," *Indian Journal of Critical Care Medicine*, vol. 21, no. 3, pp. 176–181, 2017.

[4] Y.-K. Lee, M.-Y. Huang, C.-Y. Hsu, and Y.-C. Su, "Bidirectional relationship between diabetes and acute pancreatitis: a population-based cohort study in Taiwan," *Medicine*, vol. 95, no. 2, p. e2448, 2016.

[5] A. D. Reghina, S. Craciun, and S. Fica, "Severe transient hyperglycemia in a prediabetic patient during mild acute pancreatitis," *Case Reports in Medicine*, vol. 2015, Article ID 968593, 3 pages, 2015.

[6] W. Tsuang, U. Navaneethan, L. Ruiz, J. B. Palascak, and A. Gelrud, "Hypertriglyceridemic pancreatitis: presentation and management," *The American Journal of Gastroenterology*, vol. 104, no. 4, pp. 984–991, 2009.

[7] X.-P. Zhang and H. Tian, "Pathogenesis of pancreatic encephalopathy in severe acute pancreatitis," *Hepatobiliary & Pancreatic Diseases International*, vol. 5, pp. 134–134, 2007.

[8] Y. Pan, Y. Li, L. Gao et al., "Development of a novel model of hypertriglyceridemic acute pancreatitis in mice," *Scientific RepoRts*, vol. 7, no. 1, 2017.

12

Liver Transplantation for Acute Liver Failure Attributed to Leptospirosis: A Report of Two Cases

Thibault Lebreton,[1] Fréderic Aubrun,[1] Jean-Yves Mabrut,[2] Laurent Heyer,[1] and Camille Perrin[1]

[1]Hospices Civils de Lyon, Hôpital de la Croix-Rousse, Service d'Anesthésie Réanimation, 103 Grande Rue de la Croix-Rousse, 69004 Lyon Cedex, France
[2]Hospices Civils de Lyon, Hôpital de la Croix-Rousse, Service de Chirurgie Générale, Digestive et Transplantation Hépatique et Intestinale, 103 Grande Rue de la Croix-Rousse, 69004 Lyon Cedex, France

Correspondence should be addressed to Thibault Lebreton; th.lebreton@gmail.com

Academic Editor: Gil Klinger

Background. Leptospirosis is a zoonosis caused by pathogenic spirochetes of the genus Leptospira. Although it may be limited to nonspecific fever, leptospirosis may also be responsible for neurological symptoms or fulminant diseases such as Weil's disease. Diagnosis is challenging due to the difficulty in isolating the organism and the delays required for performing the serological test. *Case Presentation.* Two cases of leptospirosis are presented here. The clinical picture differed from a real Weil's disease in the first case and from a neuro-leptospirosis in the second. However, both patients underwent liver transplantation because of the severity of the associated acute liver failure. Unfortunately, one of the cases had a fatal outcome. *Conclusion.*Antibiotic treatment for leptospirosis should not be delayed by the lack of a positive serology test for this potentially lethal disease. In the context of a history of exposure to risk factors for leptospirosis, a negative serology must be repeated 7 days to 2 weeks following the first test. Although not always present, acute liver injury may, in rare cases, require liver transplantation.

1. Introduction

It is estimated that more than 1 million severe cases of leptospirosis occur each year worldwide, with a mortality rate of 5–20% [1]. Leptospires are bacteria that colonise renal tubules of a large number of wild animals (rodents), and domestic animals (cattle, pigs, dogs) before being excreted in urine. The mode of transmission to humans can be direct (contact with infected animals), or indirect (through water and soils contaminated by infected urine) [2].

Leptospirosis demonstrates diverse clinical presentations, ranging from the anicteric febrile form, observed in the vast majority of cases, to extensive tissue damage, vasculitis that may be responsible for neurological manifestations and multiorgan failure. We report two cases of severe forms of leptospirosis with different clinical presentations that both required liver transplantation.

2. Case 1

A 23-year-old man was admitted to the Emergency Department following a 5-day history of fever with myalgia in calf muscles, jaundice, a purpuric rash on his feet, haematemesis, and anuria for 2 days.

There was no medical, surgical, or contributory medical history. The patient did not drink alcohol, smoke, or use illicit drugs. There was no travel history, but the patient reported fishing in rivers regularly and had been bitten by a ferret in the 15 days preceding presentation. Laboratory findings in the emergency ward were: haemoglobin 80 g/L, white blood cell count (WBC) 22 × 109 cells/L (neutrophils 90%), platelet count 13×10^9 cells/L, aspartate aminotransferase (AST) 174 IU/L, alanine aminotransferase (ALT) 110 IU/L, total bilirubin 28 mg/dL, international normalised ratio (INR) 2.7, serum creatinine 6 mg/dL, serum urea 106 mg/dL.

Antibiotic therapy with ceftriaxone and spiramycin was initially started after computed tomography (CT) scan of the thorax and abdomen showed diffuse micronodular interstitial syndrome. The patient was transferred to the intensive care unit due to acute liver failure and anuria that required continuous venous haemafiltration, (CVVH) therapy.

Hepatitis A, hepatitis B, and hepatitis C viruses were excluded by hepatitis-virus-panel investigation. There was no laboratory evidence of infection with Epstein-Barr virus, or Cytomegalovirus. Serum paracetamol concentration was less than 1 mg/L. Ceruloplasmin, α-1-antitrypsin, ferritin and an autoimmune screen were all unremarkable.

Based on the epidemiological context, compatible symptoms and biological results, an icterohaemorrhagic leptospirosis (Weil's disease) was suspected. This diagnosis was rapidly confirmed by positive leptospira serology combining IgM enzyme-linked immunosorbent assay method (ELISA), and microscopic agglutination test (MAT), as well as quantitative polymerase chain reaction (PCR) of blood and urine performed 7 days after the onset of symptoms. The patient was then treated with ceftriaxone alone for 2 weeks.

In the following days, the patient continued to have haematemesis and epistaxis. Liver involvement was mainly marked by cholestasis, with a maximum of total bilirubin at 65.9 mg/dL, AST at 524 IU/L, and ALT at 432 IU/L.

On the 10th day, the patient experienced haemorrhagic shock caused by bleeding from the pancreaticoduodenal artery. The patient had an asymptomatic median arcuate ligament syndrome, responsible for the development of numerous collateral fragile arteries. The haemorrhagic shock was controlled by embolisation of the pancreaticoduodenal artery.

Whilst the situation was stable, despite the persistence of liver and kidney failure, a gastroscopy was performed on the 30th day due to the appearance of melena. It found a complete ischemic necrosis of the duodenum with perforation, which was treated with a cephalic duodenopancreatectomy.

A deterioration was then noted, with major cytolysis and rapid development of acute liver failure (AST 16650 IU/L, ALT 7900 IU/L, total bilirubin 17 mg/dL, INR 3.12), requiring urgent orthotopic liver transplantation only 2 days later. Despite liver transplantation, the patient died 3 days after transplantation (36th day of hospitalisation) due to multiorgan failure and primary liver graft dysfunction.

3. Case 2

A previously healthy 60-year-old man, presented with fever, chills, and sweats, followed by an altered level of consciousness with a Glasgow coma scale score at 3. He had returned 18 days earlier from a trip to India and underwent a transrectal ultrasound guided prostate biopsy with ciprofloxacin antibiotic prophylaxis the day before. The patient was then sedated, intubated, and admitted to intensive care. The pupils were equal and he had no nuchal rigidity. Initial laboratory examination of peripheral blood showed: haemoglobin 158 g/L, white blood cell count (WBC) 13 × 109 cells/L (neutrophils 90%), platelet count 80×10^9 cells/L, AST 605 IU/L, ALT 355 IU/L, total bilirubin 3.4 mg/dL, INR 3.12, serum creatinine 2.2 mg/dL, serum urea 28 mg/dL.

Management consisted in invasive mechanical ventilation, norepinephrine infusion, and anti-infective treatment with cefotaxime, amoxicillin, and aciclovir, quickly replaced by meropenem, fosfomycin, and amikacin following the discovery of a multidrug-resistant Escherichia Coli on blood cultures.

Despite stopping the sedative infusions and a normal brain CT scan, there was no change in the level of consciousness. Furthermore, peripheral blood analysis demonstrated rapidly deteriorating acute kidney and liver failure:haemoglobin 110 g/L, white blood cell count (WBC) 15 × 109 cells/L (neutrophils 90%), platelet count 17×10^9 cells/L, AST 17000 IU/L, ALT 9500 IU/L, total bilirubin 4.7 mg/dL, INR 6.76, serum creatinine 4.5 mg/dL, serum urea 36 mg/dL.

A liver screen including serological testing for hepatitis A, B, C, HIV, herpes simplex virus, cytomegalovirus, and Epstein-Barr virus (EBV) was negative. Serum paracetamol concentration was less than 1 mg/L. Ceruloplasmin, α-1-antitrypsin, ferritin and an autoimmune screen were all negative. Dengue and other arbovirus infections were ruled out, and thick blood films were negative for malaria parasites. The initial leptospirosis serology (ELISA and MAT) was negative. Abdominal ultrasound did not demonstrate any vascular cause.

Renal replacement therapy with CVVH and hepatoprotection (*N*-acetylcysteine) were initiated. Finally, a highly urgent orthotopic liver transplantation was performed for fulminant hepatic failure, 6 days after the initial appearance of symptoms.

Following liver transplantation and cessation of sedation, whilst liver function tests and serum ammonia level returned to normal, an altered level of consciousness persisted which was associated with cerebellar ataxia, facial dyskinesia, swallowing disorders, and tremulousness of hands. Electroencephalography, cranial magnetic resonance imaging, and cerebrospinal fluid (CSF) analysis (no cells; normal glucose and proteins) were unremarkable. The diagnosis of leptospirosis with fulminant hepatitis failure and neuro-leptospirosis was finally made in view of the positivity of leptospira serology (ELISA and MAT) 2 weeks after the onset of symptoms. An Indian strain of Leptospira Hebdomadis was identified. The interrogation taught us later that the patient was led into a river whilst on an elephant ride, 3 days before his return to France. PCR performed 25 days after admission did not detect Leptospira DNA in the blood, CSF, or urine.

The clinical evolution was finally favourable, with progressive disappearance of cerebellar ataxia and improved renal function after several weeks. The patient was discharged to return home 74 days after the onset of symptoms.

4. Discussion

France, with an annual incidence between 0.5 and 1 case/100.000 inhabitants, is one of the industrialised countries with the highest incidence [3]. In nonendemic areas, travel is the main cause of leptospirosis. Other described risk factors

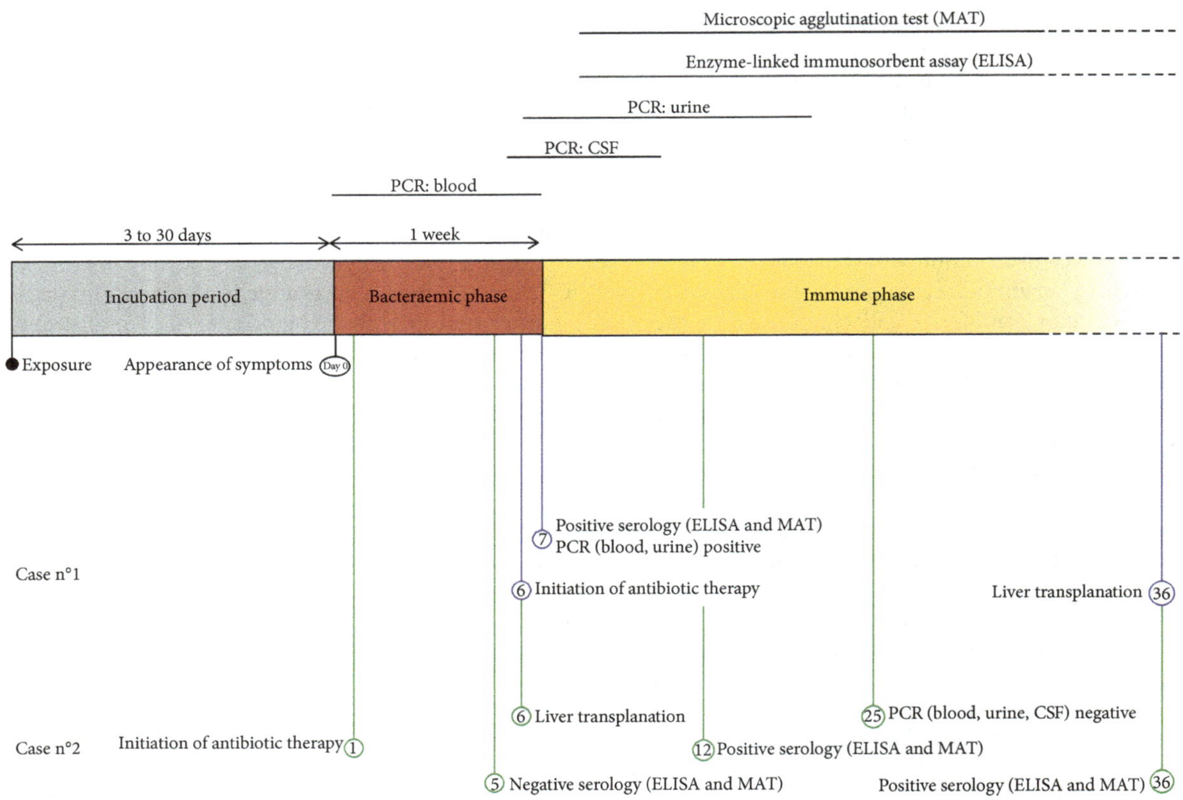

FIGURE 1: Timeline of leptospirosis management: diagnostic tests, clinical data, and test results for two cases.

are aquatic activities in potentially contaminated fresh water and some exposed professions: farmers, slaughterhouse employees, sewer workers, and gardeners. After an incubation period of 3–30 days, human leptospirosis may have diverse clinical manifestations making its diagnosis difficult. Icterohaemorrhagic leptospirosis or Weil's disease (including the major triad of acute renal failure, jaundice, and haemorrhagic diathesis) is the most severe form of the disease which carries a significant risk of mortality. Despite presenting with different symptoms, patients in the presented cases had acute liver failure requiring urgent orthotopic liver transplantation.

The first patient developed a fulminant febrile illness with jaundice, myalgia in calf muscles, acute kidney injury, and significant gastrointestinal bleeding, probably due, in part, by a median arcuate ligament syndrome. Serum bilirubin in Weil's disease is often markedly elevated with moderate elevation of transaminases and alkaline phosphatase [4]. Such findings were evident in this case, whereby serum transaminases were initially slightly raised, with a marked increase in total bilirubin which was greater than 60 mg/dL. Serum transaminase levels began to increase following arterial embolisation and cephalic duodenopancreatectomy. It is likely that the median arcuate ligament syndrome played a major role in the gastrointestinal bleeding and subsequent complications which led to the patient's death. Many collateral arteries developed to compensate for the reduced celiac artery blood flow due to extraluminal compression by the medial arcuate ligament. The vasculitis, due to leptospirosis infection, likely caused the bleeding on these already fragile collateral arteries.

For the second case, the initial symptomatology was less typical as the patient presented sudden neurological manifestations with an altered level of consciousness followed by cerebellar ataxia. The severity of the associated acute liver failure required liver transplantation. Neuro-leptospirosis occurs in around 10–15% of patients [5]. Aseptic meningoencephalitis is the most common neurological manifestation [6], but cases of myeloradiculopathy, myelopathy, and Guillain Barre syndrome have also been reported. Cerebellar involvement has also been described and is thought to affect less than 5% of cases [7]. Neurologic involvement in leptospirosis is due to capillary endothelial damage and vasculitis, and its prognosis is generally good. It is difficult to determine whether the prostate biopsy, performed the day before onset of symptoms, played a role in the clinical severity of this case. It is even more intriguing since the patient was administered ciprofloxacinas antibiotic prophylaxis, which is usually effective in leptospirosis infections.

Liver damage is common in leptospirosis infection and can present as slight disturbances in serum liver function tests or fulminant hepatic failure. Previous reports concerning pathological findings of liver disease in leptospirosis include hyperplasia of Kupffer cells, cholestasis, cell infiltration in portal areas, and sometimes extensive necrosis of hepatocytes leading to hepatic failure [8]. This has been demonstrated in these two cases, where extensive hepatocyte necrosis was identified on histopathological investigation of explanted liver, after transplantation. As demonstrated through the cases presented herein, liver injury can be rapid, important, and irreversible, sometimes leading to the death of the patient.For this reason, even in the absence of encephalopathy, every patient with a severe acute hepatitis associated with leptospirosis infection should be referred to a hospital with a transplant centre for optimal clinical management, which may include transplantation. If liver transplantation is indicated, timing will be important.

Serology is the most common test used to diagnose leptospirosis. MAT is the gold standard to detect both immunoglobulin M (IgM) and immunoglobulin G class agglutinating antibodies. However, it requires significant expertise [9]. IgM ELISA are more commonly performed as an initial screening test as they are easier to carry out, although less specific. Interpretation of serology can be complicated as the first sample is negative in half of the cases, and the test can remain negative when early antibiotic treatment is administered [10]. Therefore, negative serology does not exclude the diagnosis and must be repeated 7 days to 2 weeks later. Molecular methods detect leptospira nucleic acids in the blood in the days following the onset of clinical signs (bacteraemic phase). Leptospires then disappear from the bloodstream (immune phase) (Figure 1). PCR can sometimes detect leptospira in the CSF, and transiently in the urine, from the second week of the pathological course. In the first case, leptospirosis diagnosis was made 7 days after the appearance of the first symptoms, by positive MAT and ELISA, confirmed with PCR detection of leptospira DNA in blood and urine.In the second case, reaching a diagnosis took longer. Indeed, a first leptospira serology test, performed during the first days of hospitalisation, was negative. The diagnosis was made 12 days later by a second positive serology (ELISA and MAT). Furthermore, PCR performed on blood, CSF, and urine samples more than 3 weeks after the first symptoms did not detect leptospira DNA. The value of the various diagnostic tests therefore depends on the stage of the disease and whether the patient has received antibiotics.

Early antibiotic treatment of leptospirosis has been associated with a better prognosis [11]. Intravenous penicillin is the drug of choice, although ceftriaxone, cefotaxime, and carbapenems are also effective. Treatment duration is 5–7 days. In case of allergy to penicillin, the treatment of choice is orally administered doxycycline. Importantly, the choice of antibiotic administered does not depend on the leptospira serotype.

In conclusion, Leptospirosis infection is characterised by a generalised vasculitis responsible for a broad spectrum of clinical manifestations, including acute organ failure that can lead to death. The two reported cases presented differing clinical pictures; however, both patients experienced significant liver injury that required orthotopic liver transplantation.

Consent

Where possible, informed consent was obtained from patients for publication of these case reports.

References

[1] F. Costa, J. E. Hagan, J. Calcagno et al., "Global morbidity and mortality of leptospirosis: a systematic review," *PLoS Neglected Tropical Diseases*, vol. 9, no. 9, p. e0003898, 2015.

[2] A. R. Bharti, J. E. Nally, J. N. Ricaldi et al., "Leptospirosis: azoonoticdisease of global importance," *The Lancet Infectious Diseases*, vol. 3, no. 12, pp. 757–771, 2003.

[3] Centre national de référence de la leptospirose, "Rapport annuel d'activité," 2018, https://www.pasteur.fr/fr/file/21388/download.

[4] G. I. Gancheva, "Liver involvement in leptospirosis," *International Journal of Infectious Diseases and Therapy*, vol. 1, pp. 6–12, 2016.

[5] T. Mathew, P. Satishchandra, A. Mahadevan et al., "Neuroleptospirosis—revisited: experience from a tertiary care neurological centre from south India," *Indian Journal of Medical Research*, vol. 124, no. 2, pp. 155–162, 2006.

[6] E. Puca, J. Majko, E. Puca, E. Qyra, A. Gega, and P. Pipero, "Acute encephalitis as initial presentation of leptospirosis," *The Journal of Infection in Developing Countries*, vol. 114, pp. 361–363, 2017.

[7] R. Singh, D. Khurana, S. Mehta, A. Choudhary, G. Petluri, and V. Lal, "Cerebellar ataxia due to Leptospirosis-a case report," *BMC Infectious Diseases*, vol. 16, no. 1, p. 748, 2016.

[8] M. Shintaku, H. Itoh, and Y. Tsutsumi, "Weil's disease (leptospirosis) manifesting as fulminant hepatic failure: report of an autopsy case," *Pathology-Research and Practice*, vol. 210, no. 12, pp. 1134–1137, 2014.

[9] R. Niloofa, N. Fernando, N. L. de Silva et al., "Diagnosis of Leptospirosis: comparison between microscopic agglutination test, IgM-ELISA and IgM rapid immunochromatography test," *PloS One*, vol. 10, no. 6, p. e0129236, 2015.

[10] P. Abgueguen and E. Pichard, "Leptospiroses," *Encycl Med Chir*, pp. 1161–1164, 2006.

[11] Y. Kobayashi, "Human leptospirosis: management and prognosis," *Journal of Postgraduate Medicine*, vol. 51, no. 3, pp. 201–204, 2005.

13

Different Outcomes of "Silent Hypoxia" in Patients with COVID-19 Pneumonia

Ashani Ratnayake, Prabhashini Kumarihamy, Sujeewa Gunaratne, Hiranya Abeysinghe, Sahan Perera, and Shirley Ekanayake

District Base Hospital, Teldeniya, Sri Lanka

Correspondence should be addressed to Ashani Ratnayake; aashaniratnayake@yahoo.com

Academic Editor: Zsolt Molnár

COVID-19 has been declared a pandemic since March 2020 and it has been responsible for millions of deaths worldwide. The SARS-CoV-2 causes a spectrum of diseases mainly affecting the respiratory system. It can also complicate other systems causing thromboembolic phenomena and myocardial ischaemia. An entity of hypoxia has been described in these patients which show no clinical signs and symptoms of respiratory distress despite being extremely hypoxic. This is called silent or happy hypoxia. The exact mechanism for this is not known. We report 4 cases which had similar presentations of silent hypoxia but had different course of illness and different outcomes. All 4 patients did not show any signs of respiratory distress, but had oxygen saturation less than 82%. 3 of them needed intensive care unit support for oxygen therapy and subsequently needed noninvasive ventilation. Only one required invasive ventilation. The fourth patient did not require intensive care support. The patient who required invasive ventilation succumbed due to severe COVID pneumonia whereas the other 3 patients were discharged from the hospital. Silent hypoxemia can go undetected in COVID-19 patients particularly in the time of a pandemic. This case series highlights the importance of meticulous clinical examination including oxygen saturation measurements in suspected or confirmed patients with COVID-19. The course of illness can be different in different populations, and this needs further clinical evidence.

1. Introduction

SARS-CoV-2 virus is responsible for the spectrum of conditions in COVID-19. It is predominantly a respiratory infection that can complicate other systems. It may present with a wide spectrum of symptoms ranging from mild self-limiting upper respiratory tract infection like illness to severe pneumonia and death. The SARS-CoV-2 infection leads to severe respiratory failure in some of the patients who require advanced respiratory support. Often deterioration to this level is evident by clinically detectable respiratory distress as dyspnoea or tachypnoea. "Silent" or "apathetic" hypoxia is an entity described in patients suffering from COVID-19 pneumonia which is described as objective hypoxia in the absence of apparent respiratory distress [1, 2].

There is a certain group of patients who presents with silent hypoxia. Those patients lack proportionate clinical signs of respiratory distress, even though their chest X-rays show diffuse pneumonia and have evidence of hypoxia detectable in pulse oximetry or arterial blood gas analysis. However, sudden and rapid deterioration may occur in this subset of patients. To assess the severity of pulmonary involvement, a clinical examination should be meticulous, and adequate emphasis should be given to pulse oximetry reading and blood gas analysis. The cause of silent hypoxaemia is controversial. The outcome of these patients can also be variable, and no predictors have been identified to comment on the prognosis. We report 4 cases with silent hypoxaemia with the same presentation, but a different course of illness. The purpose of this report is to highlight the importance of "silent hypoxia" in COVID-19 patients.

2. Case 1

A 53-year-old manual labourer with a history of fever, productive cough, and sore throat for 3 days presented to a local hospital. He is a current smoker and did not have any comorbid diseases. He was diagnosed with a COVID-19 infection by a rapid antigen test and was transferred to a specialised COVID-19 treatment centre. He was not in acute distress and conversant with unlabored speech. His respiratory rate was 16/min without any dyspnoea. He had a blood pressure of 134/77 mmHg with a heart rate of 88/min. On pulse oximetry measurement, his saturation was found to be 66% on room air, and arterial oxygen partial pressure was 56 mmHg. His CXR showed bilateral patchy consolidations on admissions (Figure 1). He was admitted to the intensive care unit for oxygen therapy and required 60% O2 via a face mask. In the next 2 days, his hypoxia worsened requiring noninvasive ventilation (NIV). Subsequent chest X-rays showed gradual worsening of the air space shadowing (Figure 2). He received IV dexamethasone 6 mg daily and subcutaneous enoxaparin. He was on NIV for 48 hours which was subsequently weaned on to high flow nasal oxygen (HFNO). This was weaned off over the next 5 days. His blood investigations are given in Table 1. He had a total ICU stay for 16 days requiring intermittent oxygen therapy. Further, he had multiple episodes of silent hypoxaemia at the time of weaning from respiratory support. On discharge from ICU to ward, his saturation on room air was 90%. He was discharged from the hospital after 21 days.

3. Case 2

A 51-year-old lady with a background history of diabetes mellitus and hypertension presented to a local hospital with cough and fever for 7 days duration. She had a BMI of 39. She was transferred to a specialised COVID treatment centre after tested positive for SARS-CoV-2 rapid antigen. She denied any dyspnoea or chest pain on admission. Her respiratory rate was 20/min with a blood pressure of 155/80 mmHg and a pulse rate of 77/min. Despite the absence of signs of respiratory distress, her saturation on admission was 60% on air. Arterial blood gas revealed an arterial oxygen saturation of 51 mmHg with 26 mmHg of CO2 on room air. Her chest X-ray showed bilateral patchy consolidation (Figure 3). She was transferred to ICU for oxygen therapy. She received NIV for the first 24 hours where she became increasingly hypoxemic requiring intubation and invasive ventilation. Repeated chest X-ray showed further deterioration (Figure 4). She had a high oxygen demand ranging from 80 to 100% of oxygen and high PEEP with mechanical ventilation. She was initially on IV dexamethasone 6 mg, and after 4 doses, this was converted to IV methylprednisolone 1 g pulse therapy and continued for 3 days. Her laboratory investigations are illustrated in Table 1. She became increasingly hypoxemic and was offered prone ventilation. Careful positioning was necessary as she had a high BMI. Despite all ventilatory strategies, she succumbed on day 8 of ICU stay.

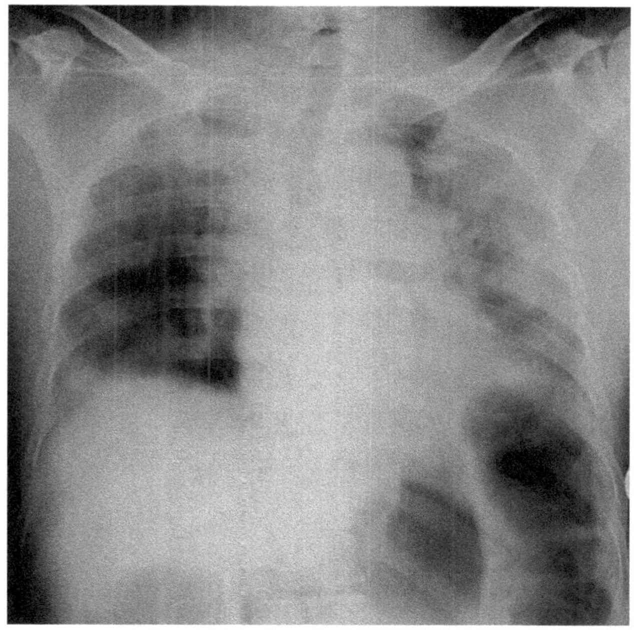

FIGURE 1: Chest radiograph of case 1 on the day of presentation with silent hypoxaemia showing extensive air space opacification involving both lungs with more changes on the left side.

4. Case 3

A 43-year-old gentleman with well-controlled diabetes, ischaemic heart disease with history of PCI to LAD 2 years back was diagnosed with COVID-19 infection and transferred to specialized COVID-19 treatment centre due to his complicated medical history. He was on clopidogrel, aspirin, and bisoprolol. On arrival, he complained of fever and cough for 2 days with a sore throat. He denied any difficulty in breathing and was not dyspnoeic at rest or on exertion. He had a blood pressure of 140/73 mmHg with a pulse rate of 68/min. On admission pulse oximetry showed a saturation of 68% on room air with a PaO_2 of 54 mmHg. He had a respiratory rate of 16/min and initial CXR showed bilateral patchy consolidations (Figure 5). The patient was sent to ICU, and high flow nasal oxygen therapy commenced with FiO2 of 70% and a flow rate of 60 L/min. He was started on IV dexamethasone 6 mg daily and continued for 10 days. The laboratory investigations are shown in Table 1. His condition deteriorated over the next 6 days and on day 6 on ICU, noninvasive ventilation was commenced. Chest X ray showed deterioration of air space opacification (Figure 6). He was treated with a single dose of IV tocilizumab 400 mg. The patients showed a rapid response to IV tocilizumab, and from day 7 onwards, the oxygen requirement was gradually declining. He was discharged on day 14 from ICU and day 19 from the hospital. He did not have any complications during the stay.

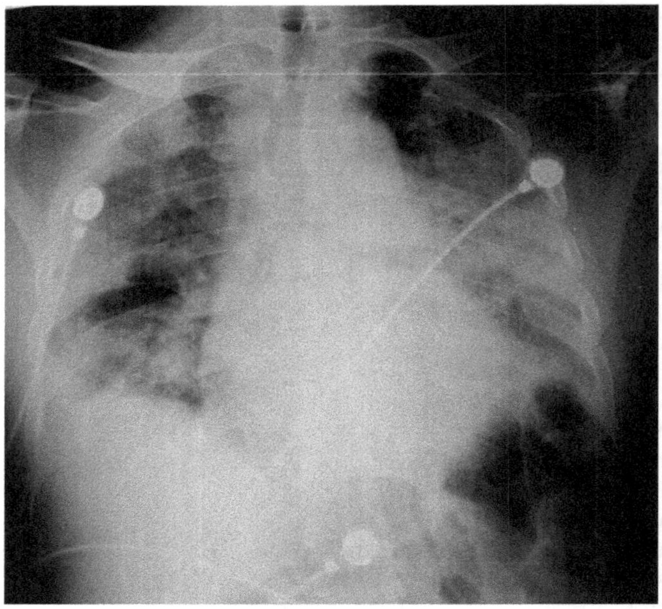

FIGURE 2: Chest radiograph of case 1 on day 3 of ICU showing progression of air space opacification in both lungs.

TABLE 1: Laboratory investigations of the patients presented with silent hypoxaemia.

	Case 1			Case 2			Case 3			Case 4		
	Day 1	Day 5	Day 10	Day 1	Day 5	Day 10	Day 1	Day 5	Day 10	Day 1	Day 5	Day 10
WBC count ($\times 10^9$/L)	18.66	13.70	11.40	12.40	11.80	N/A	13.40	12.40	11.20	9.50	9.91	10.40
N ($\times 10^9$/L)	17.28	11.54	10.20	11.60	10.20	N/A	11.30	10.30	11.70	8.73	10.5	9.10
L ($\times 10^9$/L)	0.63	1.72	1.16	1.69	1.45	N/A	0.43	1.67	1.56	0.37	1.54	1.50
E ($\times 10^9$/L)	0.04	0.03	0.13	0.03	0.04	N/A	0.04	0.05	0.03	0.04	0.20	0.30
Hb (g/dL)	12.80	12.10	13.70	10.90	8.10	N/A	13.4	14.40	14.10	11.50	11.80	11.9
Platelets (×109/mL)	289	394	231	384	247	N/A	342	356	332	315	399	366
CRP (mg/L)	190	33.60	N/A	268	162	N/A	223	112	68	31	3.34	1.80
SGOT (units/L)	16.60	20.80	21	23	88.20	N/A	35.50	31.20	32.10	35.90	37.20	N/A
SGPT (units/L)	28	22.20	20.10	15.70	110.6	N/A	32.30	30.40	30.20	37.80	23.70	N/A
Bilirubin-total (mg/dL)	0.63	0.90	0.74	0.22	0.43	N/A	0.61	N/A	0.65	0.42	N/A	N/A
Bilirubin-direct (mg/dL)	0.12	0.15	0.44	0.05	0.20	N/A	0.15	N/A	0.76	0.16	N/A	N/A
Serum creatinine (mg/dL)	1.11	1.00	1.04	0.72	1.29	N/A	0.90	0.98	0.95	9.50	0.95	N/A
Blood urea (mg/dL)	66.90	38.10	39.70	53.40	74.50	N/A	56.30	55.10	45.20	62.20	N/A	N/A
Procalcitonin (ng/mL)	3.20	N/A	N/A	0.42	1.57	N/A	0.49	0.34	N/A	0.08	N/A	N/A

N: *B*: day 1 is the day the patient was diagnosed with silent hypoxia. Case 2 did not survive 10 days; therefore, day 10 investigations were not available. N.A.: not available.

5. Case 4

A 60-year-old male with a background history of diabetes, hypertension, and ischaemic heart disease presented to the local hospital with fever, cough, and sore throat for four days. He was found to be positive for SARS-CoV-2 and was transferred to our centre for specialized COVID management. On admission, he had oxygen saturation (SpO2) of 82% on air with PaO2 of 56 mmHg with normal respiratory rate and effort. His blood pressure was 160/80, and his pulse rate was 90/min. His oxygen saturation improved to 98% on FiO2 of 40%. His CXR showed bilateral air space opacification (Figure 7). A chest X-ray repeated 2 days later showed worsening of these findings (Figure 8). He was dependent on 40% oxygen in the initial 4 days, and then, the oxygen was weaned off. He did not require admission to ICU. Laboratory findings are illustrated in Table 1. He was discharged home after 16 days of hospital stay.

6. Discussion

SARS-CoV-2 is a droplet borne virus responsible for the global pandemic of COVID-19 infection. Millions of cases

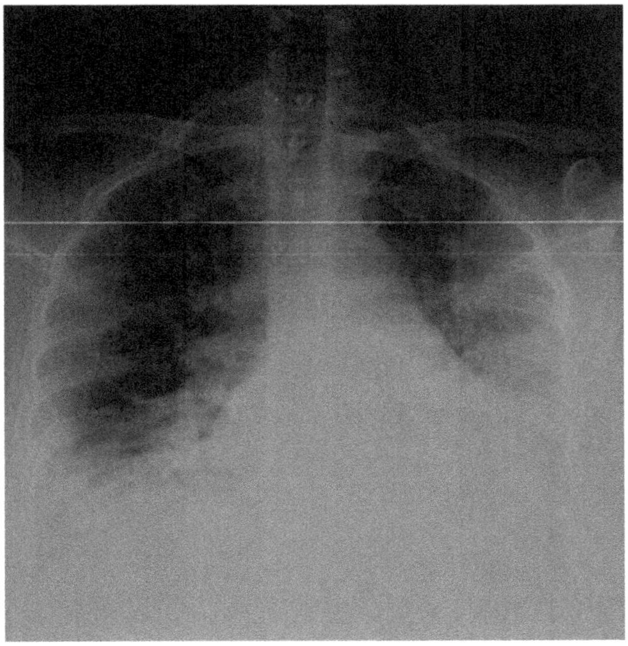

FIGURE 3: Chest radiograph of case 2 on the day of admission with silent hypoxaemia showing bilateral lower zonal opacification. There is more involvement on the left side.

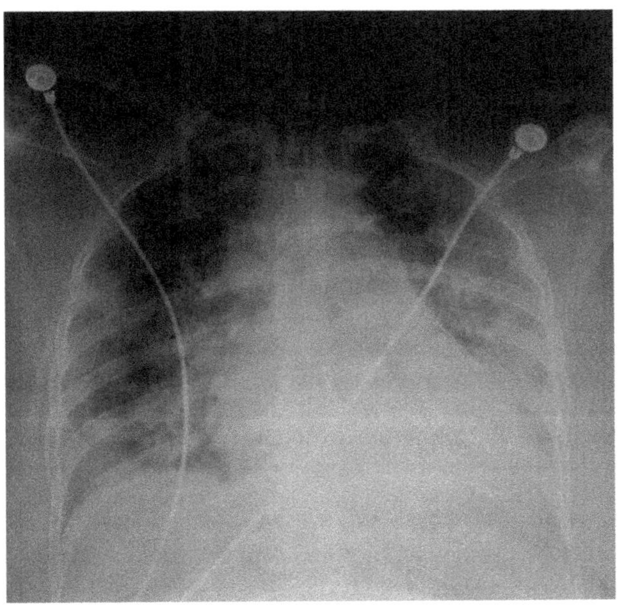

FIGURE 4: Chest X-ray of case 2 after 3 days in ICU. Endotracheal tube in situ. There is worsening of the shadowing of both lungs.

have been reported worldwide. The disease spectrum ranges from asymptomatic infection to acute respiratory distress syndrome causing death in a considerable number of patients. The course of infection can also complicate with thromboembolic phenomena, myocardial ischaemia, and secondary infections [3, 4].

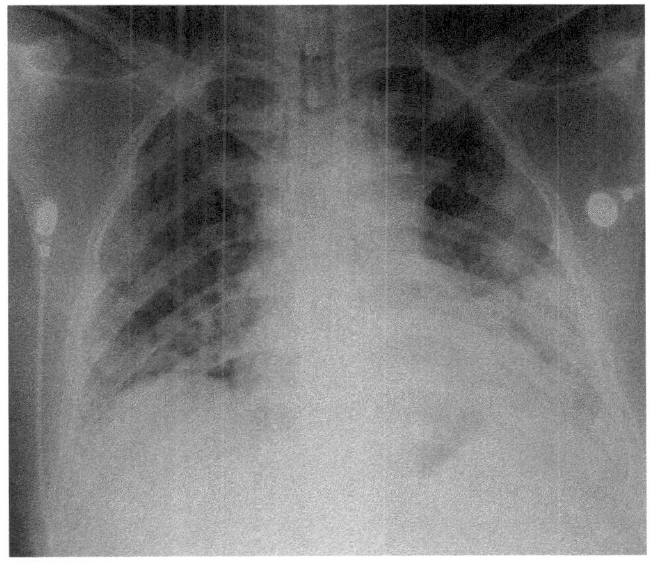

FIGURE 5: Chest radiograph of case 3 on day of the presentation with silent hypoxaemia showing widespread air space opacification in both lungs predominantly involving the lower zones.

Hypoxaemia is defined as arterial oxygen partial pressure less than 80 mmHg, and it becomes severe when it falls below 60 mmHg [5]. Hypoxaemia often accompanies signs and symptoms of respiratory distress, namely, tachypnoea and dyspnoea. In SARS-CoV-2 infection, some patients lack these clinical signs and symptoms of hypoxaemia despite alarmingly arterial oxygenation. This can only be detected by objective measurements like pulse oximetry readings and arterial blood gas measurements. This entity is called silent hypoxaemia or happy hypoxaemia, and this can be detrimental in some patients [1, 2]. Chauhan et al., hypothesized silent hypoxemia which is occurring at the initial stages of the infection, and if it is undetected and unaddressed, this persistent hypoxia contributes to a complex and vicious cycle of increased coagulopathy, cytokine storm, and ultimately more hypoxia/hypoxemia.

The exact mechanism for silent hypoxaemia is not clear. But there are several hypotheses to explain the occurrence of this entity. Most of the hypothesis is related to the preservation of the ability to remove CO2 from the body during COVID-19 infection. Pneumonia analysis of COVID-19 shows the virus causes the alveoli to collapse, reducing the oxygen level and causing hypoxia, but the reaction still enhances the normal lung ability to expel carbon dioxide. Since carbon dioxide removal is still effective, patients do not feel shortness of breath [6]. It is also proposed that intrapulmonary shunting can contribute to this. The infection causes interstitial oedema, loss of surfactant, and superimposed pressure, which induces alveolar collapse and a significant fraction of cardiac output perfusing nonaerated lung tissue. With time, increased oedema will cause alveolar collapse and dependent atelectasis, leading to increased shunting still preserving the ability to remove CO2 [7].

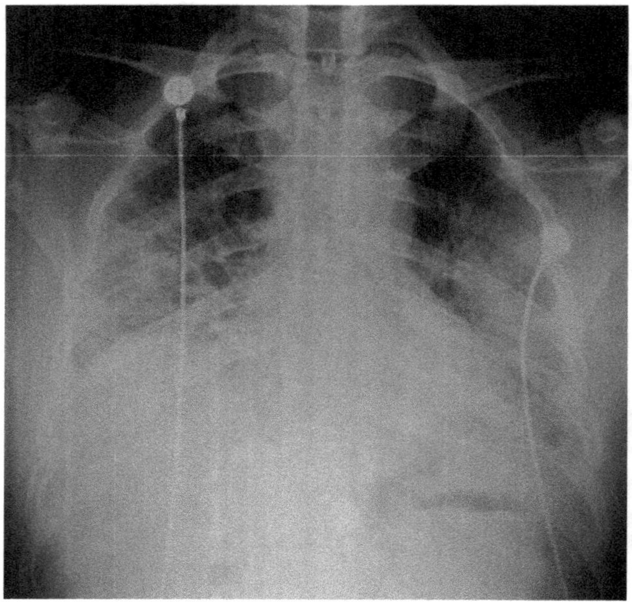

FIGURE 6: Chest radiograph of case 3 on day 3 of admission to ICU showing worsening of air space opacification in both lungs. More changes are seen on the left lung.

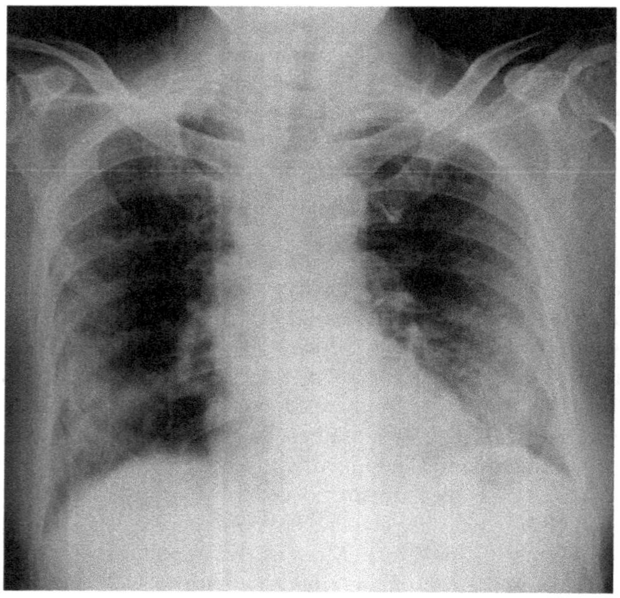

FIGURE 7: A chest radiograph of case 4 at the time of presentation with silent hypoxia showing bilateral air space opacification.

There are not enough data available to predict the clinical course or outcome in these patients with silent hypoxaemia. Chandra et al. reported a case of a 56-year-old patient who presented with silent hypoxemia who made complete recovery only with supplemental oxygen up to 15 L/min via a nonrebreather mask. He did not require ventilator support [8]. Lari et al. reported another case of a 66-year-old patient who had silent hypoxemia who eventually needed high flow oxygen therapy and NIV [9]. Similar to our first

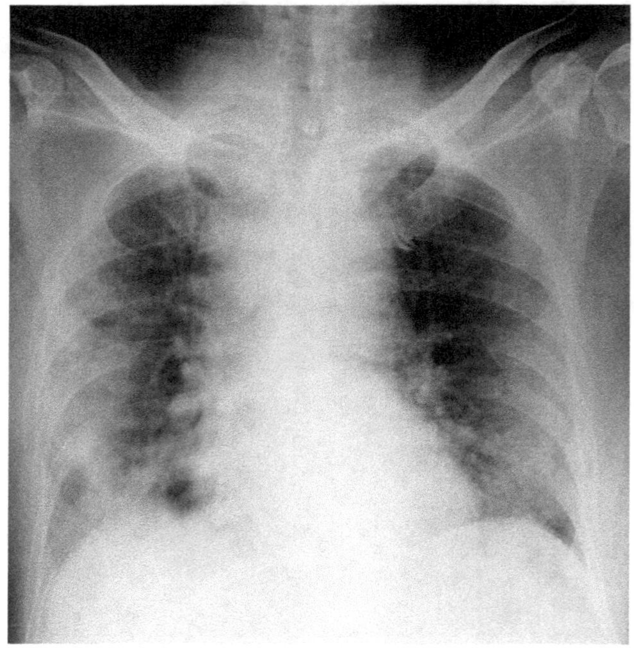

FIGURE 8: Chest radiograph of case 4 on day 2 in the ICU showing worsening of air space opacification.

patient, this patient had also shown multiple episodes of silent hypoxemia at the time of weaning from oxygen therapy. The case reported by Siswanto et al. had a worse outcome. This was a 60-year-old lady with silent hypoxaemia who needed invasive ventilation and succumbed during ICU stay [5]. Our second patient had a similar outcome.

We have reported 4 cases that we encountered who had the clinical entity of silent hypoxaemia. None of them showed apparent signs and symptoms of respiratory distress despite having alarmingly low SpO_2 level and diffuse pneumonia in CXR. Once the patients were diagnosed to have silent ischaemia, they were started on oxygen therapy. Case 1, 2, and 3 patients showed an increment in their oxygen requirement with disease progression following the diagnosis of silent hypoxaemia. In contrast the 4th patient remained on the same requirement and subsequently weaned off without the need for the ICU care. Therefore the course of illness is not similar in all patients with silent hypoxaemia. The outcome of patients was also different. Case 1 had prolonged hospital stay, and the recovery was complicated with several episodes of silent hypoxaemia while 2nd patient died after getting ARDS. The 4th patient was discharged without any complications.

All 4 patients received IV dexamethasone as a part of their treatment regimen. The third patients received IV tocilizumab when he was deteriorating rapidly. Use of tocilizumab can be commenced in hospitalized patients with COVID-19 in whom there are no signs of infection [10]. The evidence was new at the time of management of case 3, and rest of the patients were not given it as they were managed before the publication of guidelines.

Silent hypoxemia is an important entity which needs to be detected early in patients with SARS-CoV-2 infection.

However, the course of illness could be unpredictable. The exact cause of the silent hypoxaemia is also not known. In our experience, further clinical evidence is required to interpret the associations and outcome of silent hypoxemia.

7. Conclusions

Silent hypoxemia can go undetected in COVID-19 patients. This highlights the importance of meticulous clinical examination including oxygen saturation measurements in suspected or confirmed patients with COVID-19. The course of illness can be different in different populations, and this needs further clinical evidence.

Consent

No written consent has been obtained from the patients as there are no patient identifiable data included in this case series.

References

[1] A. Widysanto, T. D. Wahyuni, L. H. Simanjuntak et al., "Happy hypoxia in critical COVID-19 patient: a case report in Tangerang, Indonesia," *Physiological Reports*, vol. 8, no. 20, 2020.

[2] W. Ottestad, M. Seim, and J. O. Mæhlen, "Covid-19 med stille hypoksemi," *Tidsskr den Nor Laegeforening*, vol. 140, no. 7, 2020.

[3] A. Chauhan, R. Kaur, P. Chakrbarti, and A. Pal, ""Silent hypoxemia" leads to vicious cycle of infection, coagulopathy and cytokine storm in COVID-19: can prophylactic oxygen therapy prevent it?," *Indian Journal of Clinical Biochemistry*, vol. 15, 2021.

[4] A. Srivastava, "Blood clots in the lung may be a major cause of COVID-19 deaths," *The Hindu*, vol. 23, 2020.

[5] Siswanto, M. Gani, A. R. Fauzi et al., "Possible silent hypoxemia in a COVID-19 patient: a case report," *Annals of Medicine and Surgery*, vol. 60, pp. 583–586, 2020.

[6] J. Teo, "Early detection of silent hypoxia in Covid-19 pneumonia using smartphone pulse oximetry," *Journal of Medical Systems*, vol. 44, no. 8, p. 134, 2020.

[7] S. Dhont, E. Derom, E. Van Braeckel, P. Depuydt, and B. N. Lambrecht, "The pathophysiology of "happy" hypoxemia in COVID-19," *Respiratory Research*, vol. 21, no. 1, p. 198, 2020.

[8] A. Chandra, U. Chakraborty, J. Pal, and P. Karmakar, "Silent hypoxia: a frequently overlooked clinical entity in patients with COVID-19," *BMJ Case Reports*, vol. 13, no. 9, article e237207, 2020.

[9] A. Lari, M. Alherz, A. Nouri, L. Botras, and S. Taqi, "Caution against precaution: a case report on silent hypoxia in COVID-19," *BMJ Case Reports*, vol. 60, pp. 301–303, 2020.

[10] National institute of healthcare and Excellence, "COVID-19 rapid guideline managing COVID-19 [NICE guidelines No191]," 2021, https://www.nice.org.uk/guidance/ng191/resources/covid19-rapid-guideline-managing-covid19-pdf-51035553326.

14

Symmetrical Peripheral Gangrene: Report of Three Cases

Héctor Acosta,[1] Pau Forcada,[2] Marta Bonjorn,[2] Amer Mustafa,[2] Paul Pilares,[1] and Jordi Colomina[1]

[1]*Hospital Universitari de Santa Maria, 25198 Lleida, Spain*
[2]*Hospital Universitari Arnau de Vilanova, 25198 Lleida, Spain*

Correspondence should be addressed to Héctor Acosta; hacosta@gss.cat

Academic Editor: Kenneth S. Waxman

Symmetrical peripheral gangrene (SPG) is a rare clinical syndrome characterized by an acute onset of ischemic damage in two or more extremities without obstruction or vasculitis of supplying vessels. Body parts commonly affected include toes, hands, scrotum, and earlobes, increasing the risk of limb amputation and impairing the quality of life. The vascular injury mechanism is disseminated intravascular coagulation. SPG may manifest unpredictably in conditions associated with septic shock, low output states, vasospastic conditions, myeloproliferative disorders, or hyperviscosity syndrome. A review on the topic is presented based on a 3-case series of SPG that required amputation of fingers and toes after the administration of vasopressors in a septic shock context.

1. Introduction

Symmetrical peripheral gangrene (SPG) is a rare condition in which symmetrical ischemia and dry gangrene of the acral areas occur. Body parts commonly affected include the toes, hands, scrotum, and earlobes, increasing the risk of limb amputation and affecting the quality of life [1].

The aetiology is multifactorial but has been linked to vasopressor's use during the treatment of septic shock [1, 2]. There is consensus in the literature that early recognition of PSG, along with underlying conditions, can change significantly the treatment and the final evolution [2].

The vascular injury mechanism is disseminated intravascular coagulation (DIC) [3, 4]. Several infectious and noninfectious etiologic factors have been associated with SPG [2, 5–7]. It has been described in conditions associated with sepsis, low blood flow states, vasospastic conditions, hyperviscosity disorders, and myeloproliferative disorders [8]. The appearance of SPG related to the inappropriate use of vasopressor drugs also has been described [9].

Dopamine and norepinephrine are the first-choice drugs in septic shock cases due to their positive inotropic effects. SPG can occur with prolonged administration, especially at high infusion rates. SPG can cause catastrophic complications with high mortality rates and high frequencies of multiple limb amputations in up to 70% of surviving patients [8, 9]. We present the case of a patient with SPG associated with vasopressor use who required amputation of all fingers and toes.

2. Case Series

2.1. Case 1. A 46-year-old woman with history of uterine fibroids after elective hysterectomy presented with surgical wound infection evolving to septic shock that required admission to the intensive care unit (ICU).

During admission, the patient developed multiorgan failure, abdominal compartment syndrome, and DIC. Positive cultures for *Pseudomonas aeruginosa*, *Enterococcus faecalis*, and *Candida tropicalis* were obtained, for which intravenous antibiotics and antifungals were administered. Due to the hemodynamic instability, it was necessary to administer vasopressors to maintain systolic blood pressure and mean arterial pressure goals.

With increasing doses of 1.5 μg/kg/min of norepinephrine, the patient's lactate was 6.6 mmol/L on the same day.

On the third day of admission to the ICU, the patient underwent surgery again due to suspected abdominal compartment syndrome; twenty-four hours later, the norepinephrine dose was decreased, and a lower lactate level of 4 mmol/L was observed. On the fifth day of ICU admission, norepinephrine was withdrawn, and that same day, the presence of greyish lesions was observed on both hands, finger pads that evolved into haemorrhagic blisters on the left hand and patchy purple lesions on both feet and toes and stayed cyanosis in the heels. Radial, ulnar, pedal, and posterior tibial pulses of all extremities were normal on Doppler examination. The lesions evolved into necrotic areas at the metacarpal and phalangeal levels in both hands and distal phalangeal levels in both feet (Figure 1).

The patient received ventilatory support treatment, dialysis, and antithrombotic treatment with low molecular weight heparin, remaining in the ICU for 54 days. During necrotic lesions' delimiting time, wound care was performed with dry dressings and limbs covered with padded bandages.

In gangrenous areas, surgical amputations were performed. In the right hand, the four triphalangeal finger stumps were regularized at F1 transphalangeal level, and bone coverage with deep plane and closure by second intention was performed. In the 3rd finger, a radial pedicled flap advancement was performed, and in the thumb, regularization of the second phalanx and coverage with a Moberg-type flap was performed, leaving the matrix and part of the nail bed. Transphalangeal amputation of the 2nd and 3rd fingers was performed on the left hand associated with deep plane coverage, fingers 4th and 5th were amputated at the level of the middle phalanx, and radial flap advancement was performed on the thumb to close the cutaneous defect, maintaining part of the matrix and the nail bed. Despite the aggressiveness of the amputation surgery, the patient retains a certain ability to grip both hands and an acceptable prehension of the thumb and index on the left hand. Result of the surgeries performed can be seen in Figure 2.

Transmetatarsal amputation of the second to the fifth finger and proximal transphalangeal amputation of the first finger were performed on the left foot. On the right foot, she required complete transmetatarsal amputation plus posterior grafting.

One year later, she continued her recovery as an outpatient, presenting with right thumb nail matrix discomfort, requiring matrix surgery and sterilization, with no reports of other complications.

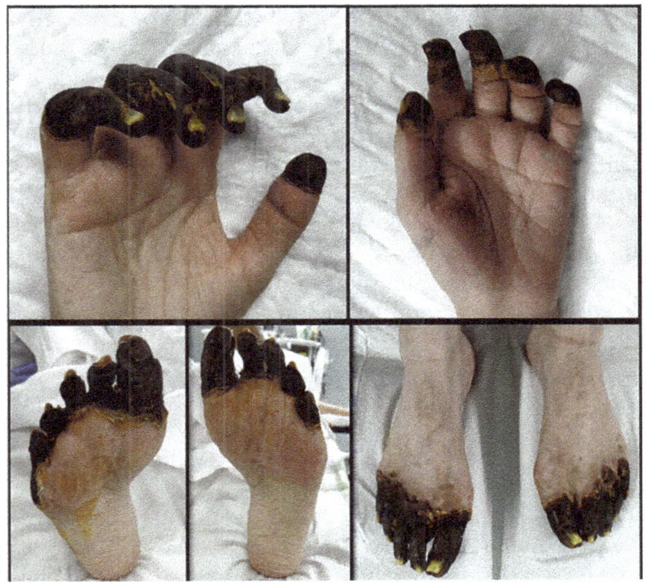

FIGURE 1: Case 1 lesions.

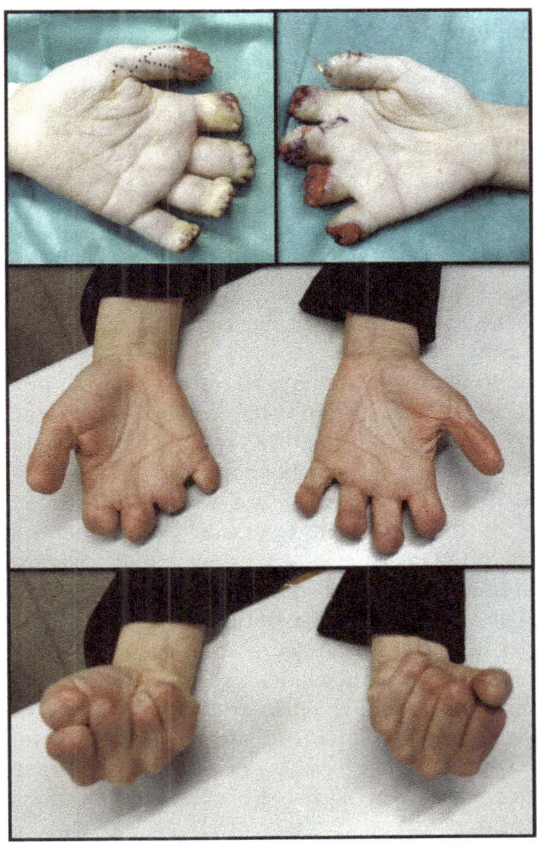

FIGURE 2: Intraoperative levels of amputation and functionality after complete wound healing.

2.2. Case 2. A 53-year-old man was in ICU after septic shock secondary to appendicitis that progressed rapidly to peritonitis and multiple organ failure with DIC.

During admission, norepinephrine administration was necessary to maintain hemodynamic stability. The patient underwent an urgent laparotomy and negative pressure therapy. Positive cultures for *E. coli* were obtained, which received targeted antibiotic treatment. Initial lactate was 6.8 mmol/L on the first day of admission. On the fourth day of admission, he presented ischemic skin lesions on the fingers of both hands and feet toes. On the left hand, nonsuppurative, dry, and well-defined necrosis stablished at the distal level of the fingers 1st, 2nd, and 3rd with proximal interphalangeal joint involvement, 4th and 5th were only affected in the pad, and also, a superficial necrotic eschar at the left dorsal hand level and wrist on its radial face appeared. On the right hand, well-defined nonsuppurative necrosis was observed in the distal ulnar aspect of the thumb with partial involvement of the finger pad, necrosis 2nd, 3rd, and 4th fingers with involvement up to PIP, finger 5 with involvement of the finger pad. Both feet presented poorly defined dry necrosis affecting all toes of both feet. For images of the described lesions, see Figure 3.

The patient received ventilatory support treatment, dialysis, and antithrombotic treatment with low molecular weight heparin, remaining in the ICU for 42 days. During the delimiting necrotic lesion time, wound care was performed with dry dressings and limbs covered with padded bandages.

The patient died on day 42.

2.3. Case 3. A 43-year-old woman with a history of acute myeloid leukaemia (AML) presented with a septic shock of abdominal origin caused by colitis, requiring admission to the ICU due to multiple organ failure and DIC.

She received treatment with norepinephrine to maintain mean blood pressure above 65 mmHg. Klebsiella and Pseudomonas were identified in the cultures, for which specific antibiotic treatment was given. Initial lactate was 11.2 mmol/L, decreasing to 1.2 mmol/L after a week, presenting thrombocytopenia for which platelet transfusion was necessary during admission. On the 12th day of admission, she was assessed for traumatology due to skin lesions on both hands with nonsuppurative dry necrosis of the tips of fingers 4th and 5th of the left hand, dry necrosis of the 5th finger of the right hand that affects up to the distal interphalangeal joint (DIP), 4th finger necrosis that affects up to the middle phalanx (F2) without reaching the joint, and 3rd finger and thumb with only of the distal fingertip involvement. There were no involvement of the toes or other acral areas in this case.

She was taken to surgery, where the necrotic tip of the 4th finger of the right hand was removed, with distal phalanx (F3) regularization and removal of the remaining nail matrix, Atasoy-type coverage was performed. In the 5th finger, the necrotic tip was removed, regularized with disarticulation at the DIP joint level and removal of cartilage remains at the distal level of F2. Fish mouth coverage type and wound closure with 5/0 monofilament. Wounds are treated and padded bandage until discharge.

After 22 days of hospitalization due to persistent fever and haemorrhagic complications, the patient presented clinical improvement and was discharged from the hospital. She is recovering on an outpatient basis with good functionality of the hand, for which she was discharged from traumatology after 6 follow-up weeks. No other complications were recorded to date.

Demographic and causal factors of the three cases summarized in Table 1. And clinical presentation and treatments are collected in Table 2.

3. Discussion

Symmetrical peripheral gangrene or purpura fulminans [10, 11] is a rare syndrome characterized by an acute onset of

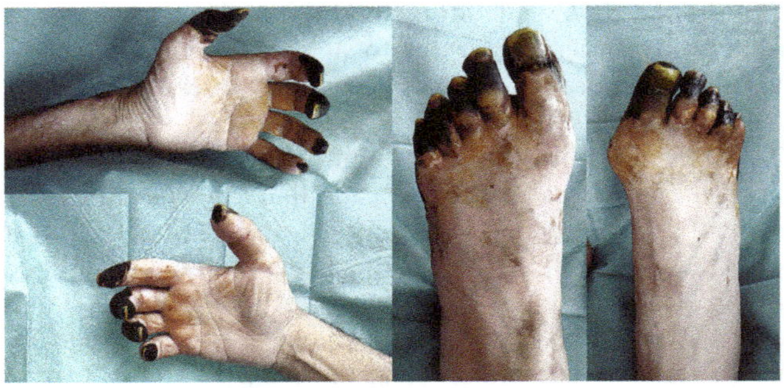

Figure 3: Case 2 lesions.

ischemic damage in peripheral acral areas without obstruction or vasculitis of the supplying vessels [1, 6].

There are no large studies that provide scientific evidence about this rare condition [8], being in this article 3 cases reported.

Altered microcirculation and vasospastic conditions with poor peripheral perfusion are the main clinical scenarios associated with SPG [1, 6, 9].

Disseminated intravascular coagulation (DIC) could be the last cause of microvascular injury. This association was first described in 1970 by Strossel and Levy [6]. The possibility that SPG may be one special cutaneous variant of DIC has been described [2].

In patients with DIC and hypovolemia, the use of vasopressor drugs like epinephrine, dopamine, and norepinephrine can cause SPG by decreasing tissue perfusion and exacerbating ischemia, leading to eventual tissue necrosis and gangrene [2, 12].

Some studies describe that the dose instead of the duration could be more important in the development of SPG and also have additive effects [2, 9, 12].

In this report, all 3 cases were caused by septic conditions [13] which lead to DIC and precise norepinephrine at curative levels developing SPG in a few days, 4 to 12.

The first suggestive sign is the presence of cold, erythematous extremities followed by dark discoloration of the skin. Ischemic changes progressing to cyanosis and hemorrhagic bullae may develop in symmetric acral distribution over the fingers and toes. In severe cases, involvement of the nose, earlobe, or scrotum can be observed [10]. Of the reported cases, two had both hands and feet involved and the 3rd only hands, no other body parts were involved.

In the first 12-24 hours, dry gangrene appears and progresses proximally with a demarcation line that develops in approximately two or three weeks [6, 8].

Laboratory tests like complete blood count with blood smear help to identify myeloproliferative or infectious alterations. D-dimer can indicate the presence of DIC. Blood biochemistry helps detect chronic pathologies. In patients with septic shock, high levels of serum lactate can be observed just before the appearance of SPG [2, 6]. In all cases, reported serum lactate was elevated from 6.6 to 11.2 mmol/L.

The initial management is hemodynamic stabilization. Early recognition of cyanosis, reversal of DIC, and

TABLE 1: Summary of the demographic and causal factors of the three cases.

Case	Sex age	Primary causal disease	Secondary casual disease	Cultures	Vasopressor	ICU days
1	M 46	Elective hysterectomy	Septic shock	*Enterococcus faecalis, Pseudomonas Aeruginosa*	Norepinephrine	54
2	F 53	Appendicitis	Septic shock	*Escherichia coli*	Norepinephrine	42
3	M 43	Colitis	Septic shock	*Klebsiella pneumoniae*	Norepinephrine	22

TABLE 2: Summary of clinical presentation and treatment of the three cases.

Case	All extremities affectation	Clamp impairment	Days from admission to onset	Treatment
1	Yes	Yes	5	All finger amputation
2	Yes	Yes	4	Death before surgery
3	No, both hands' affectation	Thumb without clamp function impairment	12	Right hand 4, 5 finger amputation

correction of hypovolemia are essential to prevent the progression to gangrene. Effective treatment of underlying pathologies like antibiotic treatment for sepsis will determine the outcome in individual cases. The use of heparin in the treatment of DIC remains controversial, although it may be useful in patients with clinically evident thromboembolism and extensive fibrin deposition. Antithrombin III alone or in association with heparin appears to be a promising agent [6].

The only definitive treatment established for gangrene of acral areas is amputation. It should be considered after the development of a clear line of demarcation, until this moment emphasis should be placed on local wound care [2]. Also, self-amputation of the gangrenous digits on very distal lesions could be seen [2, 6].

The level of amputation must be decided during surgery. Separate bone and soft tissue reconstruction leads to good results in terms of wound healing and ambulatory status [2]. In most cases of fingers, a V-Y advancement flap can be performed in either volar or a double lateral flap trying to maintain the maximum finger length, especially in thumb and index fingers used for pinch grip. Treatment in our case was amputation using different flap types like Moberg, Atasoy, or fish mouth were performed with acceptable functional results.

For the lower extremities, microsurgical techniques and the use of free flaps have been described with good functional results [14, 15]. In case one, foot amputations were performed using a skin graft in the right foot with no other complications.

4. Conclusions

SPG is a rare condition that mainly affects critical patients who require the use of inotropes such as norepinephrine. In these patients, strict surveillance of the acral areas is necessary during treatment to detect ischemic signs in time and correct the already existing DIC since the development of SPG can lead to limb amputation with serious impairment of quality of life. Treatment, once dry gangrene is established, consists of amputation of necrotic areas when they are demarcated trying to preserve functionality if possible. Clinical suspicion and early diagnosis is key improve its management.

Acknowledgments

The APC charges were covered by the Institut de Recerca Biomèdica de Lleida (IRB Lleida), Av. Alcalde Rovira Roure, 80, 25198, Lleida, Spain.

References

[1] J. Dong, L. Zhang, G. Rao, and X. Zhao, "Complicating symmetric peripheral gangrene after dopamine therapy to patients with septic shock," *Journal of Forensic Sciences*, vol. 60, no. 6, pp. 1644–1646, 2015.

[2] N. Ruffin, C. V. Vasa, S. Breakstone, and W. Axman, "Symmetrical peripheral gangrene of bilateral feet and unilateral hand after administration of vasopressors during septic shock," *Case Reports*, vol. 2018, p. bcr-2017, 2018.

[3] M. P. Davis, J. Byrd, T. Lior, and T. W. Rooke, "Symmetrical peripheral gangrene due to disseminated intravascular coagulation," *Archives of Dermatology*, vol. 137, no. 2, pp. 139-140, 2001.

[4] M. A. Molos and J. C. Hall, "Symmetrical peripheral gangrene and disseminated intravascular coagulation," *Archives of Dermatology*, vol. 121, no. 8, pp. 1057–1061, 1985.

[5] T. E. Schuh, D. Erdmann, and L. S. Levin, "Symmetrische periphere Gangrän unbekannter Ätiologie," *Die Chirurgie*, vol. 73, no. 6, pp. 638–641, 2002.

[6] B. D. Sharma, S. R. Kabra, and B. Gupta, "Symmetrical peripheral gangrene," *Tropical Doctor*, vol. 34, no. 1, pp. 2–4, 2004.

[7] S. Z. Ghafoor, E. A. MacRae, K. G. Harding, and G. K. Patel, "Symmetrical peripheral digital gangrene following severe Plasmodium falciparum malaria-induced disseminated intravascular coagulopathy," *International Wound Journal*, vol. 7, no. 5, pp. 418–422, 2010.

[8] S. K. Ghosh, D. Bandyopadhyay, and A. Ghosh, "Symmetrical peripheral gangrene: a prospective study of 14 consecutive cases in a tertiary-care hospital in eastern India," *Journal of the European Academy of Dermatology and Venereology*, vol. 24, no. 2, pp. 214–218, 2010.

[9] K. J. Jung, J. H. Nho, H. K. Cho et al., "Amputation of multiple limbs caused by use of inotropics: case report, a report of 4 cases," *Medicine (Baltimore)*, vol. 97, no. 5, p. e9800, 2018.

[10] E. Chalmers, P. Cooper, K. Forman et al., "Purpura fulminans: recognition, diagnosis and management," *Archives of Disease in Childhood*, vol. 96, no. 11, pp. 1066–1071, 2011.

[11] M. E. Colling and P. K. Bendapudi, "Purpura fulminans: mechanism and management of dysregulated hemostasis," *Transfusion Medicine Reviews*, vol. 32, no. 2, pp. 69–76, 2018.

[12] J. W. Kwon, M. K. Hong, and B. Y. Park, "Risk factors of vasopressor-induced symmetrical peripheral gangrene," *Annals of Plastic Surgery*, vol. 80, no. 6, pp. 622–627, 2018.

[13] D. Edler and T. Ihre, "Perifera gangrän vid pneumokockinfektion och disseminerad intravaskulär koagulation Peripheral gangrene in pneumococcal infections and disseminated intravascular coagulation," *Lakartidningen*, vol. 86, no. 38, p. 3142, 1989.

[14] S. Y. Lim, G. H. Kim, I. H. Sung et al., "Lower extremity salvage with thoracodorsal artery perforator free flap in condition of symmetrical peripheral gangrene," *BioMed Research International*, vol. 2018, Article ID 6508607, 8 pages, 2018.

[15] S. Rizzato, E. Kohhischeen, P. Marchica et al., "Symmetrical peripheral gangrene reconstruction after lower limb amputation," *Annali Italiani di Chirurgia*, vol. 91, pp. 432–436, 2020.

15

Ultrasound Detection of Portomesenteric Venous Gas is an Early Sign of Bowel Ischaemia in Non-Traumatic Abdominal Pain: Old Dogs, New Tricks—Four Cases Report

Mirko Di Capua[1] **Michela Tonani**[2] **and Stefano Paglia**[1]

[1]*Emergency Department, "Maggiore" Hospital of Lodi, Largo Donatori del Sangue, 1, 26900 Lodi, Italy*
[2]*Emergency Department, "Guglielmo da Saliceto" Hospital of Piacenza, Via Giuseppe Taverna, 49, 29121 Piacenza, Italy*

Correspondence should be addressed to Mirko Di Capua; mirdica@hotmail.com

Academic Editor: Silvia Natoli

Acute bowel ischemia is a severe disease often with a poor outcome. Early diagnosis can improve outcome, but atypical clinical manifestations and nonspecific laboratory and instrumental diagnostic findings may delay computed tomographic angiography (CTA). Portomesenteric venous gas (PVG), indirect sign of pneumatosis intestinalis, is considered a late finding with poor prognosis. We report four cases where PVG, easily identified through point-of-care ultrasonography (POCUS), was an early sign of bowel ischemia leading to a precocious diagnosis confirmed at CTA. In acute non-traumatic abdominal pain, an evidence of PVG could be an early ultrasonographic finding of bowel ischemia in the emergency department.

1. Introduction

Acute bowel ischemia is an uncommon cause of hospitalization, accounting for less than 1 out of 1000 admissions to hospital [1], but the overall mortality rate is approximately 70% where survivors of extensive bowel resection face lifelong disability. [2] Bowel ischemia is usually distinguished into acute mesenteric ischemia—meant as small bowel ischemia, venous mesenteric ischemia, non-occlusive mesenteric ischemia, and ischemic colitis. When hemodynamically stable ischemic colitis without gangrenous complication or perforation is suspected, colonoscopy is the gold standard and should be the first diagnostic test [3–4].

In the critical care setting, computed tomographic angiography (CTA) is considered the reference standard for diagnosis. [2]. Many authors have investigated the role of point-of-care ultrasonography (POCUS) in acute bowel ischemia [5, 6] and the European Federation of Societies for Ultrasound in Medicine and Biology (EFSUMB) recently published a position paper in intestinal emergencies. [7] Unfortunately, the intestinal ultrasonographic signs of ischemia are all nonspecific. Pneumatosis intestinalis is a well-recognized sign of bowel ischemia. It is, however, usually considered a late sign and difficult to evaluate with POCUS. Here, we describe four cases, admitted for acute non-traumatic abdominal pain, where POCUS detection of portomesenteric venous gas (PVG)—indirect sign of pneumatosis intestinalis—leads to a very early diagnosis of bowel ischemia.

2. Case 1

Male, 56 years old. He was admitted to the emergency department (ED) with mild abdominal pain and hypotension. At arrival, heart rate (HR) was 77, blood pressure (BP) 88/65 mmHg, oxygen saturation (SAT) was 98% in room air, and body temperature was 36.3°C. Venous blood gas (VBG) analysis showed a normal acid-base balance with a mild lactate increase (2.25 mmol/L, normal value <2 mmol/L). POCUS showed an altered liver ultrasound pattern due to massive air infiltration in the portal system and portal vein showed a spontaneous echo-contrast with multiple hyperechoic spots flowing in the lumen suggestive

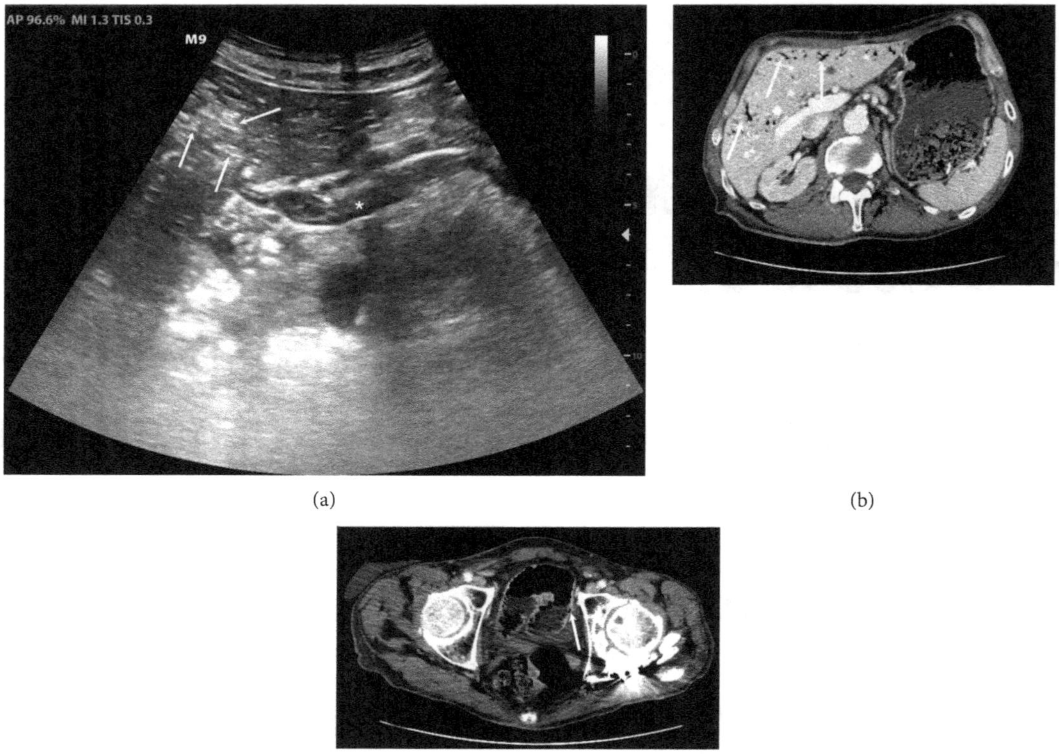

(a) (b) (c)

FIGURE 1: POCUS and CTA of case 1. (a) POCUS shows portal vein at hepatic hilum (asterisk) with multiple hyperechogenic spots into the lumen. White arrows indicate air in intrahepatic portal vessels with altered liver ultrasonographic structure. (b) A CTA scan confirms air into the liver (white arrows), while air is not easily identified into portal vein. (c) CTA confirms a little area of pneumatosis intestinalis (white arrow). POCUS stands for point-of-care ultrasonography; CTA stands for computed tomographic angiography.

of PVG (Figure 1(a)). We immediately performed a CTA that confirmed intestinal pneumatosis and diffuse air in the hepatic parenchyma (Figures 1(b) and 1(c)). The patient was admitted to the operating room and was found to have initial mesenteric ischemia due to several adhesions and a partial volvulus. Surgeons performed adhesions lysis and volvulus detorsion with success and regular post-operative progress. The patient was dismissed in 8 days.

3. Case 2

Male, 60 years old. He presented to the emergency department complaining of severe abdominal pain and vomiting. At evaluation, he presented a HR of 122 bpm, BP 112/70 mmHg, SAT 98% in room air, and body temperature of 36.3°C. Arterial blood gas (ABG) analysis showed a respiratory alkalosis and lactate within normal limits (0.95 mmol/L, normal value <2 mmol/L). Ultrasonography showed multiple hyperechogenic spots in the portal vein with altered liver ultrasonographic structure by diffuse air infiltration, compatible with PVG (Figure 2(a)). A CT angiography confirmed left colon pneumatosis and air in liver parenchyma (Figures 2(b) and 2(c)). The patient was admitted to surgery and laparotomy confirmed left colon ischemia complicated by peritonitis. Surgeons performed subtotal colectomy and an ileostomy. The patient was dismissed 30 days after surgical intervention.

4. Case 3

Female, 82 years old. She presented to the emergency department with severe acute abdominal pain, melena, and hypotension. At presentation, HR was 55 bpm, BP 80/40 mmHg, SAT 98% in ventimask with fraction of inspired oxygen of 0.4, and a body temperature of 36.2°C. A VBG showed a metabolic acidosis with hyperkalaemia (K 6.23 mmol/L), mild anaemia (haemoglobin 7.9 gr/dL), and normal lactates (1.35 mmol/L, normal value <2 mmol/L). Ultrasonography showed multiple hyperechogenic spots in the main portal vein, suggestive of PVG, and in intrahepatic portal vessels, we did not find free fluid. CT angiography confirmed intestinal pneumatosis and, moreover, showed diffuse mesenteric vascular impairment, particularly in the upper mesenteric artery. We decided not to proceed to the surgical intervention due to the high surgical risk. The patient died 16 hours after admission.

5. Case 4

Female, 88 years old. She was admitted to the emergency department complaining abdominal pain, haematochezia,

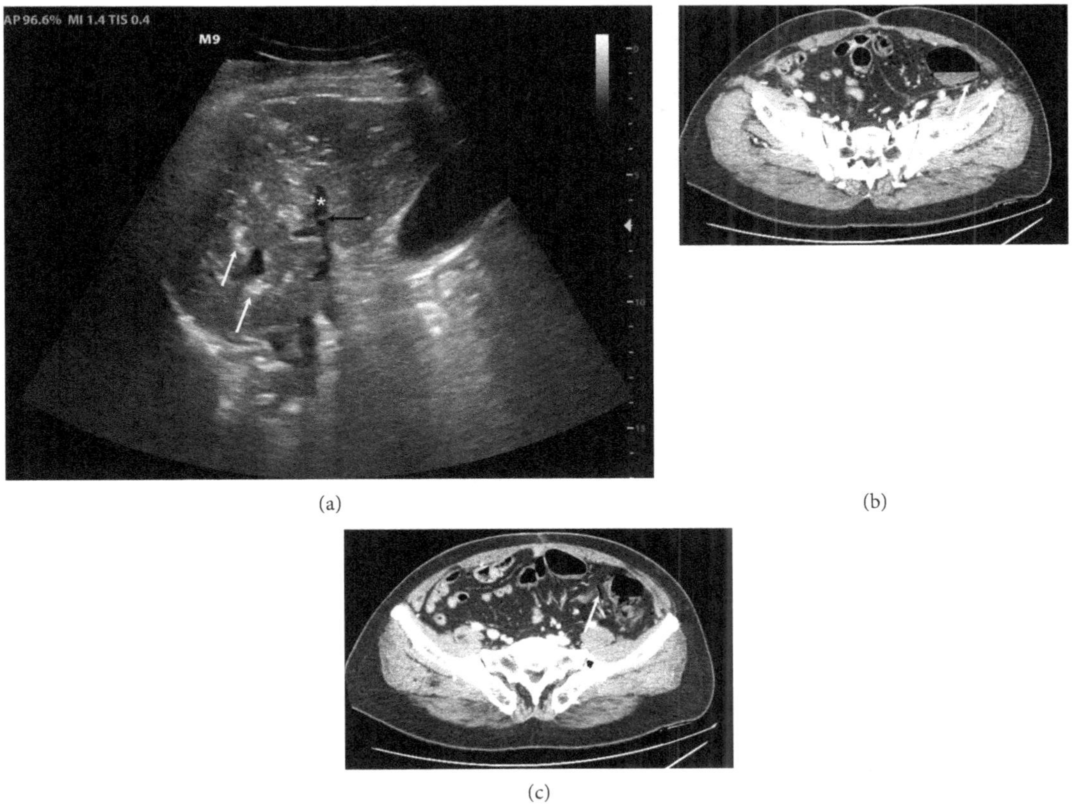

FIGURE 2: POCUS and CTA of case 2. (a) POCUS shows a right portal branch (asterisk) with some air bubbles into the lumen (black arrow). White arrows indicate some air in intrahepatic portal vessels. (b) CTA showing pneumatosis intestinalis (white arrow). (c) CTA shows the air flowing within the intestinal vessels (white arrow), as it is drained from the pneumatosis intestinalis, that will reach the portal vein. POCUS stands for point-of-care ultrasonography; CTA stands for computed tomographic angiography.

and mild fever. At presentation, she had normal parameters (heart rate, blood pressure, and saturation) and mild fever (body temperature 37.4°C). ABG lactates were within normal limits. Ultrasound showed multiple hyperechogenic spots in intra- and extrahepatic portal vessels, suggestive of PVG. We performed an abdominal CT angiography which revealed ischemic colitis of the right colon and distal ileum. She was admitted to the operating room and a hemicolectomy with ileostomy was performed. The patient was dismissed after 7 days without complications.

6. Discussion

Acute bowel ischemia remains a severe disease with an often-poor prognosis. CTA is the reference standard diagnostic technique but it requires a high index of suspicion and so it is often performed at advanced stages of the disease. On the other hand, POCUS is widely available; it is usually performed immediately at bedside after physical examination. POCUS has demonstrated a high accuracy in several cardio-thoracic and abdominal emergencies. In some cases (e.g., pneumothorax), its specificity reaches 100%, while in other diseases, such as deep vein thrombosis, POCUS is considered the reference standard. As far as bowel ischemia is concerned, duplex ultrasonography has shown relatively high accuracy—both sensitivity and specificity of 85 to 90%—in diagnosing acute mesenteric ischemia, particularly when the upper mesenteric artery is involved by a thrombosis or an embolus [8, 9]. Unfortunately, it requires high degree of expertise in ultrasonography and its accuracy seems to be lower when distal vessels are responsible for ischemia or when there is a non-occlusive intestinal ischemia. On the other hand, ruling in or out bowel ischemia with only a basic POCUS evaluation is rarely considered safe as intestinal ultrasound has nonspecific patterns in bowel ischemia and inadequate accuracy [7].

Our small case series suggests that the association of acute non-traumatic abdominal pain—not explained by other emergencies—and ultrasound detection of PVG could be an indirect sign of bowel ischemia which deserves a rapid CTA confirmation. Even if the EFSUMB position paper cite the intestinal pneumatosis as a rare and late finding associated with poor prognosis, [7] our small series shows that even adhesions and a partial volvulus caused the development of severe early PVG. This indicates that pneumatosis intestinalis, and consequently PVG, does not need massive bowel ischemia or necrosis, but could rapidly develop also in segmental and initial ischemia. POCUS detection of PVG is quite easy and does not require high competence in ultrasonography. First, duplex ultrasound is not necessary. Moreover, basic competences are sufficient to confirm PVG as air is high visible on ultrasonography and an intercostal hepatic view allows evaluation of portal vessels and liver independent of meteorism or abdominal pain. Sonography may even have a higher sensitivity than CT in detection of gas in portal peripheral branches as Maher et al. have reported cases of PVG findings with POCUS, undetectable on CT performed immediately after an ultrasound evaluation. [10] Still, the evaluation of intestinal wall, to exclude or confirm the diagnosis of intestinal ischemia, needs higher competences; there is not a specific sign of intestinal ischemia and a negative ultrasonography does not exclude intestinal ischemia. The evidence of PVG at POCUS in a patient with acute onset of abdominal non-traumatic pain and the absence of other abdominal emergencies—gallbladder stones, cholecystitis, hydronephrosis, aortic aneurysm, acute urinary retention—increase the pre-test probability of bowel ischemia and deserves an early CTA. Well-conducted studies and wider sample size are necessary to demonstrate our hypothesis.

Consent

All published material is reproduced with permission and all the patients—relatives in case 3—gave their informed consent to publish the clinical information in this article.

References

[1] W. T. Kassahun, T. Schulz, O. Richter, and J. Hauss, "Unchanged high mortality rates from acute occlusive intestinal ischemia: six year review," *Langenbeck's Archives of Surgery*, vol. 393, no. 2, pp. 163–171, 2008.

[2] Eike Sebastian Debus, "Intestinal ischemia," *International Journal of Colorectal Disease*, vol. 26, no. 9, pp. 1087–1097, 2011.

[3] L. J. Brandt and P. Feuerstadt, "Beyond low flow: how i manage ischemic colitis," *The American Journal of Gastroenterology*, vol. 111, no. 12, pp. 1672–1674, 2016.

[4] X. YuShuang, L. N. Xiong, Y. N. Li, X. Jiang, and Z. F. Xiong, "Diagnostic methods and drug therapies in patients with ischemic colitis," *International Journal of Colorectal Disease*, vol. 36, no. 1, pp. 47–56, 2021.

[5] A. Reginelli, E. A. Genovese, S. Cappabianca et al., "Intestinal ischemia: US-CT findings correlations," *Critical Ultrasound Journal*, vol. 5, no. 1, pp. 1–11, 2013.

[6] T. Ripollés, L. Simó, M. J. Martínez-Pérez, M. R. Pastor, A. Igual, and A. López, "Sonographic findings in ischemic colitis in 58 patients," *AJR. American Journal of Roentgenology*, vol. 184, no. 3, pp. 777–785, 2005.

[7] A. Hollerweger, G. Maconi, T. Ripolles et al., "Gastrointestinal ultrasound (GIUS) in intestinal emergencies-an EFSUMB position paper," *Ultraschall in der Medizin-European Journal of Ultrasound*, vol. 41, no. 6, pp. 646–657, 2020.

[8] G. L. Moneta, "Screening for mesenteric vascular insufficiency and follow-up of mesenteric artery bypass procedures," *Seminars in Vascular Surgery*, vol. 14, no. 3, pp. 186–192, 2001.

[9] A. F. AbuRahma, P. A. Stone, M. Srivastava et al., "Mesenteric/celiac duplex ultrasound interpretation criteria revisited," *Journal of Vascular Surgery*, vol. 55, no. 2, pp. 428–436, 2012.

[10] M. M. Maher, B. M. Tonra, D. E. Malone, and R. G. Gibney, "Portal venous gas: detection by gray-scale and Doppler sonography in the absence of correlative findings on computed tomography," *Abdominal Imaging*, vol. 26, no. 4, pp. 390–394, 2001.

16

A Fatal Case of Primary Amoebic Meningoencephalitis from Recreational Waters

Edward Hamaty Jr.,[1,2] Saif Faiek,[1] Minesh Nandi,[1] David Stidd,[3,4] Manish Trivedi,[5] and Hari Kandukuri[1]

[1]Department of Medicine, AtlantiCare Regional Medical Center, Atlantic City, NJ, USA
[2]Department of Critical Care, AtlantiCare Regional Medical Center, Atlantic City, NJ, USA
[3]Division of Neuroscience, AtlantiCare Regional Medical Center, Atlantic City, NJ, USA
[4]Department of Neurological Surgery, Thomas Jefferson University and Jefferson Hospital for Neuroscience, Philadelphia, PA, USA
[5]Division of Infectious Disease, AtlantiCare Regional Medical Center, Atlantic City, NJ, USA

Correspondence should be addressed to Minesh Nandi; minesh.nandi@atlanticare.org

Academic Editor: Mehmet Doganay

Background. Naegleria Fowleri is a single-cell, thermophilic amphizoid amoeba, and a rare known causative agent for primary amoebic meningoencephalitis with >97% mortality rate. The amoeba resides in freshwater lakes and ponds but can also survive in inadequately chlorinated pools and recreational waters. The mode of infection includes activities such as diving or jumping into freshwater or submerging the head under the water. Although most commonly seen in the southern United States, it is essential to keep this clinical suspicion in mind regardless of geography, as presenting symptoms can be very similar to classic bacterial meningitis. *Case Summary.* We report the first-ever case in the state of New Jersey of a 29-year-old male presented after a visit to a recreational water park in Texas five days before his presentation with altered mental status. In ICU, his ICP remained refractory to multiple therapies, including antibiotics and antivirals, external ventriculostomy drain, hypertonic saline, pentobarbital-induced coma, and bilateral hemicraniectomies. The CSF analysis revealed trophozoites indicating a protozoan infection, which we diagnosed in the neurocritical unit, and the patient was then immediately started with treatment that included amphotericin B, rifampin, azithromycin, and fluconazole. This suspicion was promptly confirmed by the Center for Disease Control (CDC). Unfortunately, despite all the aggressive intervention by the multidisciplinary team, the patient did not survive. *Conclusion.* As per the CDC, only four people out of 143 known infected individuals in the United States from 1962 to 2017 have survived. Symptoms start with a median of 5 days after exposure to contaminated water. Given the rarity of this case and its very high mortality rate, it is crucial to diagnose primary amoebic meningoencephalitis accurately as its presentation can mimic bacterial meningitis. It is vital to obtain a careful and thorough history, as it can aid in prompt diagnosis and treatment.

1. Introduction

The genus Naegleria is composed of over 30 different species made of a group of free-living ameboflagellate found in diverse habitat [1]. But only Naegleria fowleri has been isolated from the humans and a known agent for primary amoebic encephalitis. N. fowleri is a thermophilic amphizoid amoeba, single-celled microbe, commonly found around the world in warm freshwater [1]. Environmental conditions, including desiccation, salinity, and chlorination, affect their survival [2]. It can exist in a free-living state in water or soil or as a pathogen in human hosts, hence the term amphizoid. Naegleria spp. have been isolated from freshwater lakes, ponds, domestic water supplies, swimming pools, thermal pools, soil, and dust. Human disease caused by N. fowleri was first reported by Fowler and Carter in South Australia [3]. Although most commonly seen in southern states in the United States, it is essential to keep this clinical suspicion in mind regardless of geography, as presenting symptoms can be very similar to classic bacterial meningitis. Symptoms

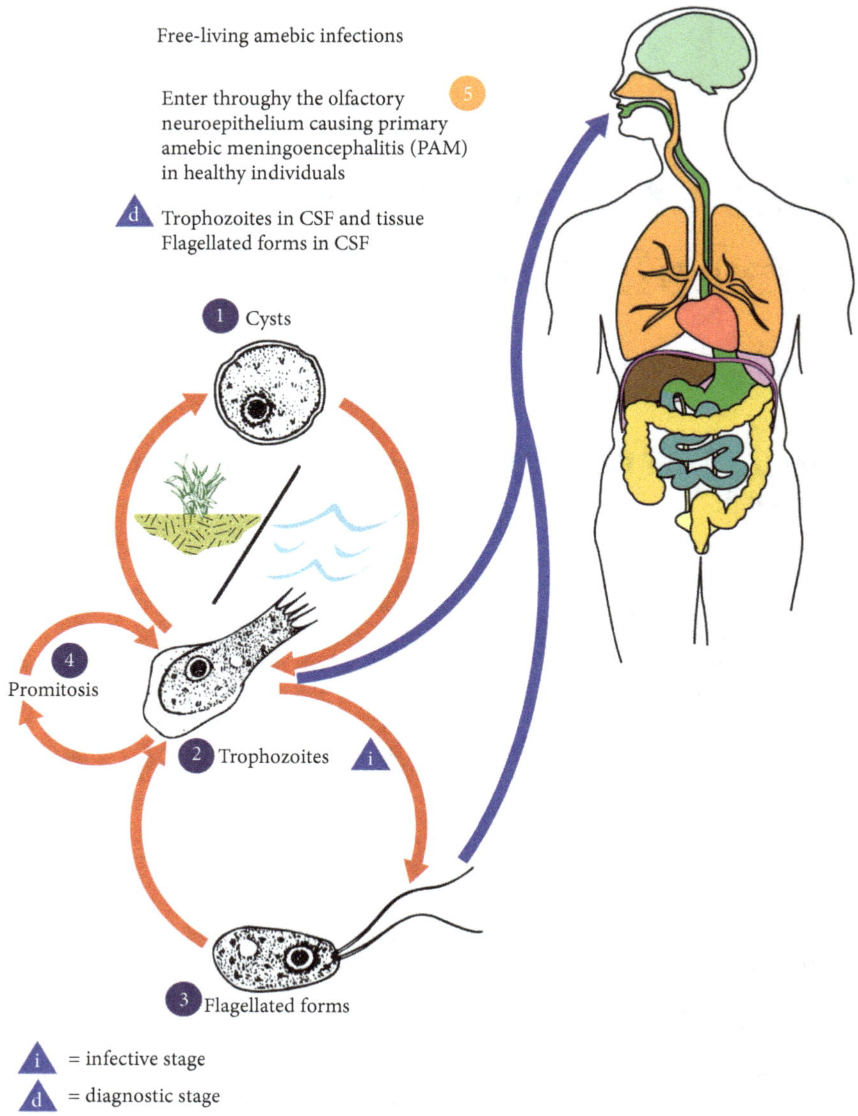

FIGURE 1: This illustration depicts the life cycle of *Naegleria fowleri*, the parasitic agents responsible for causing free-living amebic infections. Content Providers are CDC/ Alexander J. da Silva, PhD, and Melanie Moser. *N. Fowleri* has 3 stages in its life cycle: (1) cyst, (2) trophozoite, and flagellate (3). The only infective stage is the trophozoite which is 10-35 μm long with a granular appearance and a single nucleus. They replicate by binary division during which the nuclear membrane remains intact (promitosis) (4). Trophozoites infect humans or animals by penetrating the nasal tissue (5).

include fever, headaches, nausea along with nuchal rigidity, and sometimes seizures. As per the CDC, an infection can occur by recreational water activities, but not by drinking contaminated water with Naegleria. However, there have been reports of disease via nasal lavage. The majority of infections in the United States are prevalent in southern states arising in summer months, where the organism is found in geothermal water such as hot springs, lakes, poorly maintained swimming pools, and recreational waters. N. fowleri has the best growth at higher temperatures up to 115°F (46°C). The three morphological stages in the life cycle include a trophozoite, flagellate, and a cyst [4] (Figure 1). The trophozoite is the feeding and dividing stage for humans; however, the cyst can also enter through the nares and convert to trophozoites [4]. They attach to the nasal mucosa and then migrate through olfactory nerves across the cribriform plate and penetrate the brain tissue.

Through cytotoxic effects, the organism starts tissue destruction of nerve cells and ingestion of erythrocytes initiating an inflammatory response that consists of neutrophils, eosinophils, and macrophages. The pathologic mechanism includes proteinosis and possible lysis that contributes to neuronal demyelination, and destruction and lysis of erythrocytes and surrounding nerve cells [5]. As a result, neuroimaging in PAM usually shows a single focus on infection in the frontal lobe along with diffuse cerebral edema and basilar meningeal enhancement [6]. The detection method includes direct visualization under a microscope of fresh CSF samples

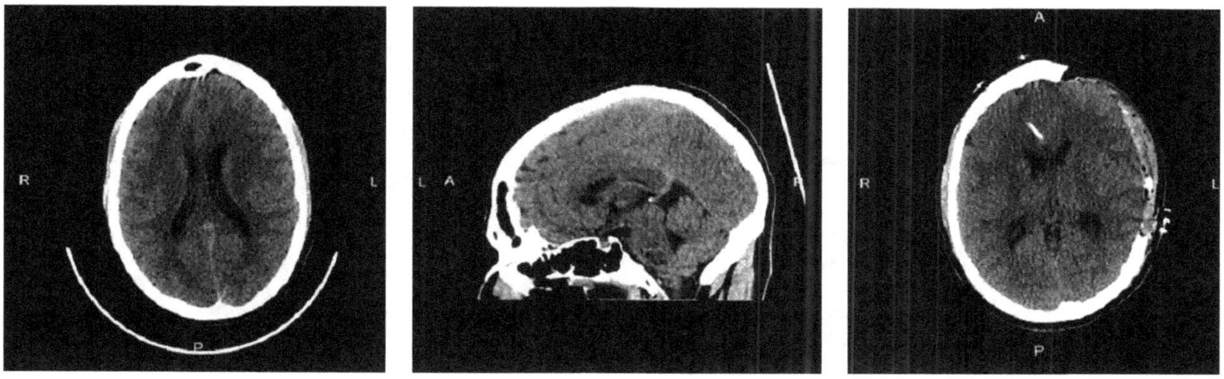

(a) (b) (c)

FIGURE 2: CAT scan on admission showing (a) axial, (b) sagittal, (c) post hemicraniectomy within 12 hrs. of admission. Note, there is diffuse sulcal effacement in (a), possibly reflecting hypoxic-ischemic encephalopathy Vs meningitis.

using Giemsa Wright or modified trichrome stain, antigen detection, PCR, or amoeba culture [7, 8]. As per the CDC, in the last ten years, out of 34 cases reported in the United States, 30 people were infected by recreational waters, and half of the examples in the U.S have occurred in Texas and Florida. Symptoms start with a median of 5 days after exposure to contaminated water. Due to the rarity of the infection and its close presentation to bacterial meningitis, 75% of diagnosis is made after the death of the patients [9].

2. Case Report

A 29-year-old Caucasian male with a past medical history of Epstein-Barr virus infection in childhood presented to AtlantiCare Regional Medical Center in New Jersey, Atlantic City division, with a sudden altered level of consciousness and fevers up to 103°F. Upon initial assessment, the patient was somnolent, altered, and not able to follow any commands. The mother provided the history given the clinical condition of the patient. She stated that the patient just returned five days ago from Texas, where he went on vacation. Also pertinent was that he worked outdoors for the New Jersey Department of Environmental Protection in water testing facility. Five days before his presentation, the patient was exposed to recreational waters at a surfing park in Waco, Texas. On physical examination, the patient was febrile and comatose with a Glasgow Coma Scale of 7. His blood pressure was 153/75 mmHg with a pulse rate of 77 beats per minute and an oral temperature of 103°F. Upon examination of lungs, abdomen, and extremities, no abnormality was noted. No features of chronic illnesses or palpable lymph nodes were appreciated. On his neurologic exam, he was altered, moving all extremities with a positive Brudzinski sign. We sedated and intubated the patient for airway protection in the emergency department and admitted him to the neurocritical care unit. A computerized tomography (CT) scan of the brain showed no evidence of acute intracranial infarction or hemorrhage; however, there was sulcal effacement concerning for hypoxic/ischemic encephalopathy versus meningitis (Figure 2). Given the patient's presentation, the suspicion was high for bacterial meningitis versus viral encephalitis. Blood cultures, serologies for West Nile virus, Rocky Mountain spotted fever, cytomegalovirus, Herpes simplex virus, Lyme's disease, and an acute Epstein-Barr virus panel were all obtained. The patient received 10 milligrams of IV dexamethasone. Vancomycin and meropenem plus acyclovir were initiated for broad-spectrum coverage. In the intensive care unit, a lumbar puncture demonstrated an opening pressure of 46 mmHg, and the procedure was aborted. We placed a right frontal external ventricular drain (EVD) that revealed an opening pressure of 15 mmHg. During this time, we collected the CSF and sent it for further studies. Cerebrospinal fluid studies showed a white cell count of 1021 cells/uL, red blood cell count of 1830 cells/uL, the glucose of 98 mg/dL, and a protein of 174 mg/dL. His peripheral white blood cell count was 11400 cells/uL (83% segmented neutrophils). The EVD was left open to drain at a pop off setting of 0 mmHg. An MRI of the brain done post admission showed no evidence of acute infarction, and the ventricular volume was normal.

On day one post admission, the patient's ICP continued to remain elevated, sustaining at 30-40 mmHg despite EVD placement and multiple interventions, including hyperventilation, hyperosmolar therapy with 3% saline, and a paralytic agent. A phenobarbital-induced coma with burst suppression was started, which initially dropped the ICP to 10 mmHg, but the ICP soon rebounded and increased to 40 mmHg. A left decompressive hemicraniectomy was then performed, which decreased the ICP to 15-20 mmHg. The patient's initial laboratory workup was still pending, including blood, fungal cultures, CSF gram stain/cultures, and viral PCR. We sent out the tick-borne disease panel, and doxycycline, azithromycin, and atovaquone were empirically added to the aforementioned antibiotic therapy.

On day two post admission, the patient's left scalp was tense, and the right frontal EVD again demonstrated elevated ICP. The elevated ICP was refractory to continued maximal medical management, and the neurosurgery team performed a right decompressive hemicraniectomy. Patient cultures and the laboratory workup, as mentioned above, were all negative. Given patient's presentation, with clinical signs and travel history, amphotericin B and fluconazole were added

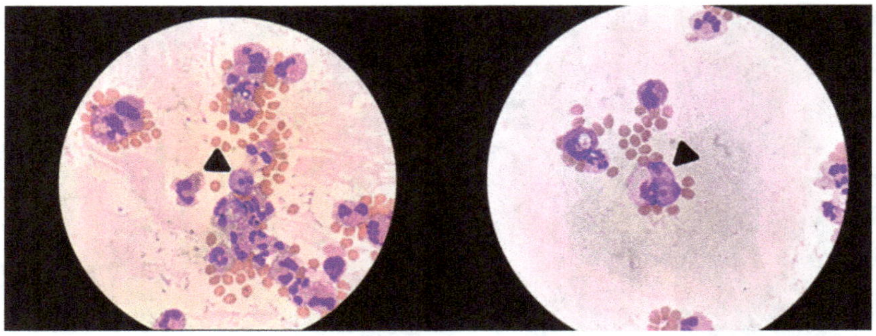

FIGURE 3: Naegleria trophozoites were rapidly identified by their large, round- to pear-shaped cells with a prominent, dark nucleus, and scattered vacuoles. Images of Naegleria fowleri on Giemsa Wright-stained CSF slides (1000x, oil immersion). Black arrowheads point to Naegleria trophozoites with a background of mostly RBC and some neutrophils.

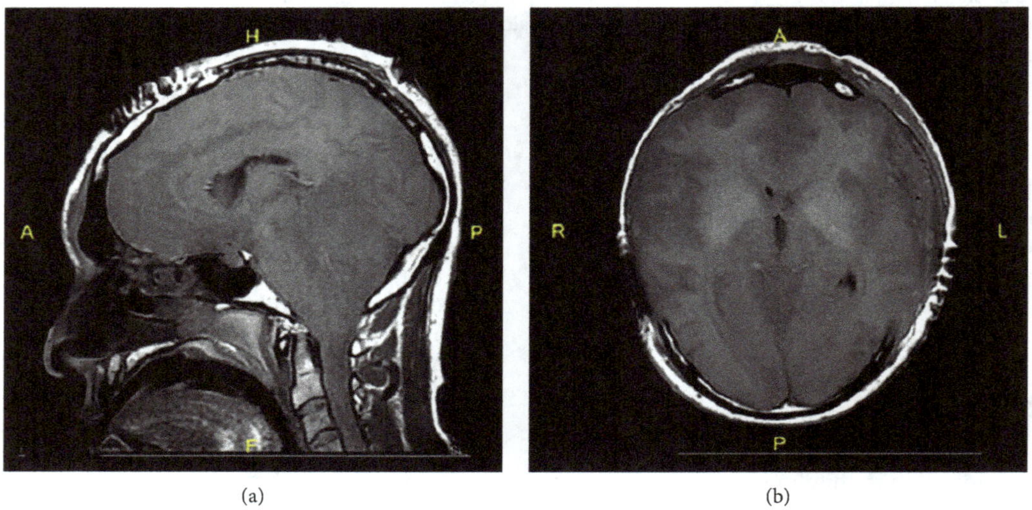

FIGURE 4: MRI post 72 hours of admission. After uncomplicated wide bilateral craniectomies. (a) The sagittal view showing transtentorial herniation with stretching and obliteration of the fourth ventricle. (b) Note on the axial view showing diffuse swelling with loss of gray white junctions and absence of ventricular space.

to the treatment and more CSF sample was sent for parasite smear to test for possible amoebic meningoencephalitis at our institution.

On the third day post admission, parasite smear results came back concerning for amoeba infection. We sent samples to the CDC, which confirmed the diagnosis of Naegleria fowleri (Figure 3). Vancomycin and acyclovir were discontinued, and we started the patient on amphotericin B, fluconazole, and azithromycin. Despite the bilateral craniectomies and other interventions, the patient's ICP remained elevated, and he started to demonstrate signs of brain death with MRI revealing transtentorial herniation without uncal or subfalcine herniation (Figure 4). The physical exam off sedation and nuclear medicine cerebral blood flow study both confirmed findings consistent with brain death, and we terminally extubated the patient.

3. Discussion

This case presents with a first-ever reported case of PAM in the state of New Jersey, and it highlights the importance of keeping a clinical suspicion in mind regardless of geographic location. The infection primarily affects younger people who are exposed to warm recreational freshwater in southern states during the summer months [10]. Increased incidence in young adults and children is likely more related to water-related activities as they are more likely to dive, submerge the head in water, or engage in water sports like water surfing, water rafting, and skiing that can force water up to the cribriform plate from the nasal cavity. The patient presented with signs including fevers, chills, photophobia, confusion, with a tripod sign that indicates respiratory distress and meningeal irritation, which required him to undergo intubation immediately as his GCS was 7.

The diagnosis of PAM is challenging because of the similarities between the presenting symptoms of PAM and other conditions, including bacterial meningitis. PAM is rapidly progressive and has a devastating disease course that usually occurs within 6-17 days after initial exposure. This can lead to death if not promptly diagnosed [11]. Specific diagnostic tools and general increased awareness of PAM are required to initiate treatment sooner. In the few cases of PAM that were successfully managed in the past, a correct and prompt diagnosis was made [12, 13]. History of water exposure is critical in diagnosing PAM. The current case presented with clinical signs and symptoms similar to previously documented cases [14, 15]. Symptoms of PAM are nonspecific symptoms and include severe headache, high-grade fever, confusion with altered level of consciousness, and neck stiffness. Death, in most cases, is due to increased intracranial pressure and herniation, as seen in our patient (Figure 4).

N. fowleri induces pore-forming proteins that cause lysis of mammalian cells on contact and secrete cytolytic molecules, including acid hydrolases, phospholipases, neuraminidases, and phospholipolytic enzymes that degrade mammalian tissue [1]. The organism also synthesizes regulatory surface proteins that confer protection to amoeba against complement-mediated lysis and other cytotoxic substances, thus evading the host immune system [1]. Laboratory findings in patients with PAM are characterized by increased leukocytes, which are predominantly polymorphonuclear cells. CSF may also be purulent with marked leukocytosis, increased protein, and reduced glucose level [14, 15]. In most cases, neuroimaging tests in the early stages of the disease did not reveal any brain abnormalities [16]. However, strong clinical suspicion of PAM with a previous history of water exposure should guide the management of the patient's presentation in the absence of bacteria or fungi and CSF specimens. Measures to avoid this fatal infection include avoiding water-related activities in freshwater lakes, rivers, or natural hot springs with high water temperatures.

Its low incidence limits effective treatments for an N. fowleri infection, and current treatment strategies are based on case reports and in vitro animal studies. Amphotericin B is a pharmacologic treatment with potential efficacy when started early. It acts by binding to ergosterol in the cell membrane with pore formation that leads to cellular lysis. In vitro studies show a concentration of at least 0.1 μg/mL is needed to suppress >90% of amoeba growth, and 0.8 mg/mL is required to achieve 100% amoebicidal capability [17, 18]. Based on this, intravenous doses of amphotericin B of 0.25 mg to1.5 mg/kg/day are recommended in adults, while doses ranging from 0.5 to 0.7 mg/kg/day is recommended in pediatric patients [18]. CDC currently recommends intravenous or intrathecal (if ICP is increased) amphotericin B at doses of 1.5 mg/kg/day in two divided doses for three days, followed by 1 mg/kg/day once daily for an additional eleven days with a total of 14 days of therapy [18]. Fluconazole, an antifungal agent, may be effective at a dose of 10 mg/kg/day daily for 28 days. Fluconazole then synergistically works with amphotericin B by inhibiting ergosterol synthesis. Also, azithromycin, the macrolide antibiotic, has in vitro activity against N. fowleri and is recommended to be used at 10 mg/kg/day once daily (maximum 500 mg daily dose) for 28 days [9]. Miltefosine, a drug effective against leishmaniasis, is another potential treatment for PAM recommended by the CDC at doses of 50 mg orally two to three times daily (based on body weight) with a maximum dose of 1.5 mg/kg/day for a total of 28 days [18]. The exact mechanism is not precise; however, it is believed to interact with phospholipids and steroid molecules in the cellular membrane.

PAM is almost always uniformly fatal. Early diagnosis and aggressive treatment are crucial for recovery. In addition to pharmacologic management against amoeba, control of high intracranial pressure, systemic inflammation, and possible induction of moderate hypothermia are a multidisciplinary approach in treating PAM [19]. Neuroprotective management principles following any cerebral insult are based on maintaining adequate cerebral perfusion, tempering oxygen consumption, and lowering ICP with mild to moderate hypothermia (32-34°C). These steps reduce reactive oxygen species formation and proinflammatory cytokines halting neuronal apoptosis [20]. Of the 143 reported PAM cases in the United States from 1962 to 2017, this is the first case reported in New Jersey. A high clinical suspicion is required to diagnose PAM for patients presenting with nonspecific symptoms similar to bacterial meningitis. History and physical exams are crucial in the diagnosis of PAM as early as possible so that appropriate treatment can be initiated, along with aggressive neurological critical care management.

References

[1] F. Marciano-Cabral and G. A. Cabral, "The immune response to Naegleria fowleri amebae and pathogenesis of infection," *FEMS Immunology & Medical Microbiology*, vol. 51, no. 2, pp. 243–259, 2007.

[2] S. L. Chang, "Resistance of pathogenic Naegleria to some common physical and chemical agents," *Applied and Environmental Microbiology*, vol. 35, no. 2, pp. 368–375, 1978.

[3] M. Fowler and R. F. Carter, "Acute pyogenic meningitis probably due to Acanthamoeba sp: a preliminary report," *British Medical Journal*, vol. 2, no. 5464, pp. 734–742, 1965.

[4] A. J. Martinez, *Free-living amoebas; natural history, prevention, diagnosis, pathology and treatment of disease*, CRC Press, Boca Raton, Florida, 1985.

[5] E. Grace, S. Asbill, and K. Virga, "Naegleria fowleri: pathogenesis, diagnosis, and treatment options," *Antimicrobial Agents and Chemotherapy*, vol. 59, no. 11, pp. 6677–6681, 2015.

[6] T. Y. Y. Ong, N. A. Khan, and R. Siddiqui, "Brain-eating amoebae: predilection sites in the brain and disease outcome," *Journal of Clinical Microbiology*, vol. 55, no. 7, pp. 1989–1997, 2017.

[7] G. S. Visvesvara, "Amebic meningoencephalitides and keratitis: challenges in diagnosis and treatment," *Current Opinion in Infectious Diseases*, vol. 23, no. 6, pp. 590–594, 2010.

[8] B. S. Robinson, P. T. Monis, and P. J. Dobson, "Rapid, sensitive, and discriminating identification of Naegleria spp. by real-time PCR and melting-curve analysis," *Applied and Environmental Microbiology*, vol. 72, no. 9, pp. 5857–5863, 2006.

[9] Centers for Disease Control and Prevention, "Investigational drug available directly from CDC for the treatment of infections with free living amebae," *MMWR. Morbidity and Mortality Weekly Report*, vol. 62, p. 666, 2013.

[10] J. S. Yoder, B. A. Eddy, G. S. Visvesvara, L. Capewell, and M. J. Beach, "The epidemiology of primary amoebic meningoencephalitis in the USA, 1962–2008," *Epidemiology and Infection*, vol. 138, no. 7, pp. 968–975, 2010.

[11] C. Lopez, P. Budge, J. Chen et al., "Primary amebic Meningoencephalitis," *Pediatric Emergency Care*, vol. 28, no. 3, pp. 272–276, 2012.

[12] J. R. Cope, D. A. Conrad, N. Cohen et al., "Use of the novel therapeutic agent miltefosine for the treatment of primary amebic meningoencephalitis: report of 1 fatal and 1 surviving case: table 1," *Clinical Infectious Diseases*, vol. 62, no. 6, pp. 774–776, 2016.

[13] A. L. Dunn, T. Reed, C. Stewart, and R. A. Levy, "*Naegleria fowleri* that induces primary amoebic meningoencephalitis: rapid diagnosis and rare case of survival in a 12-year-old caucasian girl," *Laboratory Medicine*, vol. 47, no. 2, pp. 149–154, 2016.

[14] P. E. Cogo, M. Scaglia, S. Gatti et al., "Fatal *Naegleria fowleri* meningoencephalitis, Italy," *Emerging Infectious Diseases*, vol. 10, no. 10, pp. 1835–1837, 2004.

[15] M. Fowler and R. F. Carter, "Acute pyogenic meningitis probably due to Acanthamoeba sp.: a preliminary report," *BMJ*, vol. 2, no. 5464, pp. 740–742, 1965.

[16] N. D. P. Barnett, A. M. Kaplan, R. J. Hopkin, M. A. Saubolle, and M. F. Rudinsky, "Primary amoebic meningoencephalitis with *Naegleria fowleri*: clinical review," *Pediatric Neurology*, vol. 15, no. 3, pp. 230–234, 1996.

[17] J.-H. Kim, S.-Y. Jung, Y.-J. Lee et al., "Effect of therapeutic chemical agents in vitro and on experimental meningoencephalitis due to *Naegleria fowleri*," *Antimicrobial Agents and Chemotherapy*, vol. 52, no. 11, pp. 4010–4016, 2008.

[18] Centers for Disease Control and Prevention, *N. fowleri treatment 28 May 2014*, Centers for Disease Control and Prevention, Atlanta, GA, 2014.

[19] W. M. Linam, M. Ahmed, J. R. Cope et al., "Successful treatment of an adolescent with Naegleria fowleri primary amebic meningoencephalitis," *Pediatrics*, vol. 135, no. 3, pp. e744–e748, 2015.

[20] J. E. Irazuzta, R. Pretzlaff, M. Rowin, K. Milam, F. P. Zemlan, and B. Zingarelli, "Hypothermia as an adjunctive treatment for severe bacterial meningitis," *Brain Research*, vol. 881, no. 1, pp. 88–97, 2000.

17

The Conundrum of Septic Shock Imitators in Patients with Hematologic Cancers: Case Presentation and Possible Differential Diagnoses

Giorgio Berlot,[1] Giulia Moratelli,[1] Martina Tarchini,[1] Katiuscia Battaglia,[1] Paolo Grassi,[1] Nadia Zarrillo,[2] Vincenzo Colella,[2] and Rossana Bussani[3]

[1]*Department of Anesthesia and Intensive Care, University of Trieste, Italy*
[2]*Department of Anesthesia and Intensive Care, Azienda Ospedaliera Sant'Anna e San Sebastiano di Caserta, Italy*
[3]*Department of Pathology, University of Trieste, Italy*

Correspondence should be addressed to Giorgio Berlot; berlot@inwind.it

Academic Editor: Chiara Lazzeri

The authors describe the case of a patient treated with several cycles of chemotherapy due to an advanced stage non-Hodgkin lymphoma. One daafter the last cycle, he was admitted to our Intensive Care Unit with a septic shock-like clinical picture which didn't respond to the aggressive treatment and the patient died a few hours later. The autoptical findings cast some doubts on the diagnosis, and demonstrated the presence of other factors imitating its symptoms. In this article, the mimickers of septic shock are reviewed and discussed, as some of them require an aggressive immunosuppression instead of the recommended treatment for septic shock.

1. Introduction

In the last few years, the outcome of patients with hematologic tumors has improved following the introduction of new agents directed against specific receptors exposed on the surface of the neoplastic cells or able to boost the immune capabilities against them, such as the Chimeric Antigen Receptor Modified T-cell (CAR-T) [1, 2]; consequently, an increasing number of these patients are now admitted to the Intensive Care Unit (ICU) both for the underlying disease and/or for its complications, including sepsis and septic shock (SS) [3, 4]. According to the 3rd International Consensus Definitions, this latter is considered a condition characterized by a multiple organ dysfunction (MODS) severe enough to increase the risk of death [5]; notably, this definition does not consider the following items: first of all the time course, the fulminant forms rapidly leading to MODS and death are lumped together with lesser aggressive ones than the different timeframes of SS, which can be characterized by an initial hyper-inflammatory condition switching later on to a reduced immune response, consisting of low-grade inflammatory state, hypercatabolism and the occurrence of secondary infections caused by multiple drug resistant germs and/or the reactivation of latent virus, such as Epstein–Barr virus, Cytomegalovirus (CMV) and Herpes virus [6, 7].

The classical symptoms of SS include fever or hypothermia, tachycardia, arterial hypotension, and other signs related to the MODS making the diagnosis relatively straightforward. Nevertheless, in patients with hematologic cancers causes other that SS can account for this clinical phenotype, including a life-threatening hyper-inflammation associated either to the underlying disease and/or to its treatment. The recognition and treatment of these conditions appear particularly challenging for the intensivist since (a) they are relatively uncommon; (b) they can occur in the very same circumstances of SS and the related symptoms could overlap; (c) the time course can be so fast that the clinical presentation could be represented by an overt MODS just from the onset; and, perhaps most important, (d) the mainstay of the treatment is based on an aggressive immunosuppression, which is contraindicated in SS.

TABLE 1: Time course of some blood biological variables.

Variable	Timing: ED (6 h before ICU admission)	ICU admission	+4 h	R.F.
pH	n.a.	6.97	7.06	7.38–7.42
pCO_2 (mmHg)	n.a.	68.4	53.1	35–45
PaO_2 / FIO_2 (mmHg)	n.a.	94	66	≥400
HCO_3^- (mEq/L)	n.a.	16.4	14.8	23–25
Lactate (mEq/L)	n.a.	6.7	10.8	1–2
Hb (g/dl)	14.1	12.5	13.5	13–16
WBC/ml	1820	650	350	4000–11000
Platelets /ml	131.000	89.000	14.000	180–350
IRN	n.a.	1.53	1.84	0.78–1.2
aPTTr	n.a.	0.95	2.44	0.76–1.18
Fibrinogen (mg/dl)	n.a.	272	219	180–400
D-dimer (mcg/LFEU)	n.a.	2.11	16000	<5
Glycemia (mg/dl)	132	80	72	90–110
Creatinine (mg/dl)	1.40	2.76	2.90	0.8–1.1
BUN (mg/dl)	66	80	83	15–50
ALT(U/L)	29	n.a.	65	0–40
AST (U/L)	55	n.a.	69	0–40
Amilase (U/L)	35	79	80	8–53
Ferritin mcg/m	n.a.	1750	n.a.	14–300
Triglycerydes (mg/dl)	n.a.	180	n.a.	<170
C-reactive protein (mg/dl)	36.2	142	n.a.	<5.0
Total bilirubin (mg/dl)	n.a.	0.69	0.79	0.70–1.20

ED: emergency department; R.F.: reference values; n.a.: not available; FEU: fibrinogen equivalent unit.

Hereby we describe and review a case of a patient treated for a hematologic cancer in whom the admission in ICU with the diagnosis of SS appear to have been too simplistic, because other noninfectious factors may have contributed to the MODS and to the outcome.

2. Case Description

A 53-year-old man was admitted to the Emergency Department due to 6-hour-lasting acute abdominal pain; the first CT scan demonstrated an edematous pancreatitis and a small amount of ascites; a second CT confirmed the results at 6 h from the first one. A couple of hours after hospitalization, he was transferred to our Intensive Care Unit (ICU) because he became confused, hypotensive, and anuric. The history revealed an advanced stage non-Hodgkin lymphoma (DLCBL, stage III) discovered two months before the current admission and treated with 5 cycles of Rituximab, cyclophosphamide, doxorubicin, vincristine, and prednisone (R-CHOP), the last completed the day before the admission in ICU. On a scheduled outpatient visit occurred two weeks before this hospitalization, the patient was prescribed a 10-day course of oral valganciclovir due a reactivation of CMV, but it was suspended after 7 days due to a rise of hepatic liver enzymes and the disappearance of the viral DNA. In the ICU, the patient was intubated and mechanically ventilated; lab investigations demonstrated a deep metabolic acidosis, hyperlactatemia in association with severe leukopenia, and reduced platelet count; these abnormalities worsened in the following hours (Table 1). With the clinical suspicion of SS, IV vancomycin, meropemen, and valganciclovir were initiated, along with the administration of IgM- and IgA-enriched intravenous immunoglobulins (Pentaglobin®, Biotest, Dreieich, Germany); at the same time, a renal replacement treatment was started in association with the extracorporeal removal of sepsis mediators (Cytosorb®, Aferetica, Mirandola, Italy). The arterial hypotension was unresponsive to the administration of incremental doses of fluids, norepinephrine (peaking at 2 mcg/kg/min) together with terlipressin (100 mg) and mg 200 of hydrocortisone; a continuous administration of $NaHCO_3$ failed to correct the metabolic acidosis. Despite this extremely aggressive approach, the clinical conditions further deteriorated, and the patient died six hours after the ICU admission.

At the autopsy, the liver and the spleen were enlarged and a massive purulent peritonitis was present in the absence of visceral perforations despite a severe mucosal ischemia that involved the enteric tract completely in the absence of mesenteric vascular obstructions; the pancreatic head was mildly edematous; the adrenal glands appeared hemorrhagic (Figure 1); the heart was dilated and presented a biventricular a diffuse subendocardial ischemia despite normal coronary arteries.

Microscopically, the bone marrow presented an extensive hemophagocytic lymphohistiocytosis (HLH) in the absence of residual traces of the NHL (Figure 2); an *E. coli* strain sensible to the administered antibiotics was isolated from the blood culture.

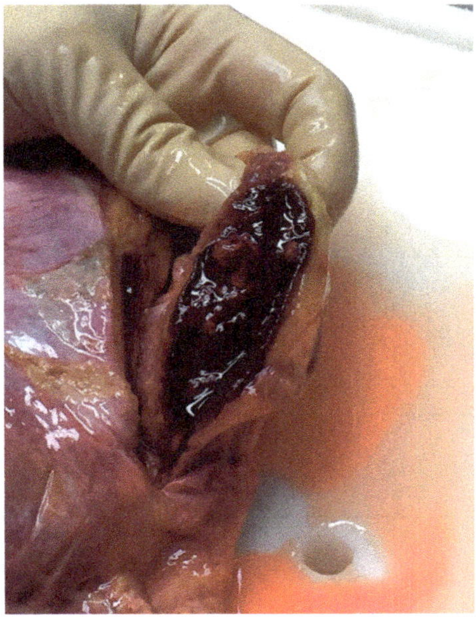

FIGURE 1: Adrenal hemorrhage.

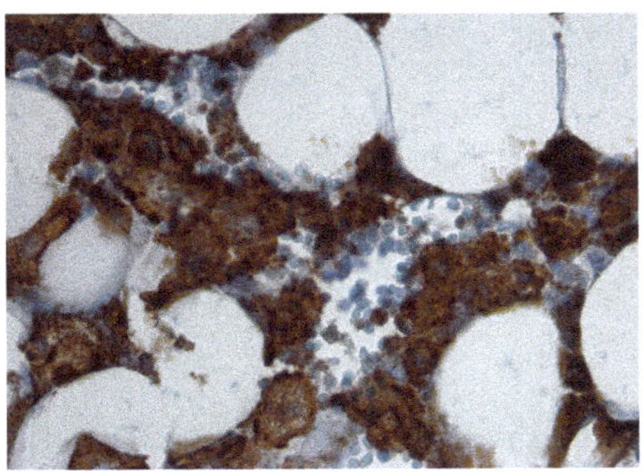

FIGURE 2: Bone marrow with extensive hemophagocytosis (CD 163, ×40).

3. Discussion

The current Surviving Sepsis Campaign (SSC) guidelines for the treatment of SS recommend the prompt administration of wide-spectrum antibiotics possibly associated with antiviral and antifungal agents in selected cases [8]. However, the diagnosis and the treatment cannot rely entirely on the microbiological findings since (a) in a high rate of cases, cultures remain sterile throughout the clinical course [9, 10]; and (b) a recent study demonstrated that in >25% of patients initially diagnosed as having SS the symptoms were caused by noninfectious diseases [11]; consequently, causes other than infections must be considered especially in the absence of any improvement despite an aggressive approach. This particularly applies to patients with hematologic tumors, in whom different factors, including the underlying disease, the related complications, and the ever-increasing use of agents interacting with the immune system can imitate SS, thus preventing the correct diagnosis and approach.

In our patient, the fulminant course of MODS could have been determined by different factors acting alone or in combination.

First, a low cardiac output (CO) could have initially occurred, determining the widespread necrosis of the enteric mucosal and the subsequent escape of bacteria and their derivates from the gut lumen, leading both the activation of septic mediators and the peritonitis. The isolation of *E. coli* in the bloodstream and the severe peritonitis in the absence of perforation supports this hypothesis, even if we could not perform an echocardiography due to the fulminating course of the MODS. The cause of the reduction of the CO is hard to identify, but it could be assumed that it was due to the anti-NHL treatment: actually, doxorubicin and the otheranthracyclines can cause a dose–dependent cardiotoxicity eventually leading to a progressive irreversible heart failure,although cases of sudden-onset cardiogenic shock have also been described [12–14]. In our patient, the cumulative dose of doxorubicin exceeded 210 mg/m^2 corresponding to an odd ratio of cardiotoxicity <7% [12]. The diffuse subendocardial ischemia observed at the post-mortem examination could be ascribed to the elevated doses of vasopressors used.

Second, although an infective trigger for the MODS is highly plausible, the further rapid deterioration of the clinical conditions despite the administration of an appropriate antibiotic treatment makes the presence of other concomitant conditions likely: actually, Vincent et al. demonstrated that in SS patients the death is associated more with a lack of improvement than with an unrelenting worsening of the clinical conditions [15]. Conversely, in our patient the MODS rapidly deteriorated since its onset and did not respond to the standard treatment of SS making the co-existence of other factors plausible.

Third, the patient underwent several cycles of a regimen that included Rituximab, a monoclonal anti-CD20 antibody largely used in the treatment of hematologic cancers and other disorders caused by chronic inflammatory conditions and an ever-increasing list of immunologic disorders [16]. The administration of rituximab has been associated with a number of early- and late-onset complications; the former include anaphylactic or allergic reactions occurring during the infusion or in the following 24 h and the latter are related to its long-term effects, including immunosuppression, renal dysfunction, and *de novo* hematologic tumors. Considering the interval from the last administration of rituximab, we guess that the profound and unresponsive hemodynamic collapse observed in our patient could be related more to the decrease of immune capabilities determined by the repeated cycles of R-CHOP than to a rituximab-induced anaphylactic reaction.

Fourth, the clinical picture could be ascribed to a hemophagocytic lymphohistiocytosis (HLH). This disturbance of the immune function exists in a familiar and in an acquired form and it is characterized by the massive production and release of inflammatory mediators caused by the dysregulated activation of T-lymphocytes, natural killer (NK)-cells, and macrophages. The familiar form is caused by the mutation of specific genes regulating the cytotoxic granule pathway leading to the impairment of the cytotoxic activity of NK cells and

TABLE 2: Diagnostic criteria of HLH.

(i) Molecular diagnosis consistent with HLH (ii) Or 5 of the following criteria	Case
(1) Fever	+
(2) Splenomegaly	+
(3) Cytopenia affecting ≥ 2 lineages	+
(a) Hemoglobin <9 g/dl	−
(b) Platelets <90.000/ml	+
(c) Neutrophils <1000/ml	+
(4) Hypertrigliceridemia and/or hypofibrinogemia	−
(a) Triglycerides >265 mg/dl	−
(b) Fibrinogen <150 mg/dl	−
(5) Hemophagocytosis in bone marrow, spleen or nodes (*)	+
(6) Low/absent NK cell activity	n.a.
(7) Ferritin ≥500 mcg/ml	+
(8) sCD25 (sIL2R) ≥2400 U/ml	n.a.

n.a: not available.

TABLE 3: HScore.

Variable	Criteria for scoring	Case
Immunosuppression	0: no 18: yes	18
Temperature (°C)	0 (<38.4) 33 (38.4–39.4) 49 (>39.4)	33
Organomegaly	0 (no) 23 (Hepatomegaly or splenomegaly) 38 (Hepatomegaly + splenomegaly)	38
n. of cytopenias	0 (1 lineage) 24 (2 lineages) 34 (3 lineages)	24
Ferritin (ng/ml)	0 (<2000) 35 (2000–6000) 50 (>6000)	0
Triglyceride (mmol/L)	0 (<1.5) 30 (1.5–4) 64 (>4)	30
Fibrinogen (g/L)	0 (>2.5) 30 (≤2.5)	30
Serum ALT	0 (<30) 19 (≥30)	19
Hemophagocytosis in B.M.	0 (no) 35 (yes)	35
Total score	**337**	**227**

B.M.: bone marrow.

cytotoxic T-lymphocytes while leaving intact the production of inflammatory cytokines, whereas in the latter the underlying mechanism is less understood and has been associated with a number of factors, including rheumatologic and autoimmune disorders, viral infections, and tumors [17]; altogether, these disorders are denominated Macrophage Activation Syndrome (MAS) and the related symptoms mime SS in its hyperinflammatory phase [18]. In both forms the stimulated cells are unable to kill the invading microorganisms, yet can activate macrophages, thus triggering a process ultimately leading to an hyperinflammatory status resembling SS due to the release of elevated amounts of IFN-γ, TNF, IL-6, IL-10 etc., [19–21]. The acquired form of HLH is increasingly recognized in SS patients undergoing bone marrow examination even if its role in influencing the outcome is still uncertain [20, 21]. As far as the underlying disorders in critically ill adult ICU patients are concerned, in a recent study HLH occurred as a complication of hematologic malignancies (57%, mainly NHL), infections (25%, mainly CMV), or a combination of both (4%) [22]. In patients with SS, it has been hypothesized that a persisting release of inflammatory mediators in response to an uncontrolled infectious trigger can prompt the occurrence of HLH that, in turn, further increase their production thus initiating a vicious cycle ultimately leading to a MOF [23]. The diagnosis of acquired HLH is based on the fulfillment of at least of 8 criteria originally established by the Histiocyte Society for the diagnosis of the congenital form (HLH 2004) (Table 2) [22]. To overcome the limitations of using this approach in the acquired HLH, a specific score (HScore) has been developed by analyzing with a logistic regression a data set of variables drawn from ICU adult patients with confirmed HLH [23] (Table 3). In our patient, despite blood levels of ferritin being relatively low (1750 mcg/ml) as compared with those reported in other studies with values exceeding 10.000 mcg/ml [20–24], both the HLH 2004 and the HScore were high enough (5 criteria and 227, respectively, corresponding to a probability of HLH ≥95%) to make the diagnosis very likely [23]. Independently from the causes, the treatment of acquired HLH consists of the administration, alone or in combination, of immunodepressant including steroids, etoposide, or cyclosporine. Due to the fulminant time course and the diagnosis of suspected SS, we did not initiate such treatment but a blood purification technique was started as a rescue treatment to remove the sepsis mediators [25]. Recently, a number of biologic agents targeting different substances involved both in different forms of MAS have been investigated, but results from clinical trials performed in acquired HLH are lacking [26–28].

Fifth, a similar stormy clinical course is described in patients with a catastrophic antiphospholipid syndrome (CAPS), which is determined by the widespread occlusion of the microvascular network by microthrombi triggered by the Lupus anticoagulant (LAC) and the anti-cardiolipin (aCL) and anti-β2-glycoprotein I (aβ2GBPI) antibodies [30]. Although the pathogenesis of CAPS is not fully clear, a number of circumstances have been associated with its occurrence, including infections, systemic lupus erythematosus, and tumors; among these latter, hematological malignancies appear particularly involved [31].The diagnosis is challenging and requires a high index of suspicion, the exclusion of other causes and the fulfillment of a number of clinical, laboratory, and pathologic criteria (Table 4). The acute treatment of CAPS

TABLE 4: Diagnostic criteria for CAPS (from [29]).

Preliminary criteria	Case
(1) Evidence of involvement of ≥3 organs, system and/or tissues	+
(2) Development of clinical manifestation simultaneously or in <1 week	+
(3) Evidence of small vessel occlusion in at least 1 organ or tissue	+
(4) Lab evidences of LAC and/or aCL and aβ2GBPI	n.a.
Definite CAPS	
(i) All 4 criteria	–
Probable CAPS	
(i) All 4 criteria, 2 organs, system and/or tissues involved	–
(ii) All 4 criteria, except for the lack of lab evidence due to the early death of patients never tested for APS	–
(iii) Criteria 1, 2, and 4	–
(iv) Criteria 1, 3, and 4 and development of a third event between one week and one month after the initial presentation despite anticoagulation	n.a.

n.a: not available.

TABLE 6: Possible therapeutic strategies.

Condition	Therapy
Septic shock	(1) Antibiotics (2) Drainage of septic foci (3) Cardiorespiratory and renal support (4) Steroids (debated) (5) Blood purification techniques
CRS (whatever cause)	(1) Treatment of the cause (2) Immunosuppression (3) Blood purification techniques
Acquired hemophagocytic lymphohistiocytosis	(1) Immunosuppression (2) Etoposide (3) Extracorporeal Blood purification
Catastrophic anti phospholipid syndrome	(1) Immunosuppression (2) IvIg (3) Anticoagulation (4) Plasmaexchange

TABLE 5: Possible differential diagnoses of fulminant MODS.

Diagnosis	Pro	Against	Likelihood
Septic shock	(1) Immusuppression (2) Blood culture positive for *E. coli*	(1) Fulminant time course of MODS (2) Not responding to standard anti-SS treatment	H
Rituximab-induced cytokine release syndrome	(1) Clinical picture resembling SIRS	(1) Interval >24 h between treatment and onset of symptoms	L
Acquired hemophagocytic lymphohistiocytosis	(1) NHL (2) Recent CMV infection (3) 5/8 preliminary diagnostic criteria fulfilled (4) Elevated HScore	none	H
Catastrophic anti phospholipid syndrome	(1) Recent NHL	(1) Diagnostic criteria unfulfilled	L
Acute adrenal failure	(1) Failed response to volume resuscitation and vasopressors (2) Autopsy findings	(1) No hyponatremia	H

H: high; L: low; I: intermediate.

consists of (1) general supportive measures (2) a rapid onset anticoagulation with iv heparin (c) a multi-faceted strategy aiming to block the production of LAC and APS or to hasten their elimination, including the administration of steroids, rituximab, plasma exchange, and immunosuppressant agents. In our patient, the absence of microvascular plugging makes the diagnosis unlikely.

Lastly, it is difficult to establish a cause-effect relationship between the adrenal hemorrhage (AH) and the MODS. Its occurrence is uncommon and is facilitated by physiological and anatomical factors including the elevated adrenal blood flow passing directly from the arteriolar network into the capillary plexus [32]. As a reassessment of the whole clinical course confirmed the absence of adrenal abnormalities at the admission CT scan, it likely occurred as a consequence of a reduced CO and SS and accounted for the failed response to vasopressors and fluid resuscitation [32, 33].

In conclusion, it is difficult if not impossible to individuate a single shooting gun responsible for the rapidly fatal MODS observed in our patient almost each potential diagnosis has its own pro- and against- factors (Table 5) as well as different and sometimes mutually exclusive approaches (Table 6); rather, it is likely that the peritonitis-induced and the SS and HLH cooperated in determining a CRS and that their combined effect led to the AH. Although the clinical presentation was suggestive also for CAPS, the biochemical and pathological findings do not confirm this diagnosis.

4. Conclusions

In patients with hematologic tumors, different factors can determine a MOF, including SS and/or other conditions associated either to the underlying disease and/or to its treatment; actually, it is hypothesizable that the prevalence of these latter will increase with a more widespread use of agents influencing the immune system such as of CAR-T. In our patient, the fulminant course can be likely ascribed to the purulent peritonitis likely determined by the massive bacterial translocation from the ischemic intestinal mucosa, although also other concomitant causes such as HLH could have triggered a massive release of inflammatory mediators. It could be advisable to measure the blood values of some related markers such as ferritin, LAC, aCL, and aβ2GBPI when the hemodynamic conditions fail to respond to a sepsis-oriented treatment in order to restrict the immunosuppressive treatment to patients with a defined diagnosis.

References

[1] F. Kroschinsky, F. Stölzel, S. von Bonin et al., "New drugs, new toxicities: severe side effects of modern targeted and immunotherapy of cancer and their management," *Critical Care*, vol. 21, no. 1, 2017.

[2] J. C. Fitzgerald, S. L. Weiss, S. L. Maude et al., "Cytokine release syndrome after chimeric antigen receptor T cell therapy for acute lymphoblastic leukemia," *Critical Care Medicine*, vol. 45, no. 2, pp. e124–e131, 2017.

[3] E. Azoulay, F. Pène, M. Darmon et al., "Managing critically ill hematology patients: time to think differently," *Blood Reviews*, vol. 29, no. 6, pp. 359–367, 2015.

[4] V. A. de Vries, M. A. C. Müller, M. S. Arbous et al., "Long-term outcome of patients with a hematologic malignancy and multiple organ failure admitted at the intensive care," *Critical Care Medicine*, vol. 47, no. 2, pp. e120–e128, 2019.

[5] M. Shankar-Hari, G. S. Phillips, M. L. Levy et al., "Developing a new definition and assessing new clinical criteria: for septic shock for the third international consensus definition for sepsis and septic shock (sepsis – 3)," *JAMA*, vol. 315, no. 8, pp. 775–787, 2016.

[6] S. J. Boomer, K. To, K. C. Chang et al., "Immunosuppression in patients who die of sepsis and multiple organ failure," *JAMA*, vol. 306, no. 23, pp. 2594–2605, 2011.

[7] R. S. Hotckiss, G. Monneret, and D. Payen, "Immunosuppression in sepsis: a novel understanding of the disorder and a new therapeutic approach," *The Lancet Infectious Diseases*, vol. 13, no. 3, pp. 260–268, 2013.

[8] A. Rhodes, L. E. Evans, W. Alhazzani et al., "Surviving Sepsis Campaign: international guidelines for management of sepsis and septic shock: 2016," *Intensive Care Medicine*, vol. 43, no. 3, pp. 304–377, 2017.

[9] J. Phua, W. J. Ngerng, K. C. See et al., "Characteristics and outcomes of culture-negative versus culture-positive severe sepsis," *Critical Care*, vol. 17, no. 5, p. R202, 2013.

[10] A. C. Heffner, J. M. Horton, M. R. Marchick, and A. E. Jones, "Etiology of illness in patients with severe sepsis admitted to hospital from the emergency department," *Clinical Infectious Diseases*, vol. 50, no. 6, pp. 814–820, 2010.

[11] D. Contou, D. Roux, S. Jochmans et al., "Septic shock with no diagnosis at 24 hours: a pragmatic multicenter prospective cohort study," *Critical Care*, vol. 20, no. 1, p. 360, 2016.

[12] S. Armenian and S. Bathia, "Predicting and preventing anthracycline-related cardiotoxicity," *American Sociey of Clinical Oncology Educational Book*, vol. 38, pp. 3–12, 2018.

[13] S. Limat, E. Daguindau, J. Y. Cahn et al., "Incidence and risk-factors of CHOP/R-CHOP-related cardiotoxicity in patients with aggressive non-Hodgkin's lymphoma," *Journal of Clinical Pharmacology and Therapeutics*, vol. 39, no. 2, pp. 168–174, 2014.

[14] M.-Y. Wu, K.-S. Liu, P.-J. Lin, Y.-K. Haung, and F.-C. Tsai, "Resuscitation of acute anthracycline-induced cardiogenic shock and refractory hypoxemia with mechanical circulatory supports: pitfalls and strategies," *Resuscitation*, vol. 80, no. 3, pp. 385–386, 2009.

[15] J.-L. Vincent, D. R. Nelson, and M. D. Williams, "Is worsening multiple organ failure the cause of death in patients with severe sepsis?," *Critical Care Medicine*, vol. 39, no. 5, pp. 1050–1055, 2011.

[16] P. M. Kasi, H. A. Tawbi, C. V. Oddis, and H. S. Kulkarni, "Clinical review: serious adverse events associated with the use of rituximab – a critical care perspective," *Critical Care*, vol. 16, no. 4, p. 231, 2012.

[17] G. Berlot, A. Tomasini, L. Zandonà, E. Leonardo, R. Bussani, and N. Zarrillo, "Fatal septic shock in a patient with hemophagocytic lymphohistiocytosis associated with an infectious mononucleosis," *Case Report in Critical Care*, vol. 2018, Article ID 9756050, 4 pages, 2018.

[18] E. Karakikke and E. J. Giamarellos-Barboulis, "Macrophage activation-like syndrome: a distinct entity leading to early death in sepsis," *Frontiers in Immunology*, vol. 10, pp. 55–59, 2019.

[19] G. Lachmann, C. Spies, T. Schenk, F. M. Brunkhorst, F. Balzer, and L. P. Rosée, "Hemophagocitic lymphohistiocytosis: potentially underdiagnosed in intensive care units," *Shock*, vol. 50, no. 2, pp. 149–155, 2018.

[20] F. Gauvin, B. Toledano, J. Champagne, and J. Lacroix, "Reactive hemophagocytic syndrome presenting as a component of multiple organ dysfunction syndrome," *Critical Care Medicine*, vol. 28, no. 9, pp. 3341–3345, 2000.

[21] S. Rivière, L. Galicier, P. Coppo et al., "Reactive hemophagocytic syndrome in adults: a retrospective analysis of 162 patients," *The American Journal of Medicine*, vol. 127, no. 11, pp. 1118–1125, 2014.

[22] A. Hayden, S. Park, D. Giustini, A. Y. Y. Lee, and L. Y. C. Chen, "Hemophagocytic syndrome (HPSs) including hemophagocytic lymphohistiocytosis (HLH) in adult: a systemic scoping review," *Blood reviews*, vol. 30, no. 6, pp. 411–420, 2016.

[23] B. Halacli, N. Uver, S. O. Halacli et al., "Investigation of hemophagocytic lymphohistiocytosis in severe sepsis patients," *Journal of Critical Care*, vol. 35, no. 1, pp. 185–190, 2016.

[24] L. Fardet, L. Galicer, O. Lambotte et al., "Development and validation of HScore, a score for the diagnosis of reactive hemophagocytic Syndrome," *Arthritis & Rheumatology*, vol. 66, no. 9, pp. 2613–2620, 2014.

[25] G. Ankawi, M. Neri, J. Zhang, A. Breglia, Z. Ricci, and C. Ronco, "Extracorporeal techniques for the treatment of critically ill patients with sepsis beyond conventional blood purification therapy: the promises and the pitfalls," *Critical Care*, vol. 22, no. 1, p. 262, 2018.

[26] N. Daver, K. McClain, C. E. Allen et al., "A consensus review on malignancy-associated hemophagocytic lymphohistiocytosis in adults," *Cancer*, vol. 123, no. 17, pp. 3229–3240, 2017.

[27] R. Ramos-Casal, P. Brito-Zerón, A. López-Guillermo, M. A. Khamashta, and X. Bosch, "Adult haemophagocytic syndrome," *The Lancet*, vol. 383, no. 9927, pp. 1503–1516, 2014.

[28] G. E. Janka and K. Lehmberg, "Hemophagocytic syndromes–an update," *Blood Reviews*, vol. 28, no. 4, pp. 135–142, 2014.

[29] R. Cervera, I. Rodríguez-pintó, and G. Espinosa, "The diagnosis and clinical management of the catastrophic antiphospholipid syndrome: a comprehensive review," *Journal of Autoimmunity*, vol. 92, pp. 1–11, 2018.

[30] W. Miesbach, R. A. Asherson, R. Cervera et al., "The role of malignancies in patients with catastrophic anti-phospholipid (Asherson's) syndrome," *Clinical Rheumatology*, vol. 26, no. 12, pp. 2109–2114, 2007.

[31] L. M. Tormos and C. A. Schandl, "The significance of adrenal hemorrhage: undiagnosed waterhouse-friedrichsen syndrome, a case series," *Journal of Forensic Science*, vol. 58, no. 4, pp. 1071–1074, 2013.

[32] S. R. Bornstein, "Predisposing factors for adrenal insufficiency," *New England Journal of Medicine*, vol. 360, no. 22, pp. 2328–2339, 2009.

[33] T. H. K. Puar, N. M. M. L. Stikkelbroeck, L. C. C. J. Smans, P. M. J. Zelissen, and Ad. R. M. M. Hermus, "Adrenal crisis: still a deadly event in the 21st century," *The American Journal of Medicine*, vol. 129, no. 3, pp. 339.e1–339.e9, 2016.

18

Right Sided Intracardiac Thrombosis during Veno-Arterial Extracorporeal Membrane Oxygenation: A Case Report and Literature Review

Anusha Ganapati Bhat,[1] **Armand Golchin**,[2]
Deepak Kumar Pasupula,[3] **and Jaime A. Hernandez-Montfort**[4]

[1]*Department of Internal Medicine, Baystate Medical Center, University of Massachusetts Medical School, Springfield, MA, USA*
[2]*Division of Critical Care Medicine, Baystate Medical Center, University of Massachusetts Medical School, Springfield, MA, USA*
[3]*Department of Internal Medicine, University of Pittsburgh Medical Center, Pittsburgh, PA, USA*
[4]*Division of Cardiology, The University of Texas Medical Branch, Galveston, TX, USA*

Correspondence should be addressed to Anusha Ganapati Bhat; anusha.bhatmd@baystatehealth.org

Academic Editor: Chiara Lazzeri

Veno-Arterial Extracorporeal Membrane Oxygenation is a common technology of the modern era used as a bridge in severe refractory cardiac and respiratory failure until definitive management is planned. However, early recognition and management of one of the most challenging complications, intracardiac thrombus, continue to remain a conundrum. The incidence of the clinical scenario is very rare. Therefore, due to the lack of literature, there are no guidelines for risk stratification, prevention, or management of intracardiac thrombus. We describe a case of massive pulmonary embolism, who developed a sudden right sided intra-cardiac thrombosis while being optimally anticoagulated on VA ECMO. We also review the literature to describe the pathophysiology, risk stratification, prevention, and management of this rare entity.

1. Introduction

Veno-Arterial Extracorporeal Membrane Oxygenation is a technology of the modern era that has progressed quickly and continues to evolve in the world of critical care. Since its initial use in 1970s for postcardiotomy cardiogenic shock, its indications have broadened to involve temporary management of severe refractory cardiac and respiratory failure until a definitive management is planned. But there have been complications associated with them. Based on Extracorporeal Life Support (ECLS) registry report 2017, intracardiac thrombus (ICT) accounts for 5-6% of all the complications of VA ECMO. To our knowledge, most of the ICT is developing while on VA ECMO involved left side or all the chambers of the heart simultaneously. We describe a case of massive pulmonary embolism, who developed a sudden right sided intra-cardiac thrombosis (ICT) while being optimally anticoagulated on VA ECMO. The incidence of the clinical scenario is very rare and reduced even more with the advancement in the ECMO technology. Therefore, due to the lack of sufficient reporting of this clinical entity, there are no guidelines for risk stratification, prevention, or management of ICT. This paper describes the risk factors and pathophysiology for development of intra-cardiac thrombus in a patient treated with VA-ECMO. We will also review the literature describing this rare entity.

2. Case Report

A 63-year-old gentleman with a past medical history of alcoholic cirrhosis presented with acute dyspnea, tachycardia, and hypotension to an outside hospital. He was found to have a massive pulmonary embolism bilaterally on Computed Tomography Angiography (CTA) chest. Additionally, there was a sizable thrombus in the right atrium partially extending through patent foramen ovale. Ultrasound Doppler of

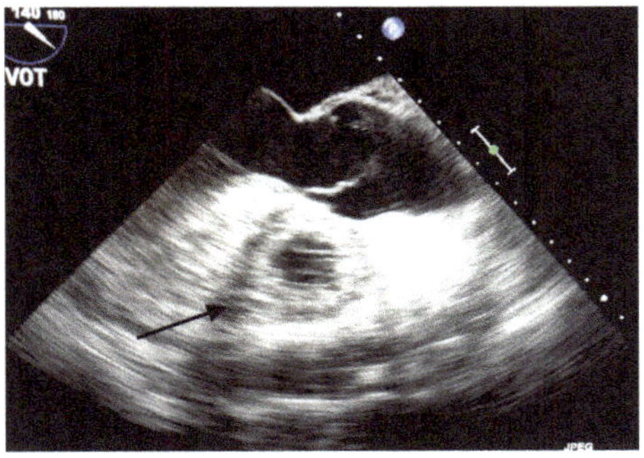

FIGURE 1: Transesophageal echocardiogram with ME AV LAX view showing extensive thrombus formation in the right ventricle.

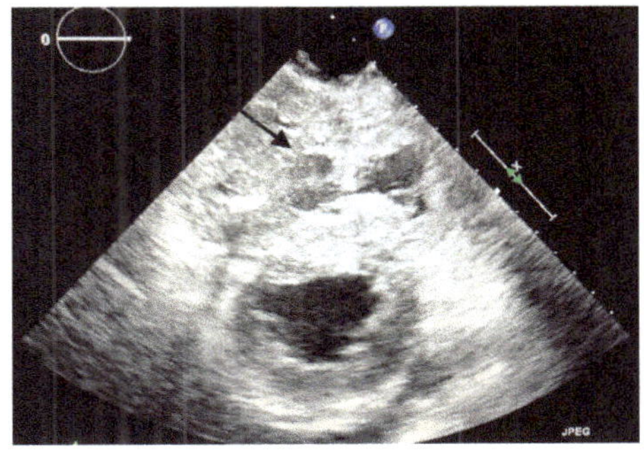

FIGURE 3: Transesophageal echocardiogram with TG SAX view showing extensive thrombus formation in the right ventricle.

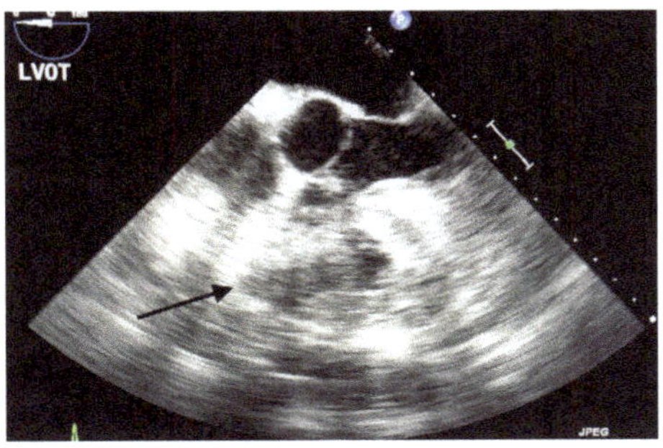

FIGURE 2: Transesophageal echocardiogram with ME 4CH view showing poor endocardial definition of the right ventricle and the thrombus.

lower extremities was negative for deep venous thrombosis. The massive PE was managed surgically for immediate stabilization with complete embolectomy followed by patent foramen ovale closure. There was no residual thrombus noted; however, CTA scan was not repeated to evaluate peripheral pulmonary artery thrombosis. Unfortunately, the procedure was complicated by postcardiotomy shock. He failed to be wean from the cardiopulmonary bypass machine and vasopressors (vasopressin, norepinephrine, and epinephrine), thus requiring central Venous-Arterial Extracorporeal Membrane Oxygenation (VA ECMO) support until recovery. Anticoagulation provided perioperatively kept his activated clotting time (ACT) greater than 300s for a few hours. Once ACT was within therapeutic range, he was reinitiated on anticoagulation with a heparin bolus of 50units/kg, followed by continuous infusion at 7.5 units/kg thereafter per ECMO management protocol of the hospital. VA ECMO settings were maintained with a flow of 4.6-4.8 L/min and sweep gas flow rate of 3-4 L/min. His mean arterial pressure was above 65 mmHg and pulmonary arterial pressure was elevated at 29-65 mmHg systolic and 7-25 mmHg diastolic.

On postoperative day 1 (POD 1) he continued to have high flow on VA ECMO, but was noted to have increasing bleed from his nasogastric tube. His hemoglobin dropped from 13.9 gm/dL to 7.5 gm/dL with a hematocrit of 21.6%. His workup was also significant for chronic unchanged thrombocytopenia of 40-50 k/mm3. At this time, systemic anticoagulation was transiently discontinued due to continued bleeding. He was managed with a transfusion of packed red blood cell, platelets, cryoprecipitate, and fresh frozen plasma over a span of 12 hours. In the meantime, he also underwent upper endoscopy, which revealed erosive esophagitis and gastric mucosal erythema, for which he received high dose intravenous proton pump inhibitors. After the completion of the blood products transfusion, his bleeding stopped. Thereafter, he was started on heparin drip at the rate of 10 units/kg/hour and managed with an activated clotting time over 200s, activated partial thromboplastin time 35-75s, and anti-Xa level 0.30-0.70 IU/ml.

His settings and flow on VA ECMO remained unchanged and he seemed to improve hemodynamically with less requirement of vasopressors in the next 24 hours. He was weaned off epinephrine. His point of care echocardiogram also revealed good cardiac activity without any visible clots. However, towards the end of POD 3, he was noted to develop worsening tachycardia, reduction in ECMO flow to 3.6L/min, and thrombosis of the mediastinal tube. Serotonin release assay for assessment of heparin induced thrombocytopenia (HIT) was negative. A bedside transesophageal echocardiogram revealed global hypokinesis and severe LV dysfunction. Additionally, there was a notably large in situ right ventricular thrombus with a posterior circumferential pericardial clot extending from 3 to 9 o'clock position surrounding the left and right ventricles. He was re-operated immediately with the removal of 1.5L blood and thrombus from the pericardium and mediastinum. There was no obvious site of bleeding noted; however repeat transesophageal echocardiogram suggested reformation of a total right ventricular thrombus, which was confirmed by a transthoracic echocardiogram. The thrombus extended to the main pulmonary artery and its branches. At this point, the family decided to pursue palliative care due to his poor prognosis and the patient expired within the next few minutes (Figures 1, 2, and 3).

3. Discussion

ECMO has been used for approximately four decades in intensive care units around the world. Over the years, there have been significant advancements in the technology resulting in improved outcomes and survival rates. Currently, VA ECMO is used for the management of cardiac arrest, cardiomyopathy, myocarditis, and congenital defect and in cardiogenic shock that are difficult to wean from cardiopulmonary bypass (CPB). However, early recognition and management of one of the most challenging complications, intracardiac thrombus, remain a conundrum.

The first case series that introduced ICT as a complication of ECMO was in 1995, where, out of 30 patients on ECMO, 6 developed ICT accounting for 20% incidence rate [1]. Mechanical clots accounted for 15.6% of all the complications and the mortality rate of thromboembolic events while on ECMO has been predicted to be 8.7% [2].

ECMO circuit is a prothrombotic stimulus since it is sensed as a foreign body physiologically. VA ECMO in particular has additional sites of thrombus formation in the heart unlike Veno-Venous ECMO (VV ECMO). Cardiac surgery causes high tissue injury, which may be worsened by further tissue injury during cannulation for vascular access. In addition, blood upon contact with the negatively charged plastic linings connecting ECMO circuit further augments Virchow's triad and sets off the coagulation cascade. In our case, the patient also had a history of alcoholic cirrhosis, which may have hindered coagulation system in the patient with subsequent massive PE in the first place. During the hospital course, his pulmonary arterial pressure (PAP) was high, indicative of evolving pulmonary hypertension as a result of PE, although we cannot ascertain if he already had developed microthrombi in his pulmonary vasculature. Thromboembolism into the blood vessels of the lungs leads to inflammation and interstitial edema subsequently leading to PH, which elevates afterload for the right heart.

Impaired right cardiac output leads to systolic dysfunction, cardiac hypokinesis, and blood stasis, ultimately resulting in ICT, which may be the most likely explanation in our case. In the setting of high prothrombotic risk factors such as coagulopathy from liver disease, additional hypercoagulability induced from multiple blood products transfusion has also been associated with increased odds of thrombosis. A systemic review by Williams et al. established risk factors for the development of ICT following CPB, where patients with surgery for over 2 hours and preexisting congestive heart failure and those undergoing blood products transfusion and antifibrinolytic administration were at a major risk. Of all the blood products, 37.5% of patients developed ICT after platelet transfusion and 27% following plasma transfusion [3].

To prevent ICT, patients are systemically anticoagulated mostly with unfractionated heparin, less frequently low molecular weight heparin, direct thrombin inhibitors, or novel anticoagulation agents, unless heparin is contraindicated. Some instances where thrombus developed while on therapeutic heparin were related to resistance to heparin, which have been partially evidenced to improve with supplemental antithrombin, but definitive evidences are scarce. Although we did not check endogenous antithrombin III level, this intervention is optional in patients undergoing cardiac surgery with CPB, the elderly, and diabetics [4–8].

Also, several advances have been made to the ECMO circuit to minimize hypercoagulability. Use of hollow microfibers to prevent direct blood-gas interactions, preventing artificial surface-blood interactions to reduce hypercoagulability, reducing turbulent flow with low-resistance oxygenators, shorter connections, and minimum circulatory volume are other interventions [9]. These changes in the technology may have reduced incidence of ECMO circuit related thrombosis, but cardiac chambers would still be at risk of forming clots due to low pressure when on VA ECMO. Therefore, systemic anticoagulation is of utmost importance, even though it is challenging as in our case due to increased bleeding potential.

Current protocol for anticoagulation is by combined measurement and assessment of activated clotting time, partial thromboplastin time, and anti-factor Xa levels to adjust anticoagulation therapy to prevent bleeding and clotting imbalance, although in our case they had poor clinical correlatability, which may indicate inappropriate estimation of anticoagulation level.

With anticoagulation, the unfortunate drawback is the risk of bleeding. Disseminated intravascular coagulation, mechanical hemolysis, gastrointestinal hemorrhage, and surgical site bleeds are accountable for up to 50.1% of all the complications from ECMO [10]. But, systemic anticoagulation is one of the key factors to ensure prevention of ICT and requires close monitoring to strike a balance between clotting and bleeding potential. Furthermore, observing pressure gradient changes in the system, timely echocardiograms, and watching for hemodynamic instability will ensure early recognition even when ICT forms.

Once ICT has developed, management options are not evidence based, but based on clinical experience and small studies. Systemic thrombolytic therapy may be fatal due to ongoing bleeds, as in our case, whereas local instillation of thrombolytics may not be helpful due to poor reachability of the medication to the site of ICT due to poor blood flow. Furthermore, inactivation of plasminogen by use of antifibrinolytics during surgery as well as dilutional drop in their levels from volume supplementation for hemodynamic stability may lead to ineffectiveness of tissue plasminogen activator [11].

Current modality used for management of ICT includes surgical thrombectomy, local thrombolysis, or usage of ventricular assist device to ensure adequate forward flow of blood to prevent new thrombus formation from stasis [12, 13]. With ICT on VA ECMO, most patients assume palliative care due to poor outcomes [14]. There is scarce data in the literature to make final conclusion about guidelines for management. But, we can try to improve risk factor predictions and manage patients based on their individual risk stratification. Future research should concentrate on conducting large scale studies for patients on VA ECMO to recognize risk factors and possible successful management of ICT to improve overall mortality outcomes.

References

[1] D. D. Muehrcke, P. M. McCarthy, R. W. Stewart et al., "Complications of extracorporeal life support systems using heparin-bound surfaces: The risk of intracardiac clot formation," *The Journal of Thoracic and Cardiovascular Surgery*, vol. 110, no. 3, pp. 843–851, 1995.

[2] A. Beiras-Fernandez, M.-A. Deutsch, S. Kainzinger et al., "Extracorporeal membrane oxygenation in 108 patients with low cardiac output-A single-center experience," *The International Journal of Artificial Organs*, vol. 34, no. 4, pp. 365–373, 2011.

[3] B. Williams, B. Wehman, M. A. Mazzeffi et al., "Acute Intracardiac Thrombosis and Pulmonary Thromboembolism After Cardiopulmonary Bypass," *Anesthesia & Analgesia*, vol. 126, no. 2, pp. 425–434, 2018.

[4] J. W. Byrnes, C. J. Swearingen, P. Prodhan, R. Fiser, and U. Dyamenahalli, "Antithrombin III supplementation on extracorporeal membrane oxygenation: Impact on heparin dose and circuit life," *ASAIO Journal*, vol. 60, no. 1, pp. 57–62, 2014.

[5] M. E. Carr, "Diabetes mellitus: a hypercoagulable state," *Journal of Diabetes and its Complications*, vol. 15, no. 1, pp. 44–54, 2001.

[6] M. G. Conlan, A. R. Folsom, A. Finch et al., "Associations of factor VIII and von Willebrand factor with age, race, sex, and risk factors for atherosclerosis. The Atherosclerosis Risk in Communities (ARIC) study," *Thrombosis and Haemostasis*, vol. 70, no. 3, pp. 380–385, 1993.

[7] V. Muedra, D. Barettino, P. D'Ocón, A. Zuñiga, and L. Moreno, "Antithrombin activity and outcomes in patients undergoing cardiac surgery with cardiopulmonary bypass," *Blood Coagulation & Fibrinolysis*, vol. 24, no. 4, pp. 454–457, 2013.

[8] M. Ranucci, A. Ditta, A. Boncilli et al., "Determinants of antithrombin consumption in cardiac operations requiring cardiopulmonary bypass," *Perfusion*, vol. 19, no. 1, pp. 47–52, 2004.

[9] D. A. Murphy, L. E. Hockings, R. K. Andrews et al., "Extracorporeal membrane oxygenation-hemostatic complications," *Transfusion Medicine Reviews*, vol. 29, no. 2, pp. 90–101, 2015.

[10] R. R. Thiagarajan, R. P. Barbaro, P. T. Rycus et al., "Extracorporeal Life Support Organization Registry International Report 2016," *ASAIO Journal*, vol. 63, no. 1, pp. 60–67, 2017.

[11] S. L. Diamond and S. Anand, "Inner clot diffusion and permeation during fibrinolysis," *Biophysical Journal*, vol. 65, no. 6, pp. 2622–2643, 1993.

[12] A. Salsano, E. Sportelli, G. M. Olivieri, N. Di Lorenzo, S. Borile, and F. Santini, "RVAD support in the setting of submassive pulmonary embolism," *Journal of Extra-Corporeal Technology*, vol. 49, no. 4, pp. 304–306, 2017.

[13] F. Sangalli, G. Greco, L. Galbiati, F. Formica, S. Calcinati, and L. Avalli, "Regional Thrombolysis with Tenecteplase During Extracorporeal Membrane Oxygenation: A New Approach for Left Ventricular Thrombosis," *Journal of Cardiac Surgery*, vol. 30, no. 6, pp. 541–543, 2015.

[14] M. Alhussein, Y. Moayedi, J. D. Posada et al., "Ventricular Thrombosis Post-Venoarterial Extracorporeal Membrane Oxygenation," *Circulation: Heart Failure*, vol. 10, no. 2, 2017.

19

Critical Illness Associated Fatal Hypoglycemia in a Nondiabetic Male

Amit Toor, Anika Toor, and Mahesh Krishnamurthy

Department of Internal Medicine, Easton Hospital, Easton, Pennsylvania, USA

Correspondence should be addressed to Amit Toor; drtooramit@gmail.com

Academic Editor: Kurt Lenz

We present here the case of a 55-year-old male who presented to the emergency department with severe abdominal pain and respiratory distress secondary to mesenteric ischemia. His critical illness on preexisting chronic kidney disease, previously undiagnosed alcoholic cirrhosis, and congestive heart failure led to a rare yet fatal consequence of refractory hypoglycemia. Critical illness associated hypoglycemia generally occurs as a result of high metabolic consumption with relative insulin excess and insufficient nutritional intake that is seen frequently in critically ill patients. This, along with reduced hepatic and renal gluconeogenesis seen in preexisting liver and renal disease, can cumulate to life-threatening hypoglycemia and is seen as a poor prognostic factor in the ICU setting.

1. Introduction

Carbohydrate metabolism and formation of glucose depends on a myriad of factors. The basic principle is dependent on nutritional intake, metabolic demand with relative insulin excess, and hepatic (to some degree also, renal) gluconeogenesis/glycogenolysis. Hypoglycemia in these nondiabetic patients can be diagnostically challenging and may indicate a poor prognosis especially in the ICU setting given severe nature of illnesses and insufficient nutritional intake. Various etiologies include medications and medication overdose, insulin producing tumors, history of gastric bypass surgery, alcohol use, critical illness, liver/renal disease, and adrenal insufficiency [1]. We present a case of a 55-year-old male with persistent, refractory hypoglycemia secondary to critical illness in the absence of Diabetes Mellitus (DM).

2. Case

A 55-year-old male with past medical history of congestive heart failure with ejection fraction of 30%, chronic kidney disease, atrial fibrillation, and alcohol abuse, presented with sudden onset of severe abdominal pain. Admission vitals were stable with the significant except oxygen saturation of 70% on room air. Labs on admission were significant for lactic acid of 5.3 mmol/L (Table 1), Acute Kidney Injury (AKI), and subtherapeutic INR of 1.5 on Coumadin. Urine toxicology screen was positive for cocaine use. CT scan of the abdomen was initially unremarkable. The patient was subsequently admitted to the ICU for severe acute hypoxic respiratory failure with potential for decompensation and clinical suspicion of mesenteric ischemia given his subtherapeutic INR in the setting of atrial fibrillation along with sudden onset of abdominal pain and elevated lactic acid without a clear cause. Cocaine abuse may have also been a contributing factor to sudden ischemia. A later repeat CT scan revealed nonspecific bowel wall thickening, and a transesophageal echocardiogram performed revealed an active left atrial thrombus, making mesenteric ischemia a higher differential. Due to the added possibility of sepsis and worsening renal function, there was no clear opportunity for surgical intervention, and conservative management was initiated through heparin drip and BiPAP showing initial clinical improvement. By hospital day 3, however, he suddenly became unresponsive. At that time, his labs revealed blood sugar of less than 10 mg/dl and worsening renal failure. The patient was aggressively managed and given multiple ampules of Dextrose 50% and infusion of Dextrose 5% was started (Table 2). Because of further decompensation of renal function, he was started

TABLE 1: Outline of pertinent lactic acid, liver enzymes, and INR throughout hospitalization.

	Day 1	Day 2	Day 3	Day 4	Day 8	Day 9	Day 10
Lactic Acid (mmol/L)	5.3	3.6	6.7	1.8	1.8	3.0	3.3
AST/ALT (U/L)	30/71	31/70	91/243	122/232	82/99	85/120	81/97
INR	1.5	1.5	2.5	2.1	3.4	6.9	4.4

TABLE 2: Outline of pertinent lowest glucose levels throughout hospitalization along with correction measures taken.

	Day 1	Day 2	Day 3	Day 4	Day 10	Day 11	Day 12	Day 13
Glucose (mg/dl)	88	78	<10	98	<30	30	46	36
Glucose/Glucagon therapy	-	-	Multiple ampules of D50 D5NS IV	D5NS IV	Multiple ampules of D50 D5NS to D10NS IV Glucagon IV	D10NS IV	D10NS IV Glucagon IV	D20NS IV Glucagon IV

D50: Dextrose 50% ampule, D5NS: Dextrose 5% in normal saline, D10NS: Dextrose 10% in normal saline, D20NS Dextrose 20% in normal saline.

on Continuous Renal Replacement Therapy (CRRT) as well. Despite these measures, his blood sugar continued to have multiple episodes reaching 40 mg/dl. His IV fluids were switched to Dextrose 10% drip and eventually to Dextrose 20% drip because of persistent episodes of hypoglycemia, also requiring intermittent IV Glucagon. The patient had no family or personal history of DM and HbA1c tested during hospitalization was 5.6%. Further testing including cortisol, pro-insulin, insulin, and C-peptide levels was within normal limits. A sulfonylurea screen was also negative. Liver function tests were within normal limits with exception of development of supratherapeutic INR of 4.4 despite not being on Coumadin, suggestive of underlying liver disease. Endoscopic Ultrasound did not reveal any pancreatic mass. The patient was subsequently transferred to a tertiary care center for further investigative work-up and management of persistent hypoglycemia. During this time, the patient had developed abdominal ascites. Paracentesis and analysis of the ascitic fluid was suggestive of underlying hepatic cirrhosis. Given the patient's history of severe alcohol abuse, it was more likely that the underlying hepatic illness was alcoholic liver cirrhosis. To confirm this, a biopsy was offered but the patient refused. It was determined that the patient's persistent hypoglycemia was likely secondary to critical illness along with and underlying background of severe hepatic and renal failure. The patient's overall prognosis was poor and his condition declined rapidly despite adequate advanced care and paracentesis. He refused any further intervention and opted for hospice care. An autopsy was not performed.

3. Discussion

The developing hypoglycemia secondary to underlying critical illness is seen in less than 1.5% of patients [2]. Despite this, there is a combination of factors that are commonly seen in the ICU setting that can contribute to its occurrence. The rise of the metabolic response in critically ill patients is seen as part of a defense mechanism in an attempt to maintain the nutritional demand of inflamed and vital organ systems [3, 4]. These mechanisms include increased sympathetic output, release of counter-regulatory pituitary and adrenal hormones, and increased rate of gluconeogenesis and glycogenolysis [5, 6]. With the development of fulminant hepatic disease and liver cirrhosis, the production of endogenous glucose is rapidly reduced. Without resolution or prevention of decompensation of hepatic disease, patients may develop hypoglycemia that is an indication of increased mortality risk. One study involving 4946 ICU patients who had developed hypoglycemia during their hospitalization revealed an in-hospital mortality of 36.6%, compared to 19.7% in nonhypoglycemic patients [7]. Acute renal failure can contribute to hypoglycemia as well. In the setting of uremia, there is reduced gluconeogenesis directly from the kidney as well as reduced production from the liver [8–10]. Also, with renal failure there is an increase in circulating insulin secondary to decreased clearance. This is generally seen when the glomerular filtration rate (GFR) is below 15–20 mL/min/1.73 m^2 [11]. In patient's receiving renal replacement therapy the sensitivity to insulin may improve, which can contribute to hypoglycemia as well [12]. In cases of severe cardiac failure in critically ill patients, it is theorized that consequent hepatic congestion may contribute to lower glucose output from the liver as well as reduced intestinal absorption [13, 14]. Alcohol abuse such as that seen in our patient also plays a major role in the development of hypoglycemia. The underlying mechanisms include alcoholic cirrhosis, malnutrition, and direct inhibition of gluconeogenesis [1]. In critically ill patients particularly in those with sepsis, adrenal insufficiency may be an important contributing factor as well. This can be screened with AM serum cortisol levels and further tested with Cosyntropin and ACTH testing [15]. Prior to attributing hypoglycemia to hepatic and renal failure in combination with severe illness, full investigative work-up should be done to exclude primary causes of hypoglycemia. This includes a complete review of patient medications and potential access to medications such as oral hypoglycemics. This can be confirmed with an oral sulfonylurea screen [1]. If insulinoma or any other form of endogenous hyperinsulinism is suspected, testing for this should be done in a fasting state if patient's status permits [1]. These tests include serum insulin, Proinsulin, and C-peptide [16]. Management of secondary hypoglycemia should be emphasized on appropriate nutritional repletion and attempted at resolution of acute illness as well as compensation for decompensated chronic diseases. There are no reliable simple equations for determination of energy requirements in such patients, given that their energy expenditures are highly variable. One of the only reliable determinants of energy expenditure and requirement is through indirect calorimetry [17]. Determination of this can guide nutritional repletion in enteral or parenteral forms. If a primary cause is identified, medical or surgical options should be explored for that specific etiology.

4. Conclusion

Patients with critical illness especially those with underlying advanced liver/renal disease, malnutrition, and advanced age may develop profound hypoglycemia even in the absence of diabetes. Recognition of malnutritional states and insufficient nutritional intake in the background of decompensated liver and kidney disease is important to prevent such life-threatening hypoglycemia. Such patients require frequent monitoring of blood sugar levels and adequate enteral or parenteral nutritional support to accommodate the increased metabolic demand and reduced gluconeogenesis. Close monitoring and prompt support for decompensated chronic illness may benefit in terms of overall survival.

Acknowledgments

This abstract was presented in 101st Annual Meeting of the Endocrine Society.

References

[1] M. E. Desimone and R. S. Weinstock, "Non-Diabetic hypoglycemia," in *Endotext*, L. J. D. Groot, G. Chrousos, K. Dungan et al., Eds., MDText.com, Inc, South Dartmouth, MA, USA, 2000.

[2] S. M. Bagshaw, R. Bellomo, M. J. Jacka et al., "The impact of early hypoglycemia and blood glucose variability on outcome in critical illness," *Critical Care*, vol. 13, no. 3, p. R91, 2009.

[3] L. Rui, "Energy metabolism in the liver," *Comprehensive Physiology*, vol. 4, no. 1, pp. 177–197, 2014.

[4] J. C. Preiser, A. R. V. Zanten, M. M. Berger et al., "Metabolic and nutritional support of critically ill patients: consensus and controversies," *Critical Care*, vol. 19, no. 1, p. 35, 2015.

[5] G. V. D. Berghe, F. D. Zegher, R. C. Baxter et al., "Neuroendocrinology of prolonged critical illness: effects of exogenous thyrotropin-releasing hormone and its combination with growth hormone secretagogues," *The Journal of Clinical Endocrinology & Metabolism*, vol. 83, no. 2, pp. 309–319, 1998.

[6] J. C. Preiser, C. Ichai, J. C. Orban, and J. Groeneveld, "Metabolic response to the stress of critical illness," *British Journal of Anaesthesia*, vol. 113, no. 6, pp. 945–954, 2014.

[7] M. Egi, R. Bellomo, E. Stachowski et al., "Hypoglycemia and outcome in critically ill patients," *Mayo Clinic Proceedings*, vol. 85, no. 3, pp. 217–224, 2010.

[8] R. Arem, "Hypoglycemia associated with renal failure," *Endocrinology and Metabolism Clinics of North America*, vol. 18, no. 1, pp. 103–121, 1989.

[9] K. Kaneko, M. Soty, C. Zitoun et al., "The role of kidney in the inter-organ coordination of endogenous glucose production during fasting," *Molecular Metabolism*, vol. 16, pp. 203–212, 2018.

[10] E. Mutel, A. Gautier-Stein, A. Abdul-Wahed et al., "Control of blood glucose in the absence of hepatic glucose production during prolonged fasting in mice: induction of renal and intestinal gluconeogenesis by glucagon," *Diabetes*, vol. 60, no. 12, pp. 3121–3131, 2011.

[11] R. H. Mak and R. A. DeFronzo, "Glucose and insulin metabolism in uremia," *Nephron*, vol. 61, no. 4, Article ID 000186953, pp. 377–382, 1992.

[12] R. A. DeFronzo, J. D. Tobin, J. W. Rowe, and R. Andres, "Glucose intolerance in uremia. Quantification of pancreatic beta cell sensitivity to glucose and tissue sensitivity to insulin," *The Journal of Clinical Investigation*, vol. 63, no. 2, pp. 425–435, 1978.

[13] G. Benzing III, W. Schubert, G. Hug, and S. Kaplan, "Simultaneous hypoglycemia and acute congestive heart failure," *Circulation*, vol. 40, pp. 209–216, 1969.

[14] S. M. Mellinkoff and P. A. Tumulty, "Hepatic hypoglycemia: its occurrence in congestive heart failure," *The New England Journal of Medicine*, vol. 247, no. 20, pp. 745–750, 1952.

[15] J. E. Fischer, T. Stallmach, and S. Fanconi, "Adrenal crisis presenting as hypoglycemic coma," *Intensive Care Medicine*, vol. 26, no. 1, pp. 105–108, 2000.

[16] P. E. Cryer, L. Axelrod, A. B. Grossman et al., "Evaluation and management of adult hypoglycemic disorders: an endocrine society clinical practice guideline," *The Journal of Clinical Endocrinology & Metabolism*, vol. 94, no. 3, pp. 709–728, 2009.

[17] S. Eghtesad, H. Poustchi, and R. Malekzadeh, "Malnutrition in liver cirrhosis: the influence of protein and sodium," *Middle East Journal of Digestive Diseases*, vol. 5, no. 2, pp. 65–75, 2013.

20

Wanting to Forget: Intrusive and Delusional Memories from Critical Illness

Lauren Doig and Kevin Solverson

Department of Critical Care Medicine, Cumming School of Medicine, University of Calgary, Calgary, Alberta, Canada

Correspondence should be addressed to Kevin Solverson; kjsolver@ucalgary.ca

Academic Editor: Joel Starkopf

Introduction. Delusional and fearful memories after critical illness are observed in up to 70% of patients post critical illness. However, they often go unrecognized after patients leave the intensive care unit (ICU). *Case Presentation.* A 40-year-old male was admitted to the ICU with community-acquired pneumonia and multiorgan failure requiring mechanical ventilation and renal replacement therapy. He developed protracted delirium and severe ICU-acquired weakness but was eventually discharged home. The patient returned to a follow-up clinic two months post-ICU discharge and revealed that he was suffering anxiety from memories in the ICU of different staff trying to harm and kill him, including being repeatedly suffocated. By providing context to the memories, the patient had significant relief in his anxiety. *Conclusions.* Intrusive memories contribute to psychological morbidity post critical illness, including posttraumatic stress disorder (PTSD) and reduced health-related quality of life. The majority of critical illness survivors do not share their intrusive or frightening memories, and therefore, most healthcare professionals are unaware of the problems they can pose. Assessment of patients' memories from the ICU is essential and may create the opportunity to help patients place memories into context and improve psychological morbidities.

1. Introduction

The mortality from critical illness is decreasing, but many patients develop multiple new and long-lasting morbidities related to critical illness. The term postintensive care syndrome (PICS) describes the physical, cognitive, and mental health comorbidities that commonly arise post critical illness [1]. Physical comorbidities that cause a reduced health-related quality of life (HRQL) as a sequela of critical illness are perhaps easy to understand because the sequelae may be readily visible and require ongoing clinical management. Perhaps as many patients also report impairments to their mental health, including depression, anxiety, and posttraumatic stress disorder (PTSD), all of which may be more difficult to recognize. An important contributor to mental health that commonly goes unrecognized is the memories patients recall from their ICU stay.

2. Case Presentation

The patient described in this report provided written consent prior to publication. A previously healthy 40-year-old Caucasian male was admitted to ICU with community-acquired pneumonia. His course was complicated by severe hypoxic respiratory failure and multiorgan dysfunction, including shock, hepatic dysfunction, delirium, and acute renal failure necessitating renal replacement therapy. He had a protracted stay due to respiratory and muscle weakness associated with critical illness myopathy confirmed by electromyography. His ICU stay was complicated by episodes of delirium necessitating the use of anxiolytics and neuroleptic medications. He was seen at an ICU follow-up visit 2 months post-discharge. Response to structured questionnaires identified significant concerns with anxiety, depression, and sleep disruption. During the clinical meeting, the patient confided of a persistent memory that one of the team members was a witch, mixing potions to poison him. His wife provided a collateral history that, although the patient was normally mild, soft-spoken, and gentle, he was singularly curt and rude to this staff member without explanation. He also had memories of a "German" man in a white "suit" that when close to him in the ICU made him feel short of breath, and the patient described subsequent disorganized frightening/disquieting dreams of the same individual. The patient was able to provide specific and explicit descriptions that permitted both individuals to be identified. He also had persistent vivid memories of forcible confinement in a cave, where he could not escape, apart from a series of white doors, none of which seemed safe or from which he could exit. The patient was provided descriptions of the staff (one a nurse with longer grey hair, the other an RT known for always wearing a buttoned white lab coat) and descriptions of their roles with possible explanations for the "memories" (the nurse mixing/administering intravenous medications; the RT suctioning the patient with associated sense of dyspnea during periods of being disconnected from the ventilator) which provided some emotional relief to the patient. The memories of specific staff slowly faded, but the vivid disquieting dreams of confinement persisted for years.

3. Discussion

The reported prevalence of delusional and hallucinatory memories from critical illness ranges from 25 to 73% [2, 3]. It is common for patients who have delusional memories also to recall factual events, but a small percentage of patients will solely recall delusional events [2]. In the critical care population, delusional memories are frequently frightening and contain persecutory themes. In this case description, the patient thought an ICU staff member was repeatedly trying to hurt him, a common presecretory theme from the ICU [4]. Wade et al. [4] describe a variety of delusional themes from patients with traumatizing memories after critical illness including purposely being poisoned, assaulted, tortured, or staff conspiring against them. The intrusive delusions and hallucinations are long-lasting and remain vivid for months after critical illness [4, 5].

ICU-acquired delirium occurs in up to 80% of the patients severely ill in the ICU [6] and is thought to be a significant risk factor for the development of delusional memories after critical illness. The presence of delirium has been associated with patients recalling fewer factual memories, and an increase in intrusive delusional memories [7]. Sedative and analgesic medications commonly used in the ICU include benzodiazepines and opioids, and they are hypothesized to have an effect on memory recall in the ICU [8]. However, a recent post hoc analysis of a randomized controlled trial of sedation protocols (light sedation versus usual care) found no difference in memory recall or the presence of delusional memories between the groups [5].

The prevalence of PTSD after critical illness ranges from 8 to 51%, and intrusive memories may be an important risk factor for its development [1]. Patients who experienced nightmares and recalled stressful memories two months after the ICU had a higher prevalence of PTSD, anxiety, and depression [3]. More than 50% of patients with PTSD six months after critical illness describe memories of panic and suffocation while in the ICU [9]. Jones et al. [10] found that patients with no factual recall of the ICU but with the presence of delusional memories scored higher on anxiety, depression, and PTSD scales in comparison to patients with factual events recalled. Wade et al. [4] found that patients with PTSD after critical illness are more likely to have intrusive memories secondary to delusions than those with intrusive memories from real or factual events.

Limited data is available on interventions to improve psychological morbidity and memories after critical illness. Jones et al. [11] studied the use of ICU diaries, documenting the patients' ICU course with written descriptions and pictures, and examined its effect on PTSD and post-ICU memories. The incidence of new PTSD was significantly reduced (5% treatment vs. 12% control) in the diary group. The authors hypothesize that the use of diaries fills in the patient's memory and may give context to delusional memories and prevent psychological distress and morbidity. As described in our case report, simply giving the patient context of their delusional memory, such as the process of endotracheal suctioning, the unpleasant symptoms it can evoke, and that no one was trying to harm him, helped the patient realize his memories were unlikely to be factual and reduced his anxiety.

The majority of patients with psychological distress related to ICU memories want to discuss these issues with a healthcare professional [4]. However, at six months after critical illness, less than 20% of patients have discussed their admission to the ICU with a primary care physician [12]. Specialized ICU follow-up clinics after critical illness are not the standard of care in most countries, leaving much of the burden of recognizing and caring for post-ICU comorbidities up to the primary health care provider. Therefore, it is crucial to increase healthcare providers' awareness of post-ICU morbidity, including memories from the ICU and the associated mental health consequences they may have so that appropriate interventions may be provided.

Consent

Consent for publication was obtained from the patient.

Authors' Contributions

LD and KS equally obtained the data for the case and wrote the manuscript.

References

[1] D. M. Needham, J. Davidson, H. Cohen et al., "Improving long-term outcomes after discharge from intensive care unit: report from a stakeholders' conference," *Critical Care Medicine*, vol. 40, no. 2, pp. 502–509, 2012.

[2] L. Orwelius, A. Teixeira-Pinto, C. Lobo, A. Costa-Pereira, and C. Granja, "The role of memories on health-related quality of life after intensive care unit care: an unforgettable controversy?," *Patient Related Outcome Measures*, vol. 7, pp. 63–71, 2016.

[3] K. A. Samuelson, D. Lundberg, and B. Fridlund, "Stressful memories and psychological distress in adult mechanically ventilated intensive care patients—a 2-month follow-up

study," *Acta Anaesthesiologica Scandinavica*, vol. 51, no. 6, pp. 671–678, 2007.

[4] D. M. Wade, C. R. Brewin, D. C. Howell, E. White, M. G. Mythen, and J. A. Weinman, "Intrusive memories of hallucinations and delusions in traumatized intensive care patients: an interview study," *British Journal of Health Psychology*, vol. 20, no. 3, pp. 613–631, 2015.

[5] L. Burry, D. Cook, M. Herridge et al., "Recall of ICU stay in patients managed with a sedation protocol or a sedation protocol with daily interruption," *Critical Care Medicine*, vol. 43, no. 10, pp. 2180–2190, 2015.

[6] T. D. Girard, P. P. Pandharipande, and E. W. Ely, "Delirium in the intensive care unit," *Critical Care*, vol. 12, Supplement 3, p. S3, 2008.

[7] H. Svenningsen, E. K. Tonnesen, P. Videbech, M. Frydenberg, D. Christensen, and I. Egerod, "Intensive care delirium—effect on memories and health-related quality of life—a follow-up study," *Journal of Clinical Nursing*, vol. 23, no. 5-6, pp. 634–644, 2014.

[8] C. R. Weinert and M. Sprenkle, "Post-ICU consequences of patient wakefulness and sedative exposure during mechanical ventilation," *Intensive Care Medicine*, vol. 34, no. 1, pp. 82–90, 2008.

[9] T. D. Girard, A. K. Shintani, J. C. Jackson et al., "Risk factors for post-traumatic stress disorder symptoms following critical illness requiring mechanical ventilation: a prospective cohort study," *Critical Care*, vol. 11, no. 1, p. R28, 2007.

[10] C. Jones, R. D. Griffiths, G. Humphris, and P. M. Skirrow, "Memory, delusions, and the development of acute posttraumatic stress disorder-related symptoms after intensive care," *Critical Care Medicine*, vol. 29, no. 3, pp. 573–580, 2001.

[11] C. Jones, C. Backman, M. Capuzzo et al., "Intensive care diaries reduce new onset post traumatic stress disorder following critical illness: a randomised, controlled trial," *Critical Care*, vol. 14, no. 5, article cc9260, p. R168, 2010.

[12] C. Granja, E. Gomes, A. Amaro et al., "Understanding posttraumatic stress disorder-related symptoms after critical care: the early illness amnesia hypothesis," *Critical Care Medicine*, vol. 36, no. 10, pp. 2801–2809, 2008.

21

Critical Care Admission of an HIV Patient with Diabetic Ketoacidosis Secondary to Pembrolizumab

John A. Cuenca,[1] Andres Laserna,[2] María P. Reyes,[1] Joseph L. Nates,[1] and Gregory H. Botz [1]

[1]Department of Critical Care & Respiratory Care, Division of Anesthesiology, Critical Care and Pain Medicine, The University of Texas MD Anderson Cancer Center, Houston, TX, USA
[2]Department of Anesthesiology and Perioperative Medicine, The University of Rochester, Rochester, New York, NY, USA

Correspondence should be addressed to Gregory H. Botz; gbotz@mdanderson.org

Academic Editor: Chiara Lazzeri

Background. Pembrolizumab is a checkpoint inhibitor that targets the programmed cell death-1 receptor (PD-1) and has shown to be effective against several malignancies, including lung cancer. However, life-threatening immune-related adverse events can result from these immunotherapy treatments. *Case presentation.* A 62-year-old man with HIV, metastatic adenocarcinoma of the lung, and no previous history of diabetes presented to the emergency department with new-onset nausea, vomiting, and generalized weakness. Glucose was 1191 mg/dl, hemoglobin A1c 11%, and potassium 6.9 mEq/L. He had metabolic acidosis with a lactate of 6.6 mmol/L and anion gap of 38 mEq/L, and ketones were detected on the urinalysis. Severe diabetic ketoacidosis was diagnosed, and the patient was admitted to the intensive care unit. Additional investigations showed low C-peptide and negative anti-glutamic acid decarboxylase antibody, anti-insulin antibody, and anti-islet-antigen 2Ab antibody. After ruling out other possible etiologies, pembrolizumab was considered to be the cause of the diabetes and ketoacidosis. *Conclusions.* Life-threatening adverse drug events associated with checkpoint inhibitors such as pembrolizumab are on the rise. We recommend to closely follow and monitor patients receiving these immunotherapies. This strategy could lead to early detection and prevention, as well as reduction of more serious life-threatening complications requiring intensive care.

1. Introduction

Many types of neoplastic cells avoid the scrutiny of the immune system through several mechanisms. One of the most studied is the overexpression of immune checkpoint proteins that are involved in the maintenance of the peripheral tolerance to self-molecules [1]. The immune checkpoint inhibitors are monoclonal antibodies that improve the ability of the immunologic system to recognize and attack tumor cells. The cytotoxic T cell and dendritic cell response against tumor cells are enhanced through the inhibition of the programmed cell death protein 1 (PD-1), programmed cell death 1 ligand (PDL-1), and cytotoxic T lymphocyte-associated antigen 4 (CTLA-4) [1]. In recent years, checkpoint inhibitors have become standard care for the treatment of several malignancies. For example, pembrolizumab targets the PD-1 protein and has been associated with better overall survival in the treatment of metastatic melanoma and advanced non-small-cell lung cancer [2, 3]. However, by decreasing immune self-tolerance, checkpoint inhibitors can enhance immune cell infiltration into normal tissues and lead to life-threatening immune-related adverse events (IR-AEs) [4]. One of the most common IR-AEs is autoimmune endocrine diseases. Insulin-dependent diabetes mellitus (IDD) has been reported as an endocrine autoimmune toxicity in patients on pembrolizumab [5]. We present a case of diabetic ketoacidosis (DKA) secondary to pembrolizumab in a patient with HIV that required intensive care management.

2. Case Presentation

A 62-year-old African-American man with a history of HIV controlled with dolutegravir, emtricitabine, and tenofovir (CD4 600 cells/mm^3 and an undetectable viral load) and a metastatic adenocarcinoma of the lung (PD-L1 80% and KRAS G12V positive) presented to the emergency department with new-onset nausea, vomiting, progressive fatigue, and generalized weakness. Two weeks before, he had received the third cycle of carboplatin, pemetrexed, and pembrolizumab. At that time, he was hemodynamically stable, tachycardic, nonfebrile, and alert. His blood glucose was 1191 mg/dl, hemoglobin A1c 11% (previously 5.3% before the first dose of pembrolizumab), serum potassium 6.9 mEq/L, 23.2 K/ul leukocytes, BUN 48 mg/dl, creatinine 2.45 mg/dl (baseline 1.12 mg/dl), and lipase levels were 17U/L. He had a metabolic acidosis with pH 7.19, $PaCO_2$ 24 mmHg, HCO_3 9 mmol/L, lactic acid 6.6 mmol/L, and anion gap 38 mEq/L, and ketones were detected on the urinalysis. The patient was admitted to the intensive care unit with presumed severe DKA of unclear etiology, possibly exacerbated by sepsis. Normal saline (NaCl 0.9%) IV hydration at a rate of 20 mL/kg/hour, 0.15 unit/kg IV bolus of insulin, followed by continuous intravenous insulin infusion at 0.1 unit/kg/hour, bicarbonate infusion, and broad-spectrum antibiotic coverage were initiated following the institutional protocol for DKA. The patient was pan-cultured for bacteria, fungi, and viruses; however, all were negative, and infection was ruled out.

A complete type 1 diabetes antibodies assay was performed. The anti-glutamic acid decarboxylase antibody (anti-GAD), anti-insulin antibody, and anti-islet-antigen 2Ab antibody were negative. C-peptide was 0.2 ng/mL (normal range: 0.5 to 2.0 ng/mL) and immunotherapy-related type 1 diabetes mellitus (T1DM) was diagnosed. The differential diagnoses were explored to find a probable etiology. Highly active antiretroviral therapy could cause hyperglycemia, but the patient had been on antiretroviral therapy for four years and had never presented with hyperglycemia. In the setting of normal serum lipase, a normal pancreatic structure in ultrasound and CT scan, and no signs of exocrine dysfunction, pancreatic insufficiency was also ruled out. In the case of new-onset T2DM, it is highly unlikely for a patient to have such rapidly progressive disease in three months. In addition, the significant rise in hemoglobin A1c after the initiation of the immunotherapy suggested a temporal association between the pembrolizumab and the development of DKA. Having ruled out other causes, new-onset IDD secondary to pembrolizumab was considered the final diagnosis.

After four days in the intensive care unit, there was a marked clinical improvement with resolution of the ketoacidosis and anion gap and control of the blood glucose. The patient was transferred to the ward and was discharged home with a subcutaneous insulin regimen. The immunotherapy was restarted after assessing the adequacy of and the compliance with the insulin regimen. He completed the fourth cycle of carboplatin, pemetrexed, and pembrolizumab and was later transitioned to the maintenance phase with pemetrexed and pembrolizumab. The endocrinology service recommended the administration of intramuscular dexamethasone as prophylaxis for an IR-AE on days 2–4 of each cycle.

3. Discussion

Diabetic ketoacidosis is a common presentation of insulin-dependent diabetes mellitus, which may be exacerbated by infection. Our patient was initially assessed for DKA in the setting of sepsis. After finding negative cultures and ruling out other common etiologies, it was concluded that the DKA was caused by an IR-AE from pembrolizumab. This has been previously described in the literature with an estimated incidence of <1% [6].

Immunotherapy-induced IDD has been classified as new-onset T1DM or worsening of preexisting T2DM. Approximately 67% of the IDD cases developed DKA as the first manifestation [5]. There are several hypotheses for the appearance of these IR-AEs. Animal studies have shown that PD-L1 expression in pancreatic beta-cells inhibits the release of cytokines from CD4+ T lymphocytes, thereby preventing the accumulation of CD8+ T lymphocyte in the pancreas [7]. Additionally, when PD-1 and PD-L1 were inhibited in diabetic mice, there was an increase in the number of self-reactive T cells in pancreatic lymph nodes [8]. Thus, the mechanism that underlies the development of immune checkpoint inhibitor-induced IDD is most likely T cell-mediated destruction of pancreatic beta-cells [5]. Interestingly, IR-AEs seem to be related to better tumor response to checkpoint inhibitors therapy [9].

A recent study evaluated nivolumab and pembrolizumab (PD-1) as an emergent cause of diabetes mellitus and found an overall incidence of new-onset IDD of 1.8%, which most frequently occurred after four cycles of the therapy. Out of the 774 patients on pembrolizumab, 11 (1.4%) had T1DM, and 6 (0.8%) had worsening of preexisting T2DM [5]. Despite unsuccessful attempts to use glucocorticoids to reverse the IDD [10], only one case has been reported with spontaneous resolution [5]. As seen in our patient, most subjects with checkpoint inhibitor-induced IDD remain permanently diabetic.

In our patient, the presentation of IR-AEs occurred in the context of an HIV infection. Until recently, most clinical trials have excluded patients with HIV requiring immunosuppressive treatment to avoid the potential risk of exacerbating the viral infection [11]. HIV infection poses an increased risk of autoimmunity [12], usually manifest as systemic lupus erythematosus, rheumatoid arthritis, Grave's disease while the immune system is still competent, or as Reiter's syndrome, psoriasis, and diffuse infiltrative lymphocytosis syndrome during the AIDS phase [13]. For this reason, it could be hypothesized that HIV patients are at increased risk to develop IR-AEs. However, HIV infection does not increase the risk of diabetes [14]. A small multicenter phase 1 clinical trial did not find evidence of IDD within an HIV population treated with pembrolizumab [15]. There was a reported case of an HIV patient who received nivolumab for Hodgkin's lymphoma and developed anti-GAD 65 positive IDD [16]. Our patient did not have detectable anti-GAD 65. These antibodies are present in up to 85% of patients with T1DM. Both patients were on highly active antiretroviral therapy, received additional cytotoxic chemotherapy, and exhibited an adequate tumor response to PD-1 inhibitors.

Due to the rise of non-AIDS defining malignancies among patients with HIV [17] and since the use of PD-1 inhibitors will continue to rise, it is essential to evaluate a possible increased risk of IR-AEs in HIV patients. Future clinical studies should assess this association.

Life-threatening adverse drug events associated with the use of checkpoint inhibitors such as pembrolizumab are becoming more prevalent. By reporting this association, we aim to raise clinicians' awareness of the vast array of these reactions. We also recommend a thorough follow-up and monitoring of patients at high risk of developing IR-AEs. Disease-specific screening should be investigated in large prospective studies. This strategy could lead to early detection and prevention, as well as reduction of more serious life-threatening complications requiring intensive care. Failing to prevent the already known complications would reduce the overall quality of care and could lead to death.

Consent

Written consent was obtained from the patient before preparing the case report.

Acknowledgments

The authors want to thank the language assistance of Mrs. Mary Ann Oler, Education Program Coordinator for the Department of Critical Care and Respiratory Care at The University of Texas MD Anderson Cancer Center.

References

[1] D. M. Pardoll, "The blockade of immune checkpoints in cancer immunotherapy," *Nature Reviews Cancer*, vol. 12, no. 4, pp. 252–264, 2012.

[2] A. Ribas, I. Puzanov, R. Dummer et al., "Pembrolizumab versus investigator-choice chemotherapy for ipilimumab-refractory melanoma (KEYNOTE-002): a randomised, controlled, phase 2 trial," *The Lancet Oncology*, vol. 16, no. 8, pp. 908–918, 2015.

[3] R. S. Herbst, P. Baas, D.-W. Kim et al., "Pembrolizumab versus docetaxel for previously treated, PD-L1-positive, advanced non-small-cell lung cancer (KEYNOTE-010): a randomised controlled trial," *The Lancet*, vol. 387, no. 10027, pp. 1540–1550, 2016.

[4] J. Naidoo, D. B. Page, B. T. Li et al., "Toxicities of the anti-PD-1 and anti-PD-L1 immune checkpoint antibodies," *Annals of Oncology*, vol. 26, no. 12, pp. 2375–2391, 2015.

[5] A. Kotwal, C. Haddox, M. Block, and Y. C. Kudva, "Immune checkpoint inhibitors: an emerging cause of insulin-dependent diabetes," *BMJ Open Diabetes Research & Care*, vol. 7, Article ID e000591, 2019.

[6] R. Barroso-Sousa, W. T. Barry, A. C. Garrido-Castro et al., "Incidence of endocrine dysfunction following the use of different immune checkpoint inhibitor regimens," *JAMA Oncology*, vol. 4, no. 2, pp. 173–182, 2018.

[7] M. E. Keir, S. C. Liang, I. Guleria et al., "Tissue expression of PD-L1 mediates peripheral T cell tolerance," *Journal of Experimental Medicine*, vol. 203, no. 4, pp. 883–895, 2006.

[8] M. J. I. Ansari, A. D. Salama, T. Chitnis et al., "The programmed death-1 (PD-1) pathway regulates autoimmune diabetes in nonobese diabetic (NOD) mice," *Journal of Experimental Medicine*, vol. 198, no. 1, pp. 63–69, 2003.

[9] M. Freeman-Keller, Y. Kim, H. Cronin, A. Richards, G. Gibney, and J. S. Weber, "Nivolumab in resected and unresectable metastatic melanoma: characteristics of immune-related adverse events and association with outcomes," *Clinical Cancer Research*, vol. 22, no. 4, pp. 886–894, 2016.

[10] J. Aleksova, P. K. H. Lau, G. Soldatos, and G. McArthur, "Glucocorticoids did not reverse type 1 diabetes mellitus secondary to pembrolizumab in a patient with metastatic melanoma," *BMJ Case Reports*, vol. 10, 2016.

[11] G. C. Persad, R. F. Little, and C. Grady, "Including persons with HIV infection in cancer clinical trials," *Journal of Clinical Oncology*, vol. 26, no. 7, pp. 1027–1032, 2008.

[12] C. M. Weyand and J. J. Goronzy, "HIV infection and rheumatic diseases - autoimmune mechanisms in immunodeficient hosts," *Journal of Rheumatology*, vol. 51, pp. 55–64, 1992.

[13] G. Zandman-Goddard and Y. Shoenfeld, *HIV and Autoimmunity*, Infect Autoimmun Elsevier, Amsterdam, Netherlands, 2004.

[14] A. A. Butt, K. McGinnis, M. C. Rodriguez-Barradas et al., "HIV infection and the risk of diabetes mellitus," *AIDS*, vol. 23, no. 10, pp. 1227–1234, 2009.

[15] T. S. Uldrick, P. H. Gonçalves, M. Abdul-Hay et al., "Assessment of the safety of pembrolizumab in patients with HIV and advanced cancer-A phase 1 study," *JAMA Oncology*, vol. 5, no. 9, pp. 1332–1339, 2019.

[16] E. Chang, G. Rivero, N. R. Patel et al., "HIV-related refractory Hodgkin lymphoma: a case report of complete response to nivolumab," *Clinical Lymphoma Myeloma and Leukemia*, vol. 18, no. 2, pp. e143–e146, 2018.

[17] A. Navarro, A. Martinez-Marti, and E. Felip, "HIV-positive patients with lung cancer: is immunotherapy a safe and active option for them?" *Journal of Thoracic Oncology*, vol. 13, no. 7, pp. 874–876, 2018.

Hopeful News for Physicians Who Involved in the Treatment of Critical Aluminum Phosphide (Rice Pill) Poisoning Patients

Fatemeh Vafapour and Moslem Sedaghattalab

Department of Internal Medicine, Yasuj University of Medical Sciences, Yasuj, Iran

Correspondence should be addressed to Moslem Sedaghattalab; moslem.sedaghattalab@gmail.com

Academic Editor: Chiara Lazzeri

Introduction. Aluminum phosphide (rice tablet) was first introduced as a pesticide in India. Rice tablets are commonly used in Iran due to their high efficacy against rodents and insects, low cost, and availability. Aluminum phosphide is a lethal poison without antidote and causes cardiocirculatory collapse and has negative inotropic cardiac effect. Human and animal studies showed that high dose insulin had positive cardiac inotropic effects. GIK (glucose, insulin, and potassium) assists heart uptake of carbohydrates that are the major fuel substrate of the myocard muscle under stressed conditions and leading to correction of acidosis, increased myocardial contractility, and peripheral vascular resistance. *Case Presentation.* In this manuscript, a young woman with aluminum phosphide poisoning was described to have presented with hypotension, hypoxemia, and severe metabolic acidosis. In contrast to our previous experiences that approximately all rice tablet poisoning patients with shock were dead despite full conservative treatment, this patient miraculously was saved with high dose intravenous regular insulin infusion and was discharged from the hospital with good condition and without any complications. *Conclusion.* Rice tablet poisoning has high fatality rate, and to date, no antidote is available. GIK is suggested as a potential life saving treatment for critical rice tablet poisoning patients with symptoms and signs of shock.

1. Introduction

Aluminum phosphide was first introduced as a pesticide in India. Rice pills are commonly used in Iran due to their high efficacy against rodents and insects, low cost, and availability. Aluminum phosphide poisoning has dramatically increased within the recent years due to its ingestion as a suicide drug. Rice tablet is a lethal poison without antidote and causes cardiocirculatory collapse and has negative inotropic cardiac effect [1].

Human and animal studies showed that high dose insulin had positive cardiac inotropic effects [2–4]. GIK assists heart uptake of carbohydrates that are the major fuel substrate of the myocard muscle under stressed conditions [5], and leading to correction of acidosis, increased myocardial contractility, and peripheral vascular resistance. High dose insulin was first introduced as a possible treatment of rice pill poisoning in 2008, although this treatment was has not proved in high power clinical randomized trials [1].

In this manuscript a young woman with aluminum phosphide poisoning was described to have presented with hypotension, hypoxemia, and severe metabolic acidosis. In contrast to our previous experiences that approximately all critical rice tablet poisoning patients with shock were dead despite full conservative treatment, this patient miraculously was saved with high dose intravenous regular insulin infusion and is discharged from the hospital with good condition.

2. Case Report

A 17-year-old young woman presented to emergency ward, Emam Sajad Hospital, Iran, with ingestion of one rice tablet 30 minutes before hospital admission, nausea, and vomiting. She also had a history of depression. Medication history was negative.

On examination, she was drowsy and Glasgow coma scale score (GCS) was 11, the body temperature, blood pressure, heart rate, oxygen saturation, and respiratory rate were

36.5°C, 80/60 mmHg, 130 beats/min, 80%, and 29 breaths/min, respectively.

Her extremities were cold, and all other examinations were normal. The patient was admitted in intensive care unit ward with hypotensive shock, severe hypoxemia; and intubation, mechanical ventilation, and other conservative treatment was initiated.

The platelet counts was 523000 (per μl), hemoglobin 12 (g/dL), and the white blood cell counts 12000 (mm^3). The alanine aminotransferase was 25 (IU/L), aspartate aminotransferase 70 (IU/L), albumin 3.4 (g/dL), alkaline phosphatase 99 (IU/L), total bilirubin 4.8 (mg/dL), conjugated bilirubin 0.3 (mg/dL), pH (potential of hydrogen) 7.12, CO_2 (Carbon dioxide) 27 (mm Hg), HCO_3 (bicarbonate) 10 (mEq/L), LDH (lactate dehydrogenase) 389 (U/ml), sodium 140 (mEq/L), potassium 3.7 (mEq/L), BUN (blood urea nitrogen) 28 (mg/dL), creatinine 0.4 (mg/dL), magnesium 2.3 (mg/dl), and blood sugar 123 (mg/dL). Other laboratory tests, such as troponin, partial thromboplastin time, prothrombin time, and blood culture were normal.

A CT (computerized tomography) scan of chest revealed mild pleural effusion. ECG (Electrocardiogram) revealed sinus tachycardia with mild and nonsignificant ST depression in inferior and lateral leads.

Treatment with sodium bicarbonate (to correct patient metabolic acidosis and to maintain serum bicarbonate above 20 mEq/L), hydrocortisone (100 mg doses at 8-hour intervals), high dose intravenous regular insulin (50 IU/hr, calculated by the formula 1 IU/kg/hr, based on previous studies (1)), potassium (maintain the serum potassium between 3.5-4.5 mEq/l), normal saline as maintenance serum therapy and loading dose for correction of hypotension, hypertonic dextrose water 50% (1 cc/kg/hr to maintain serum glucose between 100-180 mg/dL), intravenous pantoprazole for stress ulcer prophylaxis, subcutaneous enoxaparin (40 mg daily) for deep vein thrombosis prophylaxis and mechanical ventilation was initiated and the patient's symptoms and signs of hypoxemia and shock resolved completely and regular insulin was tapered after resolution of hypotension and acidosis and patient was transferred from intensive care unit ward after 4 days with good condition to general ward and was discharged from hospital without any complications.

3. Discussion

Aluminum phosphide tablets are a widely available and highly toxic without antidote. When these tablets come in contact with water, they quickly dissolve and emit phosphine gas. After ingestion of rice pill, phosphine gas is absorbed through the mucosa, causing nausea, vomiting, dyspnea, cardiac failure, refractory hypotension, and severe metabolic acidosis [6–9].

Mechanism of rice tablet toxicity includes cytochrome C oxidase inhibition by phosphine gas, oxidative injury, and lipid peroxidation that cause cellular injury. [6, 8, 9].

The most common cause of mortality in rice tablet poisoning is severe hypotension. It is commonly refractory to vasoactive agents such as norepinephrine and massive hydration with isotonic fluids such as normal saline. Other major causes of mortality in these patients are cardiogenic shock and severe metabolic acidosis, which is likely caused by cytochrome C oxidase inhibition and generalized tissue hypoperfusion. [10]

In circulatory shock, the metabolism or cellular uptake of glucose is impairing in the myocard muscle cells, resulting in a metabolic starvation, which additionally, worsens an already present toxin-induced cardiac depression. The proposed mechanism of hemodynamic benefit of high intravenous insulin and glucose is that it maximizes heart glucose uptake, enhance energy production from carbohydrates, and restitute calcium flux. The use of infusion in high dose insulin and dextrose in rice tablet poisoning was suggested after its beneficial positive inotropic heart effect in patients with severe beta-blockers and calcium channel blockers poisoning [5, 11–13].

It was determined in the study by Hassanian-Moghaddam et al. that administering high dose insulin (regular insulin 1 IU/kg/h-3 IU/kg/h followed by 0.2 to 0.5 U/kg/h with glucose and potassium) had significant effect on the decrease death in aluminum phosphide poisoning patients. Although their study has some limitations such as nonblinded randomization, low sample size (44 patients in intervention group), and dose of vasoactive support and other clinically relevant parameters were not investigated [1].

In a pilot study by Pannu et al. that administering GIK (insulin regular 0.1-0.5 IU/kg/h with glucose and potassium), they found that survival rate was significantly higher in intravenous insulin group, although their study was unblinded and had small sample size (30 patients in GIK group) and power [11].

In this manuscript a young woman with rice tablet poisoning was described to have presented with hypoxemia, severe metabolic acidosis, and hypotension. She had signs of severe shock and hypotension due to negative inotropic effect of phosphine and acidosis on heart. And her hypoxemia and metabolic acidosis were due to the inhibition of cytochrome C oxidase by phosphine and the formation of highly reactive free radicals.

In contrast to our previous experiences that approximately all critical rice tablets poisoning patients with hypoxemia and hypotension were dead, this patient at the height of disappointment was saved with high dose intravenous regular insulin and hypertonic dextrose water. Treatment with GIK, hydrocortisone, bicarbonate, mechanical ventilation, and other conservative treatment were initiated and the patient's signs of shock resolved completely and the patient was discharged from intensive care unit with good condition and without any complications.

4. Conclusion

Rice tablet poisoning has high fatality rate and to date, no antidote is available. In this manuscript a young woman with aluminum phosphide poisoning was described to have presented with hypoxemia, hypotension, and severe metabolic acidosis and successfully treated with high dose intravenous regular insulin and hypertonic dextrose, and discharged from intensive care unit with good condition. As a result, GIK is suggested as a potential life saving treatment for critical rice tablet poisoning patient with symptoms and signs of shock.

Disclosure

Informed written consent was obtained from patient before initiation of high dose insulin and for publication of this case report.

Acknowledgments

We thank skillful personnel of Emam Sajad hospital ICU who helped us in the managing of this critical patient.

References

[1] H. Hassanian-Moghaddam and N. Zamani, "Therapeutic role of hyperinsulinemia/euglycemia in aluminum phosphide poisoning," *Medicine*, vol. 95, no. 31, article e4349, 2016.

[2] W. Kerns II, D. Schroeder, C. Williams, C. Tomaszewski, and R. Raymond, "Insulin Improves Survival in a Canine Model of Acute β-Blocker Toxicity," *Annals of Emergency Medicine*, vol. 29, no. 6, pp. 748–757, 1997.

[3] I. Krukenkamp, D. Sørlie, N. Silverman, A. Pridjian, and S. Levitsky, "Direct effect of high-dose insulin on the depressed heart after beta-blockade or ischemia," *The Thoracic and Cardiovascular Surgeon*, vol. 34, no. 5, pp. 305–309, 1986.

[4] J. A. Kline, R. M. Raymond, E. D. Leonova, T. C. Williams, and J. A. Watts, "Insulin improves heart function and metabolism during non-ischemic cardiogenic shock in awake canines," *Cardiovascular Research*, vol. 34, no. 2, pp. 289–298, 1997.

[5] C. Woodward, A. Pourmand, and M. Mazer-Amirshahi, "High dose insulin therapy, an evidence based approach to beta blocker/calcium channel blocker toxicity," *DARU Journal of Pharmaceutical Sciences*, vol. 22, no. 1, pp. 1–5, 2014.

[6] Ö. Çakın, G. Tazegul, A. Gümüş, M. Cengiz, and A. Ramazanoğlu, "Incidental aluminum phosphide poisoning: case report and current management," *Folia Medica*, vol. 60, no. 3, pp. 464–467, 2018.

[7] Z. Halvaei, H. Tehrani, K. Soltaninejad, M. Abdollahi, and S. Shadnia, "Vitamin E as a novel therapy in the treatment of acute aluminum phosphide poisoning," *Turkish Journal of Medical Sciences*, vol. 47, no. 3, pp. 795–800, 2017.

[8] O. Mehrpour and S. Singh, "Rice tablet poisoning: a major concern in Iranian population," *Human and Experimental Toxicology*, vol. 29, no. 8, pp. 701-702, 2010.

[9] A. A. Moghadamnia, "An update on toxicology of aluminum phosphide," *DARU journal of Pharmaceutical Sciences*, vol. 20, no. 1, pp. 1–8, 2012.

[10] M. V. Farahani, D. Soroosh, and S. M. Marashi, "Thoughts on the current management of acute aluminum phosphide toxicity and proposals for therapy: an evidence-based review," *Indian Journal of Critical Care Medicine: Peer-Reviewed, Official Publication of Indian Society of Critical Care Medicine*, vol. 20, no. 12, pp. 724–730, 2016.

[11] A. K. Pannu, A. Bhalla, J. Gantala, N. Sharma, S. Kumar, and D. P. Dhibar, "Glucose-insulin-potassium infusion for the treatment of acute aluminum phosphide poisoning: an open-label pilot study," *Clinical Toxicology*, vol. 58, no. 10, pp. 1004–1009, 2020.

[12] K. M. Engebretsen, K. M. Kaczmarek, J. Morgan, and J. S. Holger, "High-dose insulin therapy in beta-blocker and calcium channel-blocker poisoning," *Clinical Toxicology.*, vol. 49, no. 4, pp. 277–283, 2011.

[13] J. S. Holger, S. J. Stellpflug, J. B. Cole, C. R. Harris, and K. M. Engebretsen, "High-dose insulin: a consecutive case series in toxin-induced cardiogenic shock," *Clinical Toxicology*, vol. 49, no. 7, pp. 653–658, 2011.

23

Tetanus Complicated by Dysautonomia: A Case Report and Review of Management

Nishant Sharma,[1] Si Li,[1] Metlapalli Venkata Sravanthi,[1] Dan Kazmierski,[1] Yichen Wang,[1] Amit Sharma,[2] and Pragya Dhaubhadel[2]

[1]*The Wright Center for Graduate Medical Education, 501 South Washington Avenue, Scranton, PA 18505, USA*
[2]*Geisinger Community Medical Center, 1800 Mulberry Street, Scranton, PA 18510, USA*

Correspondence should be addressed to Nishant Sharma; doctornsharma@gmail.com

Academic Editor: Mehmet Doganay

Tetanus is a life-threatening infectious neurological disorder that is now a rare disease due to the institution of wide-spread vaccination strategies. We present an uncommon case of generalized severe tetanus with consequent respiratory failure requiring mechanical ventilation, which was associated with dysautonomia. A 20-year-old unvaccinated female presented with neck stiffness and diffuse muscle spasms following a laceration sustained 3 weeks prior. She was admitted to the intensive care unit for mechanical ventilation and was treated with immunoglobulin, tetanus toxoid, metronidazole, and high doses of sedatives. She also developed dysautonomia, with alternating bradycardia and tachycardia, as well as fluctuating blood pressure. She was successfully extubated and discharged. We also review the epidemiology, pathophysiology, and management of tetanus and discuss dysautonomia in the setting of tetanus.

1. Introduction

Tetanus, a life-threatening neurological disorder involving muscle spasms caused by *Clostridium tetani*, is now a rare disease, with an annual incidence of 0.10 cases/million population in the United States [1]. We present a rare case of an unimmunized patient presenting with fulminant tetanus requiring ventilatory support, as well as severe dysautonomia. We also review the current state of disease incidence and immunization rates and summarize the management of tetanus and its complications.

2. Case Presentation

A 20-year-old unvaccinated female with a history of substance use disorder presented to the emergency department with neck stiffness and diffuse muscle spasms for three days. Her symptoms had started with neck and back stiffness three days prior and had progressed to involve other muscle groups, causing an inability to speak, swallow, or turn her head, as well as severe muscle spasms of the torso and all extremities. She had, of note, sustained a laceration on her wrist 3 weeks prior and had not sought medical evaluation. Furthermore, she was an active intravenous drug user and admitted to injecting heroin as recently as 2 days prior to presentation. Further elaboration of medical history revealed that she had never received any vaccinations because her mother "did not believe in them."

Physical examination revealed a heart rate of 85 beats min^{-1}, blood pressure of 137/65 mm Hg, respiratory rate of 23 breaths min, and a temperature of 99.5 F. She appeared ill and was in severe distress; notable findings were trismus, clenched jaw, drooling, and diffuse muscular rigidity. Wound site contractions were noted around a 5-centimeter-long laceration on the right wrist. Cardiovascular, respiratory, abdominal, and sensory examination was unremarkable. Laboratory work-up was notable for leukocytosis. Urine toxicology was positive for opiates. Computed tomography of the neck was grossly unremarkable for acute pathology.

The combination of her presentation, recent injury, and unimmunized status prompted the clinical diagnosis of generalized tetanus with subsequent administration of human tetanus immunoglobulin and tetanus toxoid and the initiation of metronidazole. The intravenous agents were administered in the antecubital vein of the same arm which had sustained the laceration. She was admitted to the intensive care unit and placed in a room with minimal auditory and visual stimuli. Diazepam, baclofen, fentanyl, and magnesium were initiated for control of muscle spasms. Shortly after admission, she developed progressive trismus and airway compromise, leading to nasotracheal intubation and initiation of mechanical ventilation. This was followed by percutaneous tracheostomy in anticipation of prolonged ventilation. Sedation proved to be challenging, requiring high doses of intravenous propofol (65 mcg/kg/min), fentanyl (200 mcg/hr), and midazolam (7 mg/hr) infusions. However, with continued supportive care, she was weaned off mechanical ventilatory support on ICU day 7. She continued to have a complicated hospital course, which was most notable for hemodynamics, with alternating tachycardia and bradycardia, and fluctuating blood pressure, attributable to autonomic dysfunction due to tetanus. Her hemodynamics stabilized with continued magnesium supplementation and supportive care. Fiberoptic laryngoscopy confirmed satisfactory airway patency, and her tracheostomy was decannulated. She was discharged after a 26-day-long hospital course, and a catch-up immunization schedule was arranged. The patient continued to have residual neck stiffness upon follow-up 6 months after discharge, which was treated conservatively with muscle relaxants.

3. Discussion

Tetanus is now a rare disease in the developed world, owing to the institution of universal vaccination policies. 23 cases of tetanus were reported in 2018 to the National Notifiable Diseases Surveillance System (NNDSS), maintained by the Center for Disease Control (CDC) [2]. Vaccination coverage, however, while high, remained incomplete—in 2017, only 83.2% of children aged 19-35 months living in the US received the full dose of the tetanus vaccine [3]. A review of vaccination coverage among adults in 2016 showed that merely 62.2% of adults over 19 years of age reported having received any tetanus toxoid containing vaccination during the preceding 10 years [4]; this figure was even lower in adults over 65 years of age: 58% [4]. Given the prevalent age of increasing vaccine skepticism, it is important that health care providers be familiar with the management of tetanus, which if left untreated has a case mortality rate approaching 100% [5]. The purpose of this presentation is to discuss the management of generalized tetanus in a community setting, in a case which was complicated by a history of substance abuse and the development of autonomic dysfunction.

Tetanus is caused by *Clostridium tetani*, a gram-positive, spore-forming, obligate anaerobe. Its spores are ubiquitous and can be found in soil, as well as the intestinal tract and feces of humans and animals. They are resilient and are incompletely destroyed by boiling. They can achieve entry into the body through disruption in the continuity of skin and, under favorable conditions, such as the anaerobic environment of devitalised tissue, germinate into toxin-producing bacteria.

The bacterium then produces two toxins: tetanolysin and tetanospasmin [6]. Tetanolysin is hypothesized to play a role in the destruction of local tissue and optimization of conditions for bacterial proliferation. Tetanospasmin disrupts synaptic neurotransmission by preventing neurotransmitter release from affected neurons. Local nerve terminals at the site of the wound are first affected, followed by hematogenous spread and retrograde axoplasmic transport, the end result being potential diffuse involvement of the nervous system. Inhibitory neurons are most affected, with the consequent inhibition of the release of gamma-aminobutyric acid (GABA) and glycine, both inhibitory neurotransmitters. It is the loss of inhibition and consequent uncontrolled efferent discharges, which lead to the syndrome of widespread muscle spasms and autonomic dysfunction that constitutes the clinical presentation of tetanus.

The incubation period of the disease is anywhere between 3 and 21 days following infection [5]. There are three categories of clinical presentation:

(1) Localized tetanus, typically seen in infections with a low toxin load, where spasms and rigidity are limited to the area around the wound

(2) Cephalic tetanus, a rare form of tetanus associated with cranial infections, which can present as cranial nerve palsies

(3) Generalized tetanus, characterized by widespread rigidity and spasms throughout the body

Early symptoms of the disease include neck stiffness and difficulty opening the mouth (lockjaw), caused by masseter muscle spasm. Facial muscles can be progressively involved, causing the distinctive facial expression associated with tetanus, risus sardonicus. Involvement of the trunk follows, with severe spasms of the back musculature, causing opisthotonus, the backward arching of the neck and back, and increased muscle tone and tonic spasms in the extremities. Autonomic involvement may also be seen and is an indicator of a poor prognosis. The sympathetic system is usually affected, with resultant tachycardia, hypertension, and vasoconstriction, but bradycardia and hypotension may also be seen. Other autonomic manifestations include increased salivation and secretions and gastric dysmotility.

There are many proposed grading systems, but the system proposed by Ablett is most commonly used (Table 1) [6].

The management of tetanus has its basis in three principles: first, the prompt neutralization of unbound toxin with the intramuscular injection of 3,000-6,000 units of human tetanus immunoglobulin. Second, the prevention of further toxin production by the administration of metronidazole, which is the antibiotic of choice. Penicillin is active against *C. tetani* but is a GABA antagonist and may be associated with convulsions [7]. Other antibiotic options include doxycycline, clindamycin, vancomycin, macrolides, and chloramphenicol. Additionally, local debridement of the wound to eradicate spores is of paramount importance.

Table 1

Grade	Severity	Symptoms
1	Mild	Mild to moderate trismus; general spasticity; no respiratory embarrassment; no spasms; little or no dysphagia.
2	Moderate	Moderate trismus; well-marked rigidity; mild to moderate but short spasms; moderate respiratory embarrassment with an increased respiratory rate greater than 30; mild dysphagia.
3	Severe	Severe trismus; generalized spasticity; reflex prolonged spasms; increased respiratory rate greater than 40; apnoeic spells; severe dysphagia; tachycardia greater than 120.
4	Very severe	Grade III and violent autonomic disturbances involving the cardiovascular system. Severe hypertension and tachycardia alternating with relative hypotension and bradycardia, either of which may be persistent.

Finally, the effect of tetanospasmin that has already achieved entry into the neuronal system must be neutralized. The patient must be placed in a room with minimal visual and auditory stimulation to avoid provoking muscle spasms. The mainstay of pharmacological treatment of diffuse muscle spasms, as seen with generalized tetanus, is administration of benzodiazepine, which increases gamma aminobutyric acid (GABA) [8]. Diazepam has been used with success but can cause prolonged sedation as well as anion gap metabolic acidosis at high doses. Midazolam appears to have fewer risks and can be used as a continuous infusion. When benzodiazepine-induced sedation proves to be inadequate, neuromuscular blockade can be instituted with agents such as pancuronium. Pancuronium inhibits the reuptake of catecholamine and can worsen autonomic instability; vecuronium is a shorter-lasting alternative which is less likely to cause cardiovascular adverse effects. Propofol, dantrolene, and intrathecal baclofen have all been reported to be of utility [9–11]. Dexmedetomidine, which has antisympathetic properties, is useful as an adjunct for sedation [8].

Autonomic dysfunction in association with generalized tetanus portends a poor prognosis [12]. Dysautonomia is not an uncommon complication of tetanus; one cross-sectional study found an incidence of 11.8% among patients who were hospitalized for tetanus [13]. Its cardiovascular manifestations are varied and range from "autonomic crises" characterized by episodes of profound hypertension and tachycardia to bradycardia, arrhythmias, and hypotension. The hyperkinetic circulatory state observed with autonomic storms has been attributed to increased sympathetic activity; there exists an elevated basal level of norepinephrine, with spikes in epinephrine during times of autonomic storms [14]. Possible mechanisms of bradycardia, as seen in our patient, are sudden withdrawal of catecholamines or increased vagal tone. The management of these cardiovascular aberrations includes the administration of combined α and β adrenergic blocking agents, such as labetolol. β-Adrenergic blocking agents should be avoided because of their potential to cause hypotension, pulmonary edema, and sudden death. There have been reports of atropine being used to alleviate cardiovascular instability [15]. Clonidine, a centrally acting α-2 agonist, reduces sympathetic outflow and may be useful in the control of sympathetic overactivity in tetanus, as demonstrated by Sutton et al. [16]. Semipermanent cardiac pacing has been shown to be useful in the management of severe bradycardia in generalized tetanus [17]. Magnesium is a presynaptic neuromuscular blocker, blocks catecholamine release from nerves, and reduces the responsiveness of receptors to catecholamines. Magnesium sulphate has been successfully used to reduce autonomic disturbance and muscle spasms [18]. One study found some success with the use of epidural blockade with bupivacaine and sufentanil, which resulted in a significant reduction in blood pressure fluctuation [19].

A special note must be made about the occurrence and management of tetanus in heroin users, such as our patient. This population appears to be at a higher risk of contracting tetanus, not only because of the potential for contaminated intravenous access sites but also because quinine, which is used to dilute heroin, may support the growth of *C. tetani* [20]. In addition, pharmacological treatment, which is a critical component of the treatment of generalized tetanus, is challenging in these patients. A high level of tolerance to sedatives is frequently encountered, necessitating the administration of high doses of multiple agents to achieve target levels of sedation. One study found nonsignificant greater total requirements for sedation and analgesia in patients with a history of substance abuse, compared to those without [21]. This patient required high doses of fentanyl, propofol, and midazolam concurrently for adequate relief of muscle spasms.

4. Conclusion

In conclusion, we present the clinical presentation and management of a severe case of tetanus complicated by autonomic dysfunction and respiratory failure requiring mechanical ventilation. We review the pathogenesis and management of this deadly disease. Tetanus is a rare disease, the management of which intensivists must be familiar with, given the prevalent era of growing vaccine skepticism and incomplete immunization.

References

[1] Centers for Disease Control and Prevention, "Tetanus surveillance - United States, 2001–2008," *Morbidity and Mortality Weekly Report (MMWR)*, vol. 60, no. 12, pp. 365–369, 2011.

[2] Centers for Disease Control and Prevention. National Notifiable Diseases Surveillance System, "Annual tables of infectious disease data," 2018, February 2020, https://www.cdc.gov/nndss/infectious-tables.html.

[3] Centers for Disease Control and Prevention, "Vaccination coverage for selected diseases among children aged 19–35 months, by race, Hispanic origin, poverty level, and location of residence in metropolitan statistical area: United States, selected years 1998–2017," February 2020, https://www.cdc.gov/nchs/hus/contents2018.htm#Table_031.

[4] Centers for Disease Control and Prevention, "Vaccination coverage among adults in the United States, National Health Interview Survey, 2016," February 2020, https://www.cdc.gov/vaccines/imz-managers/coverage/adultvaxview/pubs-resources/NHIS-2016.html#tetanus.

[5] World Health Organization, "Weekly Epidemiological Record," vol. 92, pp. 53–76, 2017, February 2020, https://www.who.int/wer/2017/wer9206/en/.

[6] T. M. Cook, R. T. Protheroe, and J. M. Handel, "Tetanus: a review of the literature," *British Journal of Anaesthesia*, vol. 87, no. 3, pp. 477–487, 2001.

[7] H. C. Johnson and A. Walker, "Intraventricular penicillin," *Journal of the American Medical Association*, vol. 127, no. 4, pp. 217–219, 1945.

[8] G. L. Maryke Spruyt and T. van den Heever, "The treatment of autonomic dysfunction in tetanus," *Southern African Journal of Critical Care*, vol. 33, no. 1, pp. 28–31, 2017.

[9] A. Borgeat, V. Popovic, and D. Schwander, "Efficiency of a continuous infusion of propofol in a patient with tetanus," *Critical Care Medicine*, vol. 19, no. 2, pp. 295-296, 1991.

[10] M. Tidyman, J. G. Prichard, R. L. Deamer, and N. Mac, "Adjunctive use of dantrolene in severe tetanus," *Anesthesia and Analgesia*, vol. 64, no. 5, pp. 538–540, 1985.

[11] N. Engrand, E. Guerot, A. Rouamba, and G. Vilain, "The efficacy of intrathecal baclofen in severe tetanus," *Anesthesiology*, vol. 90, no. 6, pp. 1773–1776., 1999.

[12] M. Wasay, B. A. Khealani, N. Talati, R. Shamsi, N. A. Syed, and N. Salahuddin, "Autonomic nervous system dysfunction predicts poor prognosis in patients with mild to moderate tetanus," *BMC Neurology*, vol. 5, no. 1, p. 2, 2005.

[13] A. Derbie, A. Amdu, A. Alamneh et al., "Clinical profile of tetanus patients attended at Felege Hiwot Referral Hospital, Northwest Ethiopia: a retrospective cross sectional study," *Springerplus*, vol. 5, no. 1, p. 892, 2016.

[14] K. Gibson, J. Bonaventure Uwineza, W. Kiviri, and J. Parlow, "Tetanus in developing countries: a case series and review," *Canadian Journal of Anaesthesia*, vol. 56, no. 4, pp. 307–315, 2009.

[15] D. Dolar, "The use of continuous atropine infusion in the management of severe tetanus," *Intensive Care Medicine*, vol. 18, no. 1, pp. 26–31, 1992.

[16] D. N. Sutton, M. R. Tremlett, T. E. Woodcock, and M. S. Nielsen, "Management of autonomic dysfunction in severe tetanus: the use of magnesium sulphate and clonidine," *Intensive Care Medicine*, vol. 16, no. 2, pp. 75–80, 1990.

[17] J. L. Millo, M. C. Culshaw, N. J. Alp, and J. B. Salmon, "Semi-permanent cardiac pacing in severe tetanus," *British Journal of Anaesthesia*, vol. 88, no. 6, p. 882, 2002.

[18] C. L. Thwaites, L. M. Yen, and H. T. Loan, "Magnesium sulphate for treatment of severe tetanus: a randomised controlled trial," *Lancet*, vol. 368, no. 9545, pp. 1436–1443, 2006.

[19] S. Bhagwanjee, A. T. Bösenberg, and D. J. Muckart, "Management of sympathetic overactivity in tetanus with epidural bupivacaine and sufentanil: experience with 11 patients," *Critical Care Medicine*, vol. 27, no. 9, pp. 1721–1725, 1999.

[20] J. Hamborsky, A. Kroger, and S. Wolfe, "Chapter 21," *Centers for Disease Control and Prevention. Epidemiology and Prevention of Vaccine-Preventable Diseases*13th edition, February 2020, https://www.cdc.gov/vaccines/pubs/pinkbook/tetanus.html.

[21] T. Ruiz-García, S. Nogué-Xarau, E. Zavala-Zegarra, A. Cirera-Guasch, and J. Ríos-Guillermo, "Need for sedation and analgesia in patients with a history of substance misuse admitted to an intensive care unit," *Nursing in Critical Care*, vol. 21, no. 6, pp. 358–366, 2016.

Life-Threatening Intrapulmonary Hemorrhage due to Vancomycin-Induced Thrombocytopenia: A Case Report

Haneen Abdalhadi,[1] Yazan Fahmawi,[1] Abhijin Das,[1,2] and Brian Fouty[1,3]

[1]*Department of Internal Medicine, University of South Alabama, Mobile, AL, USA*
[2]*Division of Nephrology, University of South Alabama, Mobile, AL, USA*
[3]*Division of Pulmonary and Critical Care, University of South Alabama, Mobile, AL, USA*

Correspondence should be addressed to Haneen Abdalhadi; habdalhadi@health.southalabama.edu

Academic Editor: Gil Klinger

Thrombocytopenia is a rare and sometimes life-threatening complication of Vancomycin. A 52-year-old male patient with acute kidney injury was treated with Vancomycin for ventilator-associated pneumonia. Three days later, his platelets decreased from 172×10^9/L to 3×10^9/L over a 36-hour period. The patient developed significant intrapulmonary bleeding leading to profound hypoxemia. Workup was negative for thrombotic thrombocytopenic purpura, disseminated intravascular coagulopathy, atypical hemolytic uremic syndrome, heparin-induced thrombocytopenia, and autoimmune diseases. All recently started medications were discontinued, and the patient was started empirically on methylprednisolone and intravenous immunoglobulin. The patient's platelets increased, and his airway bleeding stopped within 48 hours; his platelet count returned to normal by 18 days. Vancomycin-dependent anti-platelet antibodies were identified in the patient's serum by flow cytometry. Thrombocytopenia is an underrecognized complication of Vancomycin that can lead to life-threating bleeding. Stopping Vancomycin may be sufficient to reverse the thrombocytopenia in patients with normal renal function, but more aggressive measures such as steroids, IVIG, and dialysis may be required to stop bleeding and reverse thrombocytopenia in patients with underlying kidney injury who cannot effectively excrete Vancomycin.

1. Introduction

Vancomycin is a glycopeptide antibiotic commonly used to treat severe gram-positive bacterial infections, especially those caused by methicillin-resistant *Staphylococcus aureus* and coagulase-negative *Staphylococci* [1]. Nephrotoxicity, ototoxicity, red-man syndrome, and reversible neutropenia are well-known side effects of Vancomycin [2–4]. Thrombocytopenia is a less commonly described complication of Vancomycin that is frequently overlooked by physicians likely due to the presence of other potential causes of thrombocytopenia in critically ill patients, such as sepsis and concomitant heparin use. The lack of an easily available point-of-care assay makes it a difficult diagnosis to confirm. Herein, we present a case of severe symptomatic Vancomycin-induced thrombocytopenia (VIT) that was confirmed by identifying Vancomycin-dependent anti-platelet antibodies in the patient's serum.

2. Case Presentation

A 52-year-old Caucasian male with diabetes mellitus, hypertension, and coronary artery disease was initially admitted to the Intensive Care Unit for pulmonary edema secondary to hypertensive emergency with a blood pressure of 254/157 mmHg. He required intubation for acute hypoxemic respiratory failure. The patient developed acute kidney failure (AKI) in the hospital. Workup for his AKI, including renal ultrasound and serologies, failed to identify a specific cause for his AKI. There was no evidence of vasculitis clinically or on renal biopsy. He was begun on hemodialysis. During this entire period, his platelet count was normal.

He developed a ventilator-associated pneumonia and was begun on empiric Vancomycin and Meropenem; no pathogen was ever identified in the patient's sputum or blood. Three days after starting these antibiotics, his platelets decreased precipitously from 172×10^9/L to 3×10^9/L over a 36-hour period (Figure 1). No schistocytes were seen on the peripheral smear, and there was no clinical evidence of hemolysis. Additional studies to evaluate for thrombotic thrombocytopenic purpura, disseminated intravascular coagulopathy, atypical hemolytic uremic syndrome, heparin-induced thrombocytopenia, and autoimmune diseases were performed; all came back negative. The patient's platelet count decreased to $1 \times 10^3/\mu$L despite multiple platelet transfusions. The patient developed an intrapulmonary hemorrhage and became severely hypoxemic despite receiving 100% oxygen. A presumptive diagnosis of drug-induced immune thrombocytopenia was made. All medications that had been recently started, including Vancomycin and Meropenem, were discontinued. Due to his life-threatening airway bleeding, the patient was treated with high-dose methylprednisolone (500 mg/day) and a five-day course of intravenous immunoglobulin (IVIG). His platelet count began to increase 48 hours after steroids were begun, and his intrapulmonary bleeding resolved with improvement in his oxygenation. After 7 days, his platelet count was 160×10^9/L. The platelet count decreased to less than 100×10^9/L after methylprednisolone was stopped. Therefore, it was restarted for an additional 10 days. Incubation of the patient's serum with platelets from normal donors resulted in the binding of IgG and IgM antibodies in the presence of Vancomycin, but not in its absence, supporting a diagnosis of Vancomycin-induced thrombocytopenia (VIT).

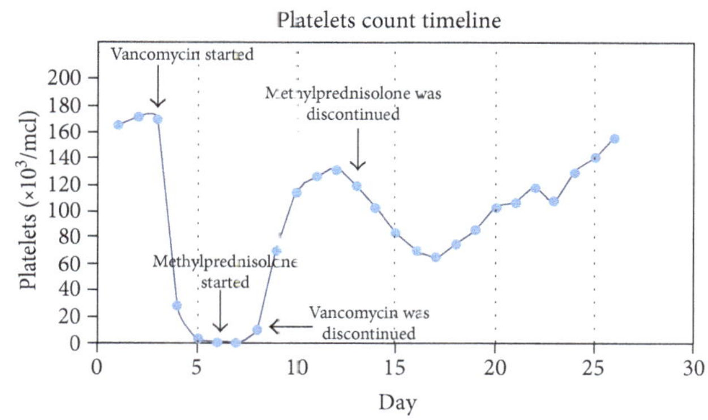

FIGURE 1: The platelets trend during patient hospitalization.

3. Discussion

Thrombocytopenia is an underrecognized complication of Vancomycin that can lead to life-threatening bleeding. Early recognition is important because discontinuation of Vancomycin is required for its resolution. The pathophysiology behind VIT is not completely understood. *Ex vivo* assays demonstrate that the antibodies bind platelets only in the presence of Vancomycin [5] as has been described for other drugs such as quinine and quinidine [6]. It has been proposed that Vancomycin acts as a hapten, binding to the platelet's surface glycoprotein IIb and/or IIIa leading to antibody formation [7]. An alternative explanation suggests that the drug binds initially to circulating antibodies (not to the large protein carrier as is classically described for the generation of hapten-specific antibodies), changing the antibody's configuration so that it can more tightly bind the platelet's αIIb/β3 integrin (GPIIa/IIIb) [8]. Whatever the sequence of initiating events, these antibodies, in the continued presence of Vancomycin, coat platelets leading to complement activation and platelet destruction [9]. Unlike heparin-induced thrombocytopenia which can cause both bleeding and thrombosis, Vancomycin-induced thrombocytopenia only increases the risk of bleeding [10]. One published case series of VIT indicated that one-third of the patients experienced severe bleeding, but none had thrombosis [5]. This is consistent with the described patient who developed a life-threatening intrapulmonary hemorrhage, but without any evidence of venous or arterial thrombosis.

Reports suggest that at least 6 days are needed after an initial Vancomycin exposure to develop VIT with a mean of 8 days to reach platelet nadir after first exposure [5, 7]. However, the interval can be significantly shorter in cases of reexposure to Vancomycin [11–13]. In the described patient, thrombocytopenia started within 3 days of receiving Vancomycin raising the possibility that this was not a primary, but an anamnestic antibody response due to prior treatment with Vancomycin. A review of the patient's chart did not reveal previous treatment with Vancomycin during his current hospitalization, but the presence of both IgM and IgG antiplatelet antibodies suggests he may have previously been exposed to this antibiotic at an outside hospital.

The normalization of the platelet count in VIT is thought to require a decrease in serum Vancomycin levels below the threshold necessary to activate the anti-platelet antibodies [14]. A mean of 7.2 days between drug discontinuation and a platelet count greater than 150×10^9/L (off steroids) has been reported [5]. In contrast, this patient's platelets did not stay above 150×10^9/L off steroids until 18 days after Vancomycin discontinuation. His prolonged duration of thrombocytopenia was likely due to decreased Vancomycin clearance due to the patient's acute kidney injury. Dialysis was paused when his platelets decreased to less than 10×10^9/L due to concerns over potential bleeding; this may have prolonged the patient's thrombocytopenia since it allowed the Vancomycin to remain in the patient's serum longer than had we continued dialysis. Although treatments such as IVIG, plasma exchange, platelets transfusion, and steroid have shown minimal benefits in previously published reports [5], we chose to empirically treat the patient with steroids and IVIG due to his intrapulmonary hemorrhage. His airway bleeding stopped, and his platelets began to increase 48 hours after beginning steroids, at a time when his Vancomycin trough was still 10 micrograms/ml, suggesting that the steroids and/or IVIG may have been helpful.

The assay for Vancomycin-dependent antibodies is a flow cytometry-based detection of drug-dependent platelet antibodies; it is a send-out test done by Versiti Wisconsin Inc. and, at present, cannot be used to diagnose VIT in the acute setting. Therefore, awareness that Vancomycin can cause thrombocytopenia is the first line of defense for diagnosing this condition.

References

[1] C. Vidal, A. González Quintela, and R. Fuente, "Toxic epidermal necrolysis due to vancomycin," *Annals of Allergy*, vol. 68, no. 4, pp. 345–347, 1992.

[2] J. Marraffa, R. Guharoy, D. Duggan, F. Rose, and S. Nazeer, "Vancomycin-induced thrombocytopenia: a case proven with rechallenge," *American College of Clinical Pharmacy Journal*, vol. 23, no. 9, pp. 1195–1198, 2003.

[3] J. C. Kuruppu, T. P. le, and C. U. Tuazon, "Vancomycin-associated thrombocytopenia: case report and review of the literature," *American Journal of Hematology*, vol. 60, no. 3, pp. 249-250, 1999.

[4] R. H. Aster, "Drug-induced immune cytopenias," *Toxicology*, vol. 209, no. 2, pp. 149–153, 2005.

[5] A. Von Drygalski, B. R. Curtis, D. W. Bougie et al., "Vancomycin-induced immune thrombocytopenia," *The New England Journal of Medicine*, vol. 356, no. 9, pp. 904–910, 2007.

[6] T. Kunicki, N. Russell, A. T. Nurden, R. H. Aster, and J. P. Caen, "Further studies of the human platelet receptor for quinine-and quinine-dependent antibodies," *The Journal of Immunology*, vol. 126, no. 2, pp. 398–402, 1981.

[7] M. Mohammadi, Z. Jahangard-Rafsanjani, A. Sarayani, M. Hadjibabaei, and M. Taghizadeh-Ghehi, "Vancomycin-induced thrombocytopenia: a narrative review," *Drug Safety Journal*, vol. 40, no. 1, pp. 49–59, 2017.

[8] D. W. Bougie, J. Peterson, M. Rasmussen, and R. H. J. B. Aster, "Mechanism of quinine-dependent monoclonal antibody binding to platelet glycoprotein IIb/IIIa," *The Journal of the American Society of Hematology*, vol. 126, no. 18, pp. 2146–2152, 2015.

[9] M. T. Rondina, A. Walker, and R. C. Pendleton, "Drug-induced thrombocytopenia for the hospitalist physician with a focus on heparin-induced thrombocytopenia," *Hospital Practice Journal*, vol. 38, no. 2, pp. 19–28, 2010.

[10] D. A. Zinkovsky and M. S. Antonopoulos, "Heparin-induced thrombocytopenia: overview and treatment," *Pharmacy and therapeutics journal*, vol. 33, no. 11, 2008.

[11] P. Mizon, V. Kiefel, L. Mannessier, C. Mueller-Eckhardt, and J. Goudemand, "Thrombocytopenia induced by vancomycin-dependent platelet antibody," *Vox Sang Journal*, vol. 73, no. 1, pp. 49–51, 1997.

[12] M. A. Ruggero, O. Abdelghany, and J. E. Topal, "Vancomycin-induced thrombocytopenia without isolation of a drug-dependent antibody," *Pharmacotherapy Journal*, vol. 32, no. 11, pp. e321–e325, 2012.

[13] G. J. Zenon, R. M. Cadle, and R. J. Hamill, "Vancomycin-induced thrombocytopenia," *Archives of Internal Medicine*, vol. 151, no. 5, pp. 995-996, 1991.

[14] B. R. Curtis, J. G. McFarland, G. G. Wu, G. P. Visentin, and R. H. Aster, "Antibodies in sulfonamide-induced immune thrombocytopenia recognize calcium-dependent epitopes on the glycoprotein IIb/IIIa complex," *Blood*, vol. 84, no. 1, pp. 176–183, 1994.

25

COVID-19-Associated Coagulopathy: A Case Report of Thrombosis despite Therapeutic Anticoagulation

Habiba Hussain,[1] **Matthew Sehring,**[2] **and Bhagat Singh Aulakh**[2]

[1]*Department of Internal Medicine, University of Illinois College of Medicine at Peoria, Peoria, IL, USA*
[2]*Department of Pulmonary & Critical Care Medicine, University of Illinois College of Medicine at Peoria, Peoria, IL, USA*

Correspondence should be addressed to Habiba Hussain; hhussain@uic.edu

Academic Editor: Mehmet Doganay

The Coronavirus disease (COVID-19) pandemic, caused by Severe Acute Respiratory Syndrome Coronavirus 2 (SARS-CoV-2), has led to tremendous morbidity and mortality. Various inflammatory markers have been monitored and considered to be associated with disease prognosis. One of the major sources of comorbidity involved has been development of thrombosis alongside the infection. This prothrombotic phenomenon considered, COVID-19-associated coagulopathy (CAC), has been the center of discussion in dealing with this infection. There still remains ambiguity regarding management guidelines for thromboprophylaxis dosing and therapeutic anticoagulation. We present a case of severe SARS-CoV-2 infection complicated by thrombosis despite therapeutic anticoagulation contributing to prolonged intensive care unit and hospital stay.

1. Introduction

The COVID-19 pandemic has led to tremendous morbidity and mortality. SARS-CoV-2 is a positive sense single-stranded RNA virus genome with an envelope surrounded by surface glycoprotein, spike or S protein, responsible for tropism towards angiotensin-converting enzyme 2 (ACE2) receptor of human respiratory epithelium [1]. Increasing evidence of postmortem findings for microvascular and thromboembolic phenomenon seen in patients with COVID-19 prompted the discussion for the role and extent of venous thromboembolic (VTE) prophylaxis [1, 2].

2. Case Description

A 59-year-old male with a past medical history of 30-pack per year tobacco abuse and a recent history of vaping presented with fever, cough, shortness of breath, and generalized fatigue. He was found in acute hypoxic respiratory failure requiring mechanical ventilation (pressure-regulated volume control (PRVC) mode, respiratory rate (RR) 16/minute, tidal volume (TV) 480 mL, positive end expiratory pressure (PEEP) 7 centimeters of water, fractional inspiratory oxygen (FiO_2) 80%, and partial arterial oxygen (PaO_2/FiO_2) < 100). He was further noted to be in septic shock likely secondary to pneumonia as chest X-ray (CXR) showed bilateral pulmonary opacities (Figure 1). He received empiric therapy for community-acquired pneumonia with ceftriaxone and azithromycin. Repeat CXR upon worsening symptoms showed increased bilateral diffuse opacities concerning for acute respiratory distress syndrome (ARDS) (Figure 2). During his acute decompensation, testing for SARS-CoV-2 resulted positive. In an effort to optimize respiratory status with available modalities at the time he received diuresis, hydroxychloroquine and trial of prone positioning.

Meanwhile, in light of hypercoagulable pattern observed in SARS-CoV-2 infections, he was maintained on adequate VTE prophylaxis with enoxaparin 40 mg daily (sequential organ failure assessment: SOFA score 5, sepsis-induced coagulopathy: SIC score 2) [1, 2]. During the course of intensive care unit (ICU) stay, he occasionally developed leukocytosis (peak 24,000 with neutrophilic predominance), C-reactive protein (CRP) peak at 37.4 mg/dL, and ferritin peak at 589 ng/mL. The most remarkable feature noted was an

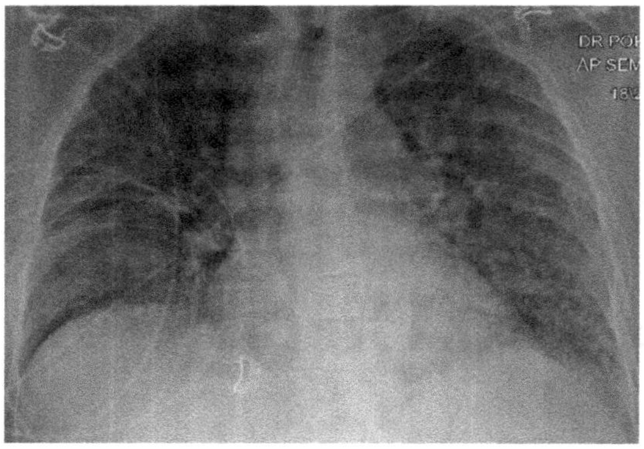

FIGURE 1: Initial bilateral pulmonary opacities.

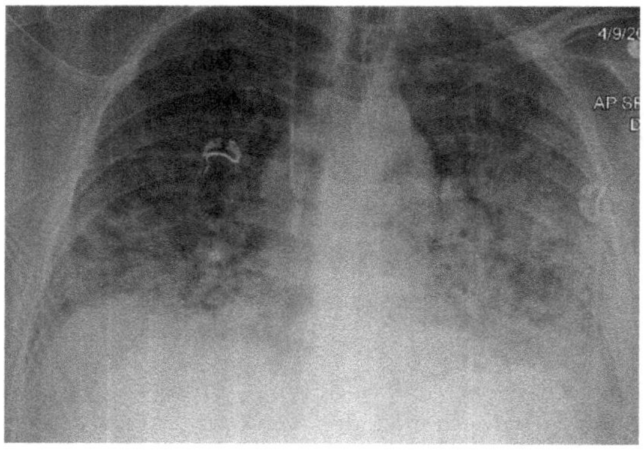

FIGURE 2: Worsening bilateral diffuse opacities.

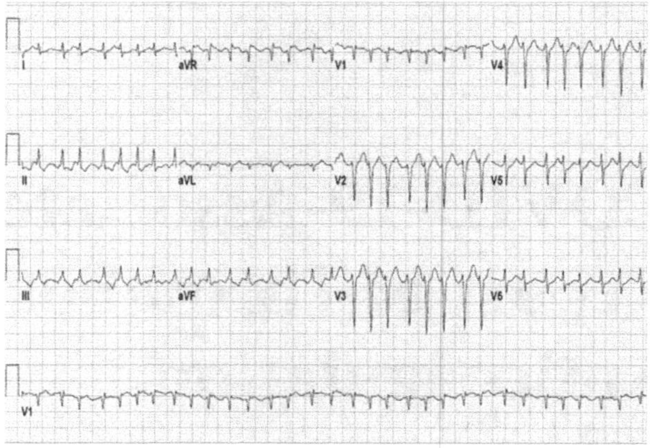

FIGURE 3: Supraventricular tachycardia with ventricular rate > 190 bpm.

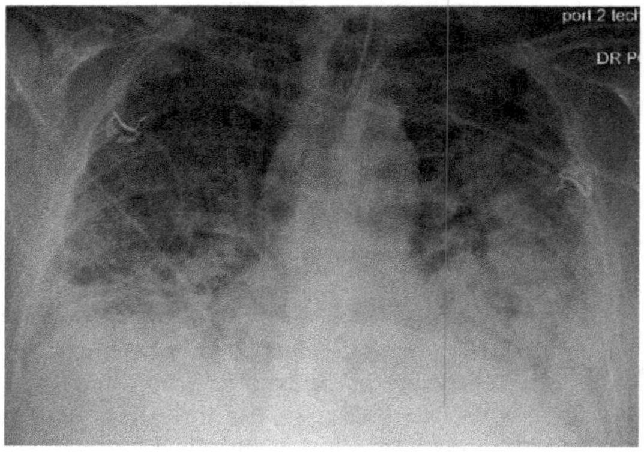

FIGURE 4: Diffuse bilateral airspace opacities with dense opacification in the left midlung.

elevated D-dimer > 20 mcg/mL on the day of presentation, declining to 8.76 mcg/mL the next day and thereafter improved to plateau around 3-5 mcg/mL. Due to failure of improvement, requiring increased vasopressor and ventilatory support, he received empiric treatment for superimposed ventilator-associated pneumonia and immunomodulation with the interleukin 6 (IL6) inhibitor tocilizumab which showed transient clinical improvement. He again worsened to developed unstable supraventricular tachycardia (SVT) requiring electrical cardioversion for return to sinus rhythm (Figure 3). With the knowledge of elevated D-dimer, worsening oxygenation, and new unstable arrhythmia indicative of microvascular thrombosis depicting end-organ dysfunction, he was empirically started on therapeutic dosing of enoxaparin maintaining target anti-Xa level (enoxaparin increased from 40 mg daily to 90 mg twice daily on day 14 of admission, while the d-Dimer was 5.68 mcg/mL). His mechanical ventilatory support requirements continued to rise (higher PEEP 18-20 cm water and FiO_2 80-90%) despite treatment and therapeutic anticoagulation; hence, he was started on convalescent plasma and high-dose steroids on day 27 of admission (Figure 4). Following a long course of critical illness, he was able to be weaned off of vasopressors and ventilatory support. Eventually, he was tested and found negative for COVID-19 for the first time on day 33 of admission, with a repeat negative test three days later. In an effort to transition off therapeutic anticoagulation dosing after being tested negative, he underwent computed tomography with angiography (CTA) which showed bilateral subsegmental pulmonary emboli, lower lobe traction bronchiectasis, fibrotic changes, and diffuse subpleural cysts. He was also noted to have multiple thick-walled cavitary lesions in the right middle lobe, bilateral bases, and left basilar cavitary abscess 5.4 × 3.5 cm (Figures 5 and 6). With the evidence of new bilateral segmental pulmonary emboli, he was transitioned from therapeutic enoxaparin to apixaban 5 mg twice daily for around 6 months until further evaluation.

3. Discussion

Implication of SARS-CoV-2 infection with thromboembolism or disseminated intravascular coagulation (DIC) has been extrapolated from sepsis-induced coagulopathy (SIC). The cause is thought to be triggered by a host inflammatory reaction leading to consumptive coagulopathy, since the virus itself is not known to have a procoagulant effect [1]. Preliminary data emerging from Wuhan, China, and Netherlands have demonstrated evidence of coagulopathy with abnormal parameters such as prothrombin time, activated prothrombin time, D-dimer, fibrinogen, ESR, CRP, thrombocytopenia, and IL6 levels [1–7]. This propensity of abnormal

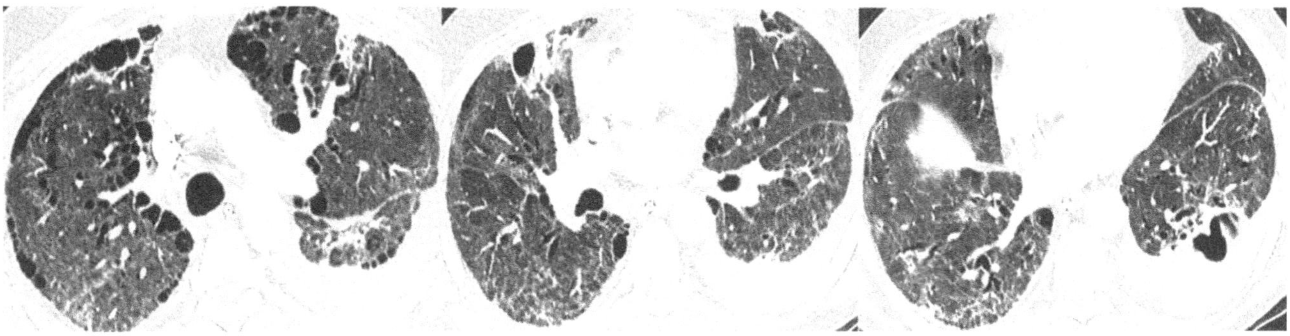

Figure 5: Bilateral lower lobe traction bronchiectasis, evidence of emphysema, post ARDS fibrosis with interlobar septal thickening from recent viral infection, diffuse subpleural cysts, multiple thick-walled cavitary lesions concerning for bacterial superinfection with intrapulmonary abscesses in the lower lobes.

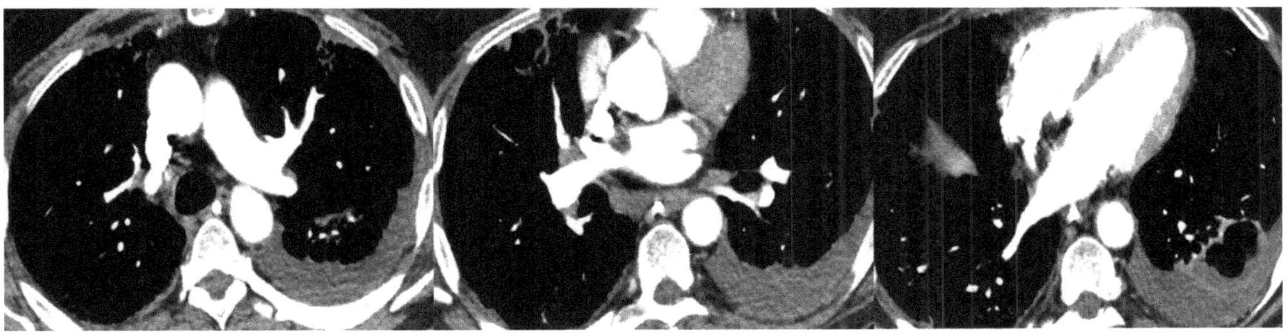

Figure 6: Filling defects in the right lower lobe, right middle lobe, and left upper lobe subsegmental arteries.

values is seen more predominantly in ICU patients dealing with severe SARS-CoV-2 infection (respiratory rate > 30/minute, saturation < 93% on room air, and partial pressure of arterial oxygen/fraction of inspired oxygen PaO_2/FiO_2 < 300 mmHg) [1]. The International Society on Thrombosis and Haemostasis (ISTH) devised SIC score for diagnosis and evaluation for risk of transition to DIC [1]. Elevated levels of D-dimer have been associated with increased mortality risk [2, 8–10]. Thromboprophylactic heparin used in patients with severe COVID-19 showed decreased mortality in patients with SIC score > 4 and patients with D-dimer > 3 mcg/mL likely by mitigating the risk of microvascular thrombosis or pulmonary embolism. However, it is imperative to note that underlying cytokine storm in addition to coagulation activation also contributes to elevated levels of D-dimer, as against solely a thromboembolic phenomenon [1]. Our case and reports from data available from Netherlands and France suggest higher propensity of pulmonary embolism in the intensive care unit with SARS-CoV-2 infection while patients received standard dose of VTE prophylaxis [1, 11]. This has prompted a shift in practice for increase to intermediate dosing VTE prophylaxis with enoxaparin (0.5 mg/kg twice daily) or heparin (7500 U three times daily) [1, 11–13].

SIC score has been based on the effect of inflammatory storm which is expected to resolve with the treatment of sepsis, therefore indicating likely benefit with transient prophylaxis. However, SARS-CoV-2 infection in the setting of absence of definitive treatment has a more prolonged course hence longer duration of anticipated inflammatory storm. With reported cases of thrombosis despite receiving VTE prophylaxis and continued challenge in the availability of appropriate imaging in SARS-CoV-2 infection, it raises concern for the need of empiric therapeutic anticoagulation in select cases. This is in effort to overcome the development of microvascular thrombosis and end-organ dysfunction [1, 2]. Therapeutic anticoagulation is currently only considered in the setting of new worsening respiratory status with evidence of right heart strain or thrombosis on extremity duplex.

We present the case of a patient with severe SARS-CoV-2 infection requiring around 25 days of ventilatory support who had presented with significantly elevated level of D-dimer > 20 mcg/mL. He was maintained on VTE prophylaxis since initial presentation and was switched to empiric therapeutic anticoagulation (day 14 of admission) upon development of worsened respiratory decline and new unstable arrhythmia. He remained on enoxaparin 90 mg twice daily for the majority of ICU stay. Despite receiving therapeutic anticoagulation, he was noted to develop bilateral pulmonary emboli likely contributing to protracted ICU course. This presentation raises concerns regarding severity of cytokine storm as evidenced from the marked elevation of D-dimer, fibrinogen, CRP, and ferritin levels and its effect on COVID-19-associated coagulopathy. This also questions the benefit of VTE prophylactic dosing in preventing microvascular thrombosis or end-organ dysfunction in severe SARS-CoV-2 infection where therapeutic anticoagulation may also be unable to prevent thrombosis.

References

[1] J. M. Connors and J. H. Levy, "COVID-19 and its implications for thrombosis and anticoagulation," *Blood*, vol. 135, no. 23, pp. 2033–2040, 2020.

[2] M. Levi, J. Thachil, T. Iba, and J. H. Levy, "Coagulation abnormalities and thrombosis in patients with COVID-19," *The Lancet Haematology*, vol. 7, no. 6, pp. e438–e440, 2020.

[3] F. J. S. H. Woei-A-Jin, W. E. van der Starre, M. E. T. Tesselaar et al., "Procoagulant tissue factor activity on microparticles is associated with disease severity and bacteremia in febrile urinary tract infections," *Thrombosis Research*, vol. 133, no. 5, pp. 799–803, 2014.

[4] G. Chen, W. G. Di Wu, Y. Cao et al., "Clinical and immunologic features in severe and moderate coronavirus disease 2019," *The Journal of Clinical Investigation*, vol. 130, no. article 137244, 2020.

[5] C. Huang, Y. Wang, X. Li et al., "Clinical features of patients infected with 2019 novel coronavirus in Wuhan, China," *The Lancet*, vol. 395, no. 10223, pp. 497–506, 2020.

[6] M. Levi and M. Scully, "How I treat disseminated intravascular coagulation," *Blood*, vol. 131, no. 8, pp. 845–854, 2018.

[7] G. Lippi, L. Bonfanti, C. Saccenti, and G. Cervellin, "Causes of elevated D-dimer in patients admitted to a large urban emergency department," *European Journal of Internal Medicine*, vol. 25, no. 1, pp. 45–48, 2014.

[8] N. Tang, D. Li, X. Wang, and Z. Sun, "Abnormal coagulation parameters are associated with poor prognosis in patients with novel coronavirus pneumonia," *Journal of Thrombosis and Haemostasis*, vol. 18, no. 4, pp. 844–847, 2020.

[9] W. J. Guan, Z. Y. Ni, Y. Hu et al., "Clinical characteristics of coronavirus disease 2019 in China," *The New England Journal of Medicine*, vol. 382, no. 18, pp. 1708–1720, 2020.

[10] F. Zhou, T. Yu, R. du et al., "Clinical course and risk factors for mortality of adult inpatients with COVID-19 in Wuhan, China: a retrospective cohort study," *The Lancet*, vol. 395, no. 10229, pp. 1054–1062, 2020.

[11] J. Poissy, J. Goutay, M. Caplan et al., "Pulmonary embolism in patients with COVID-19," *Circulation*, vol. 142, no. 2, pp. 184–186, 2020.

[12] C. J. Pannucci, K. I. Fleming, K. Holoyda, L. Moulton, A. M. Prazak, and T. K. Varghese Jr., "Enoxaparin 40 mg per day is inadequate for venous thromboembolism prophylaxis after thoracic surgical procedure," *The Annals of Thoracic Surgery*, vol. 106, no. 2, pp. 404–411, 2018.

[13] T. F. Wang, P. E. Milligan, C. A. Wong, E. N. Deal, M. S. Thoelke, and B. F. Gage, "Efficacy and safety of high-dose thromboprophylaxis in morbidly obese inpatients," *Thrombosis and Haemostasis*, vol. 111, pp. 88–93, 2014.

Flecainide Toxicity Secondary to Accidental Overdose: A Pediatric Case Report of Two Brothers

Sarah E. Gardner Yelton[1] **James B. Leonard**[2] **Caridad M. de la Uz,**[3] **Rajeev S. Wadia**[1] **and Sean S. Barnes**[1]

[1]*Department of Anesthesia and Critical Care Medicine, Charlotte R. Bloomberg Children's Center, Johns Hopkins University School of Medicine, Baltimore, Maryland, USA*
[2]*Maryland Poison Center, Baltimore, Maryland, USA*
[3]*Department of Pediatrics, Division of Pediatric Cardiology, Charlotte R. Bloomberg Children's Center, Johns Hopkins University School of Medicine, Baltimore, Maryland, USA*

Correspondence should be addressed to Sarah E. Gardner Yelton; sgardn19@jhmi.edu

Academic Editor: Tuuli Metsvaht

Flecainide is a class 1C antiarrhythmic with a narrow therapeutic window and thereby a high-risk medication for causing acute toxicity. Dysrhythmias secondary to flecainide ingestion are often refractory to antiarrhythmics and cardioversion, and patients commonly require extracorporeal support. We review the successful resuscitation of two brothers aged 2 and 4 who presented two years apart with unstable wide-complex tachyarrhythmia suspicious for severe flecainide toxicity. Each patient received sodium bicarbonate and 20% intravenous lipid emulsion with a full recovery. While extracorporeal support is often required following flecainide ingestion, we present two cases where it was avoided due to aggressive multimodal management with sodium bicarbonate, electrolyte repletion, and 20% intravenous lipid emulsion. In addition, avoidance of agitation-induced tachycardia may be beneficial.

1. Introduction

Flecainide is a class 1C antiarrhythmic commonly used in pediatrics to treat refractory supraventricular arrhythmias [1]. It has a narrow therapeutic index with goal trough levels ranging from 0.2 μg/mL to 1 μg/mL but toxic levels as low as 0.7 μg/mL and a mortality rate of approximately 22.5% [1–3]. Maximum recommended pediatric daily dosing is 200 mg/m^2/day [1]. Flecainide blocks fast sodium channels to slow cardiac conduction, therefore widening the QRS complex and prolonging both the QT and PR intervals [1]. Signs of serious intoxication include altered mental status, seizures, hypotension, ventricular tachydysrhythmia, severe bradycardia, and AV block [1]. Patients with structural heart disease are particularly vulnerable to arrhythmias [4]. Although there are some reports of successful cardioversion with usual therapies (i.e., amiodarone, lidocaine, and defibrillation), flecainide-induced dysrhythmias are often refractory to these treatments [5, 6]. Alternative therapies include sodium bicarbonate, 20% intravenous lipid emulsion (ILE), and progression to extracorporeal support. However, there are no randomized controlled trials to support these treatments, and neither sodium bicarbonate nor ILE is approved by the Food and Drug Administration for the indication of flecainide overdose [1]. We describe the clinical presentation of two children with flecainide toxicity and review their life-saving resuscitation.

2. Case Presentation

Informed parental consent was obtained to report the following cases.

2.1. Case 1. Child 1 is a 4-year-old male with permanent junctional reciprocating tachycardia (PJRT) on flecainide maintenance therapy (30 mg every 8 hours). He presented to the emergency department three hours after an unwitnessed ingestion of approximately 2 g of flecainide with alternating bradycardia and wide complex tachyarrhythmia (Figure 1(a)), altered mental status, hypotension, and poor perfusion. Presenting heart rate varied from 60 beats per minute (BPM) to 160 BPM, blood pressure was 50/30 mmHg with weak central pulses. Although the patient was breathing spontaneously with oxygen saturations of 100% on a nonrebreather mask, he was responsive only to pain. Initial pH was 7.13 with a pCO_2 of 71 mmHg and a serum bicarbonate level of 23 mmol/L. Flecainide trough level on arrival was 5.6 μg/mL (therapeutic range 0.2 μg/mL to 1 μg/mL). Synchronized cardioversion was performed three times (0.5 J/kg, 1 J/kg, 2 J/kg), and 1-2 mEq/kg 8.4% sodium bicarbonate boluses were given three times, resulting in conversion to sinus rhythm with widened QRS (Figure 1(b)). The patient was transferred to the pediatric intensive care unit (PICU) with consultation from the local poison center.

On admission to the PICU, the patient's heart rate was 160 BPM with no other changes to his physical exam or vital signs. He was intubated and mechanically ventilated with extracorporeal support and a pediatric cardiac electrophysiology consultant immediately available. The patient's serum potassium was 2.5 mEq/L; ionized calcium was 0.9 mmol/L with otherwise normal electrolytes. Sodium bicarbonate boluses were given in 1-2 mEq/kg increments for QRS > 100 ms to maintain a goal pH of 7.5. He was initiated on a sodium bicarbonate infusion at a rate of 1 mEq/kg/hr which continued until the following morning. Serum calcium and potassium were replaced and magnesium given for treatment of the wide complex arrhythmia. Due to continued dysrhythmia and hemodynamic instability despite the above treatments, the child received 1.5 mL/kg 20% ILE bolus followed by a 0.25 mL/kg/min infusion. Following, the child had successful conversion to a sinus rhythm at a rate of 80 BPM with a wide QRS, blood pressure of 90/60 mmHg, and improved perfusion and mental status. The ILE infusion was weaned and completely discontinued after two hours. The child continued to have intermittent runs of pleomorphic ventricular tachycardia with agitation while mechanically ventilated. These episodes of agitation-induced tachycardia were successfully treated with an appropriate sedative dose. Following hemodynamic stability, the child was extubated after 36 hours, at which time the QRS had completely normalized. The patient's serum flecainide level had decreased to 0.3 μg/mL, and his home dose of flecainide restarted. He was discharged home on the same maintenance dose of 30 mg every 8 hours.

2.2. Case 2. Child 2, a 2-year-old male with history of fetal supraventricular tachycardia (resolved), presented to the emergency department with seizure-like activity, altered mental status, bradycardia, and hypotension. Although serum flecainide concentrations were not obtained, the patient's mother reported finding the child near his brother's (child 1) empty flecainide bottle, estimating approximately a 400 mg ingestion 45 minutes prior to presentation. This occurred two years following his brother's hospitalization. On arrival to the hospital, his heart rate was 70 BPM, blood pressure 70/30 mmHg with faint central pulses, and capillary refill time of 4 seconds. He was breathing spontaneously with an oxygen saturation of 100% on a nonrebreather mask. He was responsive only to pain. Presenting pH was 7.2 with a pCO_2 of 63 mmHg and a serum bicarbonate level of 24 mmol/L. After receiving 1 mg/kg lidocaine bolus with no effect, he was given three 0.5 mEq/kg sodium bicarbonate boluses resulting in wide complex tachycardia (Figure 1(c)). He was then transferred to the PICU. The local poison center was consulted.

On admission to the PICU, the patient's heart rate was 150 BPM with a blood pressure of 64/40 mmHg but otherwise no change in his physical exam or vital signs. The child was intubated and mechanically ventilated with extracorporeal support and a pediatric cardiac electrophysiologist immediately available, as above. Sodium bicarbonate boluses were given in 1-2 mEq/kg increments for QRS > 100 ms to maintain a goal pH of 7.5. Serum potassium was 3.3 mEq/L, and ionized calcium was 0.91 mmol/L, both of which were repleted. All other electrolytes were normal. A 50 mg/kg intravenous dose of magnesium sulfate was given for the wide complex tachyarrhythmia with brief conversion to sinus rhythm (Figure 1(d)).

An isoproterenol infusion was initiated in an attempt to suppress recurrent ventricular tachycardia at 0.1 mcg/kg/min, resulting in persistent widening of the QRS, so the infusion was stopped. He also received 1 mEq/kg 3% hypertonic saline. Due to continued dysrhythmia and hemodynamic instability despite the above interventions, the child received 1.5 mL/kg 20% ILE bolus followed by a 0.25 mL/kg/min infusion. He required a second bolus of 1.5 mL/kg 20% ILE due to persistent hypotension, followed by an increase in the infusion rate to 0.5 mL/kg/min. With the above interventions, the child had successful conversion to a sinus rhythm at a rate of 90 BPM with a wide QRS, blood pressure of 100/50 mmHg, strong pulses, and capillary refill time of 2 seconds. The ILE infusion was weaned and completely discontinued after two hours. Similar to his brother, the patient continued to have intermittent runs of pleomorphic ventricular tachycardia with agitation while mechanically ventilated, which resolved with appropriate sedative dosing. Following hemodynamic stability, child 2 was extubated after 24 hours of mechanical ventilation with no remaining sedative requirement. Complete normalization of the QRS took approximately 36 hours. Child protective services was notified in both cases, and a safety plan for discharge was determined.

3. Discussion

Management of flecainide toxicity can be challenging. We described the presentation and successful treatment of two children, which precluded the need for extracorporeal support. In cases of severe intoxication and hemodynamic instability, we recommend an integrated approach with sodium bicarbonate, normalization of electrolytes, ILE, avoidance of agitation, mechanical ventilatory support, and immediate availability of extracorporeal support.

Sodium bicarbonate can be used as monotherapy and is commonly given as the first line treatment for QRS > 100 ms in increments of 1-2 mEq/kg [1, 7–9]. It increases the

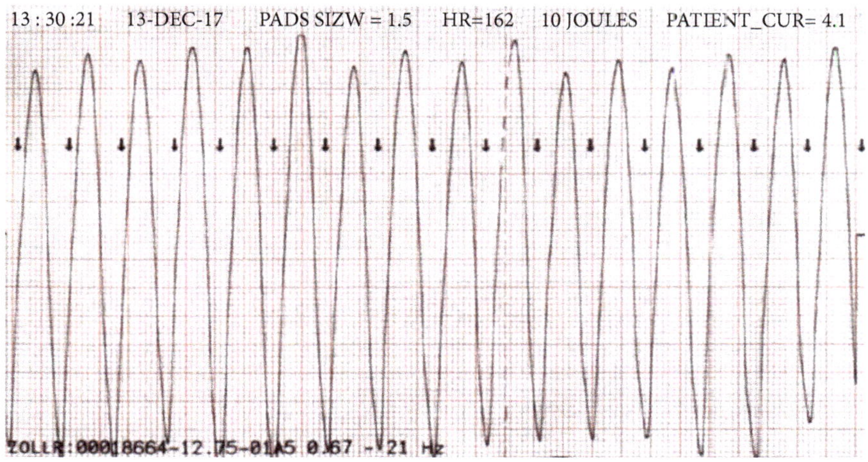

(a)

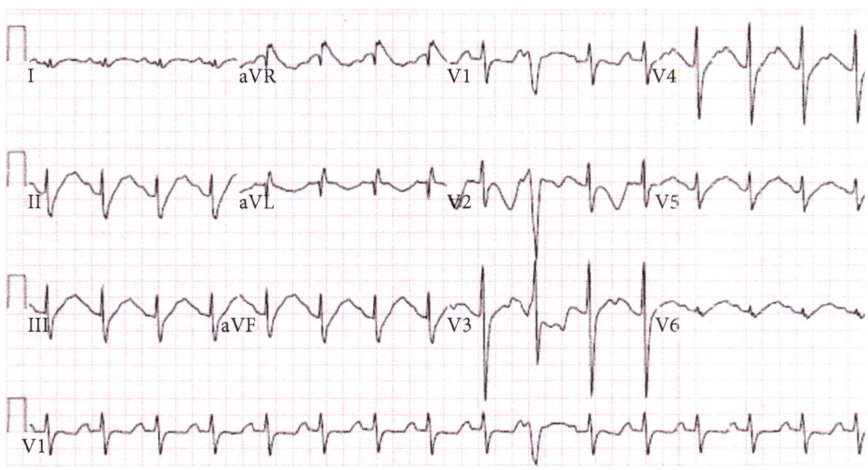

(b)

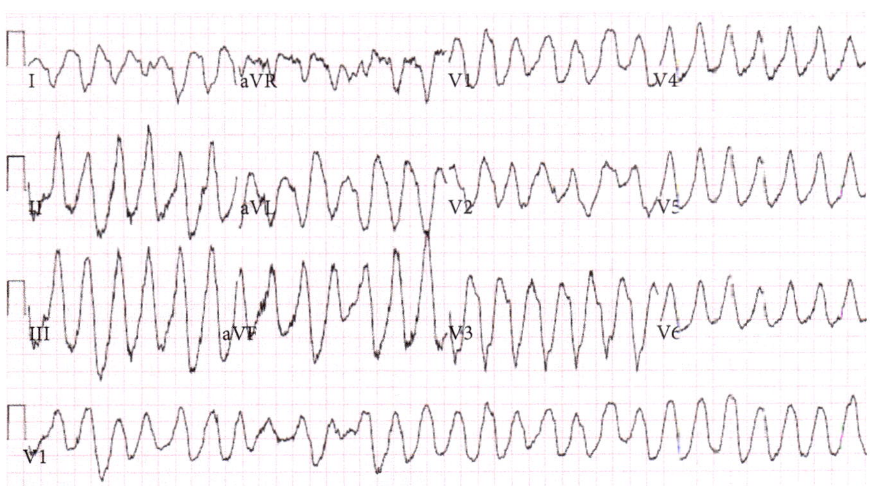

(c)

Figure 1: Continued.

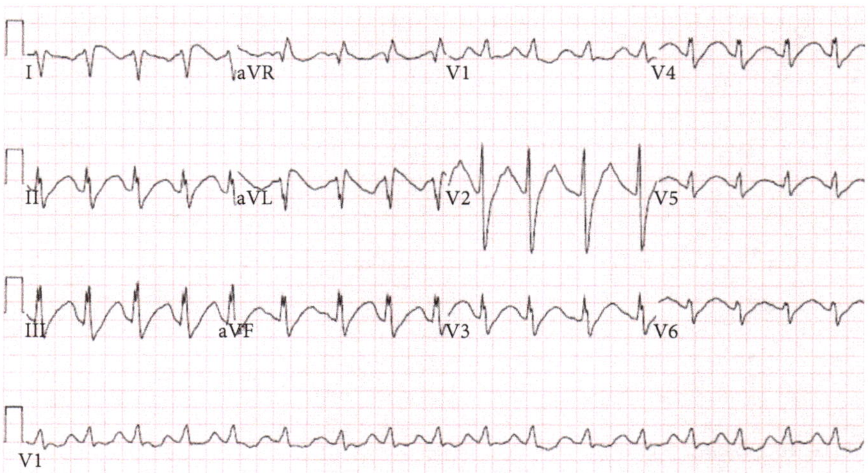

(d)

FIGURE 1: (a) Child 1 rhythm strip on presentation. (b) Child 1 electrocardiogram (EKG) on pediatric intensive care unit admission. (c) Child 2 EKG in emergency department. (d) Child 2 EKG following magnesium administration.

TABLE 1: 20% intravenous lipid emulsion dosing recommendations [20–24].

Initial dosing	Infusion	Refractory	Maximum dosing
1.5 mL/kg 20% ILE as IV bolus over 2-3 minutes	0.25 mL/kg/min for 60 min	If continued instability after 3-5 minutes of infusion, repeat initial bolus dose and increase infusion to 0.5 mL/kg/min. Can give additional bolus doses for clinical deterioration.	Continue infusion for 10 minutes after circulatory stability is achieved. 10-12 mL/kg cumulative dosing within first 30 minutes of administration.

availability of extracellular sodium to compete with flecainide for binding sodium channels and raises the serum pH to increase the electrochemical gradient across cell membranes [10]. In animal models, sodium bicarbonate decreases QRS prolongation caused by flecainide and improves survival when compared with normal saline [11, 12]. Although child 1 received a bicarbonate infusion, administering serial bolus doses is considered more effective. Alkalization of the urine following bicarbonate administration may delay clearance of flecainide, so adjunctive therapies have been proposed [1]. Limited data supports the use of 3% hypertonic saline as an adjunct to sodium bicarbonate administration [13]. Additionally, isoproterenol has been used to reverse toxic effects of flecainide by increasing inward sodium current [14].

The rationale for using intravenous lipid emulsion (ILE) in flecainide toxicity is extrapolated from its use in the treatment for regional anesthetic drug toxicity [15, 16]. Similar to flecainide, regional anesthetic drugs (i.e., bupivacaine and ropivacaine) are also lipophilic and block sodium channels. ILE creates a "lipid sink" that removes any lipophilic drug from the intravascular space by incorporating it into the fat globules of the lipid, thus sequestering it from the remainder of the body [15, 17, 18]. Additionally, it increases inotropy [19]. In a systematic review, Jamaty et al. recommend ILE for local anesthetic toxicity in the setting of neurologic or cardiovascular deterioration, in addition to hemodynamic instability from intoxication from other fat-soluble drugs, after other supportive measures and antidotes have been unsuccessful [20]. In the case of flecainide ingestion, collaborative guidelines from several toxicology societies give ILE use a neutral recommendation if cardiac arrest or potential life-threatening ingestion is present and recommend against its use for non-life-threatening ingestions [21, 22]. Most commonly cited dosing is reported in Table 1. There have been reports of fat emboli, pancreatitis, and acute respiratory distress syndrome with administration of large doses of ILE and decreasing the infusion rate followed by ILE discontinuation as soon as hemodynamic stability is achieved is suggested [20–24]. The most common side effect, which occurred in our case, is lipemia, which can interfere with serum analysis and complicates laboratory interpretation [20].

Rhythm response to normalization of electrolytes has been reported, and as per pediatric advanced life support recommendations, magnesium should be administered for polymorphic ventricular tachycardia [1, 25, 26]. Extracorporeal support is commonly required for unstable refractory arrhythmias to support hemodynamics until drug clearance can occur [27, 28]. Flecainide clearance can be prolonged as the average half-life is 20 hours, and failure to provide hemodynamic support can result in death or permanent neurologic injury. The volume of distribution of flecainide precludes the use of dialysis and hemoperfusion for removal and is therefore not recommended [29].

Both children had progressive widening of the QRS complex with tachycardia in the setting of agitation during the first 12 hours postingestion. This association of tachycardia and QRS prolongation has been described in both human and animal models with maintenance flecainide doses, even in the absence of toxicity [30–32]. At a higher heart rate, more sodium channels are normally open, and since flecainide preferentially blocks open channels, its effects may be exacerbated [31]. To our knowledge, no other case reports describe induction of wide-complex tachycardia with agitation. In both children, this arrhythmia was successfully reversed with administration of sedation.

4. Conclusions

Flecainide ingestions can cause wide complex tachyarrhythmias and hemodynamic collapse refractory to typical management, often requiring extracorporeal support. While we cannot conclude with certainty if one treatment was solely responsible for the improvement observed in our patients, we do provide validation for a multimodal treatment approach to flecainide toxicity, preventing the need for extracorporeal support. Flecainide toxicity should be treated with sodium bicarbonate boluses; electrolyte repletion, with particular attention to magnesium: intravenous lipid emulsion; judicious administration of sedatives to avoid tachycardia from agitation; and if needed extracorporeal support.

Consent

Written consent from caregiver obtained for case publication.

eferences

I IBM Micromedex® DRUGDEX® (electronic version), *Flecainide*, IBM Watson Health/EBSCO Information Services, Greenwood Village, Colorado; Cambridge, Massachusetts, USA, 2021, https://www.dynamedex.com.

'. Tamargo, J. Y. Le Heuzey, and P. Mabo, "Narrow therapeutic ndex drugs: a clinical pharmacological consideration to flecaiide," *European Journal of Clinical Pharmacology*, vol. 71,). 5, pp. 549–567, 2015.

Koppel, U. Oberdisse, and G. Heinemeyer, "Clinical course 1 outcome in class IC antiarrhythmic overdose," *Journal of :icology: Clinical Toxicology*, vol. 28, no. 4, pp. 433–444, 0.

:anu, D. Agostini, G. Grollier, A. Belin, B. Valette, and J. C. :r, "Proarrhythmic effects of antiarrhythmic drugs," *La e de Médecine Interne*, vol. 16, no. 8, pp. 602–607, 1995.

'gers and P. N. Board, "Amiodarone used in successful itation after near-fatal flecainide overdose," *Resuscita-* ɔl. 53, no. 1, pp. 105–108, 2002.

ıley, J. Bourke, and A. Gascoigne, "Survival in a case of ·atening flecainide overdose," *Intensive Care Medicine*, no. 7, pp. 740–742, 1998.

'se and C. J. Banks, "Pediatric flecainide toxicity from a 'ose," *The American Journal of Emergency Medicine*, o. 9, pp. 2095.e1–2095.e2, 2012.

P. Garrett, and C. Anstey, "Managing cardiovascular n severe flecainide overdose without recourse to ›real therapy," *Emergency Medicine Australasia*, . 2, pp. 155–159, 2007.

[9] D. H. Jang, R. S. Hoffman, and L. S. Nelson, "A case of near-fatal flecainide overdose in a neonate successfully treated with sodium bicarbonate," *The Journal of Emergency Medicine*, vol. 44, no. 4, pp. 781–783, 2013.

[10] S. Ranger, R. Sheldon, B. Fermini, and S. Nattel, "Modulation of flecainide's cardiac sodium channel blocking actions by extracellular sodium: a possible cellular mechanism for the action of sodium salts in flecainide cardiotoxicity," *The Journal of Pharmacology and Experimental Therapeutics*, vol. 264, no. 3, pp. 1160–1167, 1993.

[11] D. E. Keyler and P. R. Pentel, "Hypertonic sodium bicarbonate partially reverses QRS prolongation due to flecainide in rats," *Life Sciences*, vol. 45, no. 17, pp. 1575–1580, 1989.

[12] D. M. Salerno, M. M. Murakami, R. B. Johnston, D. E. Keyler, and P. R. Pentel, "Reversal of flecainide-induced ventricular arrhythmia by hypertonic sodium bicarbonate in dogs," *The American Journal of Emergency Medicine*, vol. 13, no. 3, pp. 285–293, 1995.

[13] L. Tortora and G. Canning, "Severe flecainide toxicity with cardiac arrest treated with 3% hypertonic saline in addition to standard sodium bicarbonate therapy," *Journal of Medical Toxicology*, vol. 15, 2019.

[14] B. Avitall, J. W. Hare, P. Tchou, M. Jazayeri, and M. Akhtar, "Flecainide toxicity: reversal of drug effects by isoproterenol infusion," *Journal of Cardiovascular Electrophysiology*, vol. 2, no. 5, pp. 431–440, 1991.

[15] G. L. Weinberg, T. VadeBoncouer, G. A. Ramaraju, M. F. Garcia-Amaro, and M. J. Cwik, "Pretreatment or resuscitation with a lipid infusion shifts the dose-response to bupivacaine-induced asystole in rats," *Anesthesiology*, vol. 88, no. 4, pp. 1071–1075, 1998.

[16] M. A. Rosenblatt, M. Abel, G. W. Fischer, C. J. Itzkovich, and J. B. Eisenkraft, "Successful use of a 20% lipid emulsion to resuscitate a patient after a presumed bupivacaine-related cardiac arrest," *Anesthesiology*, vol. 105, no. 1, pp. 217-218, 2006.

[17] J. F. Butterworth IV, "Models and mechanisms of local anesthetic cardiac toxicity: a review," *Regional Anesthesia and Pain Medicine*, vol. 35, no. 2, pp. 167–176, 2010.

[18] J. Picard and T. Meek, "Lipid emulsion to treat overdose of local anaesthetic: the gift of the glob," *Anaesthesia*, vol. 61, no. 2, pp. 107–109, 2006.

[19] M. R. Fettiplace, R. Ripper, K. Lis et al., "Rapid cardiotonic effects of lipid emulsion infusion," *Critical Care Medicine*, vol. 41, no. 8, pp. e156–e162, 2013.

[20] C. Jamaty, B. Bailey, A. Larocque, E. Notebaert, K. Sanogo, and J. M. Chauny, "Lipid emulsions in the treatment of acute poisoning: a systematic review of human and animal studies," *Clinical Toxicology (Philadelphia, Pa.)*, vol. 48, no. 1, pp. 1-27, 2010.

[21] American College of Medical Toxicology, "ACMT position statement: guidance for the use of intravenous lipid emulsion," *Journal of Medical Toxicology*, vol. 13, no. 1, pp. 124-125, 2017.

[22] S. Gosselin, L. C. Hoegberg, R. S. Hoffman et al., "Evidence-based recommendations on the use of intravenous lipid emulsion therapy in poisoning," *Clinical Toxicology*, vol. 54, no. 10, pp. 899–923, 2016.

[23] G. Weinberg, "LipidRescue," 2020, http://www.lipidrescue.org.

[24] G. Cave, W. Harrop-Griffiths, M. Harvey et al., "AAGBI safety guideline: management of severe local anaesthetic toxicity," 2020, http://www.aagbi.org/sites/default/files/la_toxicity_2010_0.pdf.

[25] A. Khavandi and P. R. Walker, "Flecainide cardiotoxicity precipitated by electrolyte imbalance. Caution with thiazide diuretics," *Emergency Medicine Journal*, vol. 24, no. 5, 2007.

[26] R. Ohki, M. Takahashi, O. Mizuno et al., "Torsades de pointes ventricular tachycardia induced by mosapride and flecainide in the presence of hypokalemia," *Pacing and Clinical Electrophysiology*, vol. 24, no. 1, pp. 119–121, 2001.

[27] N. de Schryver, P. Hantson, V. Haufroid, and M. Dechamps, "Cardiogenic shock in a hemodialyzed patient on flecainide: treatment with intravenous fat emulsion, extracorporeal cardiac life support, and CytoSorb® hemoadsorption," *Case Reports in Cardiology*, vol. 2019, Article ID 1905871, 5 pages, 2019.

[28] S. Sivalingam, V. Gadiraju, M. Hariharan, A. R. Atreya, J. E. Flack, and H. Aziz, "Flecainide toxicity — treatment with intravenous fat emulsion and extra corporeal life support," *Acute Cardiac Care*, vol. 15, no. 4, pp. 91-92, 2013.

[29] R. Wurzberger, E. Witter, H. Avenhaus, H. Hennemann, and J. U. Becker, "Hemoperfusion in flecainide poisoning," *Klinische Wochenschrift*, vol. 64, no. 9, pp. 442–444, 1986.

[30] C. Cros, M. Skinner, J. Moors, P. Lainee, and J. P. Valentin, "Detecting drug-induced prolongation of the QRS complex: new insights for cardiac safety assessment," *Toxicology and Applied Pharmacology*, vol. 265, no. 2, pp. 200–208, 2012.

[31] T. Sadanaga, S. Ogawa, Y. Okada et al., "Clinical evaluation of the use-dependent QRS prolongation and the reverse use-dependent QT prolongation of class I and class III antiarrhythmic agents and their value in predicting efficacy," *American Heart Journal*, vol. 126, no. 1, pp. 114–121, 1993.

[32] M. A. Valentino, A. Panakos, L. Ragupathi, J. Williams, and B. B. Pavri, "Flecainide toxicity: a case report and systematic review of its electrocardiographic patterns and management," *Cardiovascular Toxicology*, vol. 17, no. 3, pp. 260–266, 2017.

27

Euglycemic Diabetic Ketoacidosis in Pregnancy: A Case Report and Review of Current Literature

Johnny F. Jaber[1] **Matthew Standley,**[1] **and Raju Reddy**[2]

[1]*Division of Internal Medicine, University of Florida College of Medicine, Gainesville, FL, USA*
[2]*Division of Pulmonary, Critical Care and Sleep Medicine, University of Florida College of Medicine, Gainesville, FL, USA*

Correspondence should be addressed to Raju Reddy; raju.reddy@medicine.ufl.edu

Academic Editor: Kenneth S. Waxman

Diabetic ketoacidosis (DKA) in pregnancy is associated with high fetal mortality rates. A small percentage of DKA occurs in the absence of high glucose levels seen in traditional DKA. Prompt recognition and management is crucial. We report a case of a 30-year-old pregnant woman with type 1 diabetes mellitus admitted with euglycemic DKA (blood glucose <200 mg/dL). Initial laboratory testing revealed a severe anion gap acidosis with pH 7.11, anion gap 23, elevated β-hydroxybutyric acid of 9.60 mmol/L, and a blood glucose of 183 mg/dL—surprisingly low given her severe acidosis. The ketoacidosis persisted despite high doses of glucose and insulin infusions. Due to nonresolving acidosis, her hospital course was complicated by spontaneous intrauterine fetal demise. Euglycemia and severe acidosis continued to persist until delivery of fetus and placenta occurred. It was observed that the insulin sensitivity dramatically increased after delivery of fetus and placenta leading to rapid correction of ketoacidosis. This case highlights that severe ketonemia can occur despite the absence of severely elevated glucose levels. We discuss the mechanism that leads to this pathophysiologic state and summarize previously published case reports about euglycemic DKA in pregnancy.

1. Introduction

Euglycemic diabetic ketoacidosis (EDKA) is a biochemical triad consisting of blood glucose level less than 200 mg/dL, increased anion gap metabolic acidosis, and ketonemia [1]. The incidence of EDKA is reportedly between 0.8% and 1.1% of all pregnant DKA cases [2]. Euglycemia presents a diagnostic challenge often leading providers to believe ketoacidosis is less severe. As a result, EDKA can frequently go unrecognized. Prompt recognition of EDKA is critical in pregnancy, since fetal demise can be as high as 35% without appropriate treatment [3]. We report a case of EDKA in the third trimester of pregnancy and discuss the management challenges in a patient with euglycemia and a high ketone burden. We also summarize other reported cases of EDKA (Table 1).

2. Case Presentation

A 30-year-old gravida 2 para 0101 (0 full term, 1 preterm, 0 abortions, and 1 live child) woman at 32 weeks, 3 days gestation presented to our hospital with a two-day history of nausea and vomiting. Her prior medical history included type 1 diabetes mellitus on continuous glucose monitoring and insulin pump. She has had a history of prior episodes of diabetic ketoacidosis requiring hospitalization; however, as her home glucose readings were only marginally elevated at 100–200 mg/dL, she did not think to present to the hospital sooner than she did. Upon initial examination in the emergency department, she appeared uncomfortable with Kussmaul breathing. Fetal heart monitoring showed absent variability and recurrent late decelerations. Her initial admission laboratory results showed a blood glucose of 183 mg/dL, acidosis with an anion gap of 23, pH 7.11, β-hydroxybutyric acid (β-HA) 9.6 mmol/L (normal 0.02–0.27 mmol/L), and lactate 0.65 mmol/L (normal 0.3–1.5 mmol/L). The patient was admitted to the high risk obstetrics service for further management of her acidosis and resulting fetal distress. As the patient was initially euglycemic, insulin infusion was initiated at 2 units/h as per the institution's DKA protocol. After four liters of bolus intravenous fluids, a maintenance fluid rate of 5% dextrose/0.45% NaCl solution at 250 mL/h was initiated.

TABLE 1: Summary of literature describing cases of euglycemic diabetic ketoacidosis in pregnant mothers.

Authors	Age (years)	Diabetic history	Gestational age	Admission blood glucose (mg/dL)	Outcome of mother	Outcome of fetus
Bryant et al. [18]	Describes three cases of diabetic ketoacidosis in pregnant patients with admission glucose <200 mg/dL. No specifics about the three cases are given					
Cardonell et al. [19]	33	Type 2 diabetes mellitus	Third trimester, 35 weeks	134	Discharged home	Emergent C-section at 35 weeks
Chico et al. [14]	29	Type 1 diabetes mellitus	Third trimester, 34 weeks	87	Discharged home	Nonemergent C-section at 34 weeks
Clark et al. [20]	34	Gestational diabetes	Third trimester, 36 weeks	140	Discharged home	Nonemergent C-section at 36 weeks
Cullen et al. [21]	Describes four cases of diabetic ketoacidosis in pregnant patients with admission glucose <200 mg/dL. No specifics about the four cases are given					
Darbhamulla et al. [22]	30	Gestational diabetes	Third trimester, 33 weeks	95	Discharged home	Elective C-section at 39 weeks
Franke et al. [15]	23	Gestational diabetes	Third trimester, 32 weeks	127	Discharged home	Delivery at 38 weeks
Frise et al. [23]	40	Gestational diabetes	Third trimester, 35 weeks	52–85	Discharged home	Emergent C-section at 35 weeks
Guo et al. [4]	29	Unknown	Third trimester, 32 weeks	124	Discharged home	Delivery at 38 weeks
Kamalakannan et al. [24]	28	Type 1 diabetes mellitus	Third trimester, 36 weeks	234	Discharged home	Intrauterine fetal demise
Karpate et al. [25]	25	Unknown	Third trimester, 37 weeks	103	Discharged home	Delivery at 37 weeks
Lucero and Chapela [13]	22	Type 1 diabetes mellitus	First trimester, unknown weeks	153	Discharged home	Unknown
Madaan et al. [26]	30	Type 2 diabetes mellitus	Third trimester, 36 weeks	75–155	Discharged home	Elective C-section at 38 weeks
Madaan et al. [26]	23	Gestational diabetes	Third trimester, 34 weeks	89–164	Discharged home	Emergent C-section at 37 weeks
Montoro et al. [27]	Describes two cases of diabetic ketoacidosis in pregnant patients with admission glucose <200 mg/dL. No specifics about the two cases are given					
Napoli et al. [16]	26	Type 1 diabetes mellitus	Third trimester, 34 weeks	211	Discharged home	Elective C-section at 34 weeks
Oliver et al. [28]	29	Type 1 diabetes mellitus	Third trimester, 28 weeks	245	Discharged home	Elective C-section at 34 weeks
Rivas et al. [29]	39	Gestational diabetes	Third trimester, 32 weeks	120	Discharged home	Emergent C-section at 32 weeks
Tarif and Al Badr [30]	37	Type 2 diabetes mellitus	Third trimester, 35 weeks	77	Discharged home	Unknown
Yu et al. [31]	30	Type 2 diabetes mellitus	Third trimester, 28 weeks	121	Discharged home	Elective C-section at 36 weeks

Approximately four hours after admission, the patient's euglycemia continued to persist with serum glucose readings averaging 165 mg/dL (Figure 1). Given this euglycemia, the obstetrics team continued to cautiously titrate the patient's insulin drip. Over the next hour, her acidosis progressively worsened with a blood pH nadir of 6.97. Fetal heart tracings continually deteriorated. Unfortunately, the patient was not a surgical candidate for emergent fetal delivery due to her severe acidosis. Bicarbonate containing maintenance fluids were not utilized; however, a total of seven ampules of bicarbonate were administered to the patient throughout her hospitalization to attempt to stabilize the fetus, though bicarbonate containing drips were never initiated. The obstetrics team at this time consulted the medical intensive care unit (MICU) for assistance with further management. At this time, the MICU team consulted endocrinology for assistance with management. The patient's fluids were changed to a 10% dextrose containing fluids at 250 mL/h with the goal of intensifying the insulin infusion to correct the ketoacidosis. Despite this, however, the patient's respiratory status declined to the point of requiring intubation and mechanical ventilation. Approximately eight hours after admission, the fetal heart rate became difficult to detect, and intrauterine fetal demise was declared.

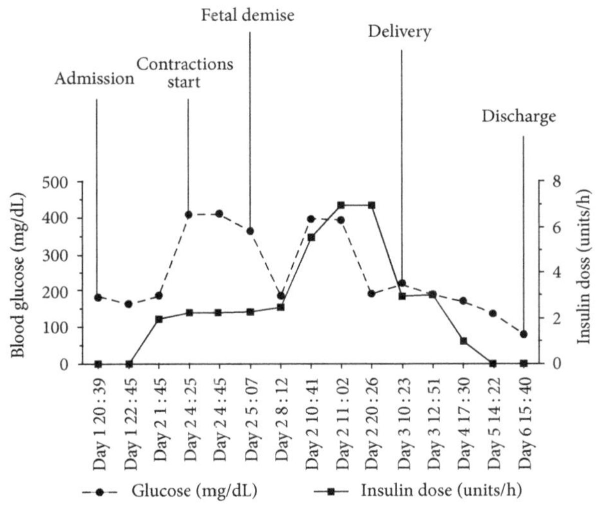

FIGURE 1: Blood glucose levels and insulin drip rates throughout the patient's hospitalization by day and time of significant events.

Despite fetal demise, the patient's insulin requirements were still larger than expected at 7 units/h. Endocrinology believed that this was secondary to the placental hormones still in the patient's circulation causing significant peripheral insulin resistance. It was determined that until delivery occurred, the patient would continue to have significant insulin resistance. As soon as one hour after delivery, the patient's insulin sensitivity rapidly improved, and glucose sequestration by the placental circulation disappeared. Acidosis began to rapidly improve. Her glucose now ranged between 200 mg/dL and 400 mg/dL. Her insulin drip was rapidly weaned to 3 units/h, pH continued to rise to 7.33, and the anion gap closed to 7 (Figure 1). The patient was extubated on hospital day 2, and was discharged home three days later without any further events.

3. Discussion

EDKA during pregnancy is an obstetric and medical emergency. It is characterized by a state of marked insulin resistance, severe electrolyte derangement, and only marginal elevation of serum glucose. Early recognition and management are crucial, since prolonged ketosis is associated with neurologic complications, and even death in the fetus.

The incidence of DKA is higher in pregnant patients compared to nonpregnant patients, 8.9% vs. 3.1%, respectively [4]. A number of physiologic changes occur in pregnancy predisposing one to severe ketoacidosis [4]. This occurs via multiple mechanisms, the first being marked insulin resistance during pregnancy from several hormones including human placental lactogen, placental insulinase, and progesterone. These hormones peak in the second and third trimesters and can inhibit the effects of maternal insulin resulting in relative insulin deficiency [4]. This could explain why DKA is most common during the second and third trimesters (Table 1). To compensate for the increased insulin resistance, insulin production increases with advancing gestational age [5]. In our case, it is likely that the mother had relative insulin deficiency in the setting of an acute illness and underlying insulin resistance leading to ketosis. Other contributory factors for increased incidence of DKA in pregnancy include lower serum bicarbonate levels (19–20 mEq/L), which occur as a compensatory mechanism for pregnancy-induced respiratory alkalosis.

The mechanism underlying ketosis in pregnancy is similar to that of nonpregnant patients. Ketosis occurs much more rapidly in diabetic patients that are pregnant. In the third trimester alone, the maternal metabolic rate increases by an average of 30% compared to prepregnancy [6]. As a result, even short periods of starvation in pregnant patients predispose them to developing ketosis. Metzger et al. showed that pregnant patients had higher levels of free fatty acids and β-HA after a 12 h fast compared to nonpregnant patients [7]. This might serve as a mechanism to provide nutrition to the fetus during periods of decreased caloric intake. In our case, the patient had decreased oral intake for 36 h prior to presentation. The relative insulin deficiency, prolonged starvation, and upregulation of counterregulatory hormones were the likely driving factors for the severe ketonemia observed in our patient.

Not only does ketosis occur much more rapidly in pregnant diabetic patients, it also occurs at much lower serum glucose levels compared to nonpregnant patients [4]. The proposed mechanisms are as follows. First, placental glucose transporters (GLUT-1, GLUT-4, and GLUT-9) are increased during pregnancy. Among those on insulin therapy, placental expression of these receptors is increased even further [8]. As a result of increased placental glucose transporters, maternal levels may be only marginally elevated despite a high ketone burden. Second, euglycemia may also occur due to the physiologic hemodilution that occurs due to increased plasma volume in pregnancy [9]. Third, glomerular filtration rate can increase by 60% from the first trimester to around 4 weeks postpartum, contributing to an osmotic diuresis and thus, absence of marked hyperglycemia despite a high ketone burden [10].

DKA during pregnancy is associated with multiple immediate and late fetal complications. Immediate complications include high fetal mortality rates at 27%–35%, decreased uterine perfusion, fetal hypoxia, and recurrent late decelerations [3, 11, 12]. Our patient had multiple late decelerations on presentation likely reflecting the severity and duration of acidosis. Generally, it is recommended to continue the pregnancy while attempts are made to identify and correct the physiologic derangement. Typically, once the acidosis is corrected, fetal abnormalities improve [4, 12–16]. Emergent cesarean delivery should only be attempted if the maternal condition worsens, but this is associated with high maternal morbidity and mortality. Long term effects of ketoacidosis include impaired brain development. One study found an inverse relationship with maternal ketonemia and mental development index scores (lower scores indicating inadequate development) at two years of age [17]. Prevention remains a key aspect of managing diabetic pregnant patients. Women should be counseled on checking serum ketones in cases of acute illness or if blood glucose levels begin to rise above their baseline.

4. Conclusions

Despite a normal presenting blood glucose level, it is imperative to have a high suspicion for ketoacidosis in an acidotic pregnant patient with diabetes mellitus or gestational diabetes. Placental sequestration of blood glucose can make DKA a diagnostic and therapeutic challenge. Serum ketones must be checked in any diabetic patient during periods of illness. High doses of insulin may be required despite euglycemia to correct acidosis and ketonemia.

Our case highlights the diagnostic and treatment challenges associated with EDKA, and its accompanying complications including fetal demise. The mainstay of treatment remains early recognition and timely administration of fluids, carbohydrates, and insulin.

References

[1] A. E. Kitabchi, G. E. Umpierrez, J. M. Miles, and J. N. Fisher, "Hyperglycemic crises in adult patients with diabetes," *Diabetes Care*, vol. 32, no. 7, pp. 1335–1343, 2009.

[2] S. P. Chauhan, K. G. Perry, B. N. McLaughlin, W. E. Roberts, C. A. Sullivan, and J. C. Morrison, "Diabetic ketoacidosis complicating pregnancy," *Journal of Perinatology*, vol. 16, no. 3 Pt 1, pp. 173–175, 1996.

[3] M. G. Dalfra, S. Burlina, G. Sartore, and A. Lapolla, "Ketoacidosis in diabetic pregnancy," *The Journal of Maternal-Fetal and Neonatal Medicine*, vol. 29, no. 2016, pp. 2889–2895, 2016.

[4] R.-X. Guo, L.-Z. Yang, L.-X. Li, and X.-P. Zhao, "Diabetic ketoacidosis in pregnancy tends to occur at lower blood glucose levels: case-control study and a case report of euglycemic diabetic ketoacidosis in pregnancy," *Journal of Obstetrics and Gynaecology Research*, vol. 34, no. 3, pp. 324–330, 2008.

[5] P. M. Catalano, N. M. Drago, and S. B. Amini, "Longitudinal changes in pancreatic β-cell function and metabolic clearance rate of insulin in pregnant women with normal and abnormal glucose tolerance," *Diabetes Care*, vol. 21, no. 3, pp. 403–408, 1998.

[6] M. Lof, H. Olausson, K. Bostrom, B. Janerot-Sjöberg, A. Sohlstrom, and E. Forsum, "Changes in basal metabolic rate during pregnancy in relation to changes in body weight and composition, cardiac output, insulin-like growth factor I, and thyroid hormones and in relation to fetal growth," *The American Journal of Clinical Nutrition*, vol. 81, no. 3, pp. 678–685, 2005.

[7] B. E. Metzger, V. Ravnikar, R. A. Vileisis, and N. Freinkel, ""Accelerated starvation" and the skipped breakfast in late normal pregnancy," *The Lancet*, vol. 319, no. 8272, pp. 588–592, 1982.

[8] P. J. Stanirowski, D. Szukiewicz, M. Pyzlak, N. Abdalla, W. Sawicki, and K. Cendrowski, "Impact of pre-gestational and gestational diabetes mellitus on the expression of glucose transporters GLUT-1, GLUT-4 and GLUT-9 in human term placenta," *Endocrine*, vol. 55, no. 3, pp. 799–808, 2017.

[9] S. de Haas, C. Ghossein-Doha, S. M. J. van Kuijk, J. van Drongelen, and M. E. A. Spaanderman, "Physiological adaptation of maternal plasma volume during pregnancy: a systematic review and meta-analysis," *Ultrasound in Obstetrics & Gynecology*, vol. 49, no. 2, pp. 177–187, 2017.

[10] P. Moran, P. H. Baylis, M. D. Lindheimer, and J. M. Davison, "Glomerular ultrafiltration in normal and pre-eclamptic pregnancy," *Journal of the American Society of Nephrology*, vol. 14, no. 3, pp. 648–652, 2003.

[11] M. B. Schneider, G. E. Umpierrez, R. D. Ramsey, W. C. Mabie, and K. A. Bennett, "Pregnancy complicated by diabetic ketoacidosis: maternal and fetal outcomes," *Diabetes Care*, vol. 26, no. 3, pp. 958–959, 2003.

[12] Y. Takahashi, I. Kawabata, A. Shinohara, and T. Tamaya, "Transient fetal blood flow redistribution induced by maternal diabetic ketoacidosis diagnosed by Doppler ultrasonography," *Prenatal Diagnosis*, vol. 20, no. 6, pp. 524–525, 2000.

[13] P. Lucero and S. Chapela, "Euglycemic diabetic ketoacidosis in the ICU: 3 case reports and review of literature," *Case Reports in Critical Care*, vol. 2018, Article ID 1747850, 6 pages, 2018.

[14] M. Chico, S. N. Levine, and D. F. Lewis, "Normoglycemic diabetic ketoacidosis in pregnancy," *Journal of Perinatology*, vol. 28, no. 4, pp. 310–312, 2008.

[15] B. Franke, D. Carr, and M. H. Hatem, "A case of euglycaemic diabetic ketoacidosis in pregnancy," *Diabetic Medicine*, vol. 18, no. 10, pp. 858–859, 2001.

[16] A. Napoli, M. Framarino, A. Colatrella et al., "Eating disorders and diabetic ketoacidosis in a pregnant woman with type 1 diabetes: a case report," *Eating and Weight Disorders - Studies on Anorexia, Bulimia and Obesity*, vol. 16, no. 2, pp. e146–e149, 2011.

[17] T. Rizzo, B. E. Metzger, W. J. Burns, and K. Burns, "Correlations between antepartum maternal metabolism and intelligence of offspring," *New England Journal of Medicine*, vol. 325, no. 13, pp. 911–916, 1991.

[18] S. N. Bryant, C. L. Herrera, D. B. Nelson, and F. G. Cunningham, "Diabetic ketoacidosis complicating pregnancy," *Journal of Neonatal-Perinatal Medicine*, vol. 10, no. 1, pp. 17–23, 2017.

[19] B. L. Cardonell, B. A. Marks, and M. H. Entrup, "Normoglycemic diabetic ketoacidosis in a pregnant patient with type II diabetes mellitus presenting for emergent cesarean delivery," *A & A Case Reports*, vol. 6, no. 8, pp. 228–229, 2016.

[20] J. D. A. Clark, A. McConnell, and M. Hartog, "Normoglycaemic ketoacidosis in a woman with gestational diabetes," *Diabetic Medicine*, vol. 8, no. 4, pp. 388–389, 1991.

[21] M. T. Cullen, E. A. Reece, C. J. Homko, and E. Sivan, "The changing presentations of diabetic ketoacidosis during pregnancy," *American Journal of Perinatology*, vol. 13, no. 7, pp. 449–451, 1996.

[22] S. Darbhamulla, N. Shah, and P. Bosio, "Euglycaemic ketoacidosis in a patient with gestational diabetes," *European Journal of Obstetrics & Gynecology and Reproductive Biology*, vol. 163, no. 1, pp. 118–119, 2012.

[23] C. J. Frise, L. Mackillop, K. Joash, and C. Williamson, "Starvation ketoacidosis in pregnancy," *European Journal of Obstetrics & Gynecology and Reproductive Biology*, vol. 167, no. 1, pp. 1–7, 2013.

[24] D. Kamalakannan, V. Baskar, D. M. Barton, and T. A. M. Abdu, "Diabetic ketoacidosis in pregnancy," *Postgraduate Medical Journal*, vol. 79, no. 934, pp. 454–457, 2003.

[25] S. J. Karpate, H. Morsi, M. Shehmar, J. Dale, and C. Patel, "Euglycemic ketoacidosis in pregnancy and its management: case report and review of literature," *European Journal of Obstetrics & Gynecology and Reproductive Biology*, vol. 171, no. 2, pp. 386–387, 2013.

[26] M. Madaan, K. Aggarwal, R. Sharma, and S. S. Trivedi, "Diabetic ketoacidosis occurring with lower blood glucose levels in pregnancy: a report of two cases," *Journal of Reproductive Medicine*, vol. 57, no. 9-10, pp. 452–455, 2012.

[27] M. N. Montoro, V. P. Myers, J. H. Mestman, Y. Xu, B. G. Anderson, and S. H. Golde, "Outcome of pregnancy in diabetic ketoacidosis," *American Journal of Perinatology*, vol. 10, no. 1, pp. 17–20, 1993.

[28] R. Oliver, P. Jagadeesan, R. J. Howard, and K. Nikookam, "Euglycaemic diabetic ketoacidosis in pregnancy: an unusual presentation," *Journal of Obstetrics and Gynaecology*, vol. 27, no. 3, 308 pages, 2007.

[29] M. M. Rivas, P. Z. Belmar, P. A. Durruty, L. M. Sanhueza, and G. S. López, "Normoglycemic diabetic ketoacidosis in pregnancy. Report of one case," *Revista médica de Chile*, vol. 144, no. 10, pp. 1360–1364, 2016.

[30] N. Tarif and W. Al Badr, "Euglycemic diabetic ketoacidosis in pregnancy," *Saudi Journal of Kidney Disease and Transplantation*, vol. 18, no. 4, pp. 590–593, 2007.

[31] X. Yu, S. Zhang, and L. Zhang, "Newer perspectives of mechanisms for euglycemic diabetic ketoacidosis," *International Journal of Endocrinology*, vol. 2018, Article ID 7074868, 8 pages, 2018.

Coccidioidomycosis of the Vocal Cords Presenting in Sepsis

Curtis Converse,[1] **Atish Dey**,[1] **Samuel Decker**,[2] **Sarkis Arabian**,[1] **and Michael Neeki**[2]

[1]*Department of Internal Medicine, Arrowhead Regional Medical Center, Colton, CA, USA*
[2]*Department of Emergency Medicine, Arrowhead Regional Medical Center, Colton, CA, USA*

Correspondence should be addressed to Curtis Converse; conversecu@armc.sbcounty.gov

Academic Editor: Mehmet Doganay

Coccidioidomycosis is a predominantly pulmonary disease caused by species of *Coccidioides*, a fungus endemic to the American Southwest. Most cases involve exclusively pulmonary manifestations while less than one percent present with disseminated infection, usually with meningeal or skin involvement. In this case, a patient with a history of odynophagia, sore throat, productive cough, weight loss, and abnormalities on chest radiograph presented with sepsis and diabetic ketoacidosis. During admission, the patient underwent bronchoscopy with resulting tissue and bronchoalveolar lavage samples positive for *Coccidioides immitis*, later supported by confirmatory serum studies. This case illustrates a rare presentation of vocal fold involvement without direct invasion from a continuous site and highlights the importance of a high index of suspicion for disseminated coccidioidomycosis with prompt antifungal treatment in order to avoid the very high morbidity and mortality in such cases.

1. Introduction

Coccidioidomycosis is a fungal disease that may cause pulmonary or disseminated infection [1, 2]. The distributions of the causative dimorphic fungi, *Coccidioides immitis and C. posadasii*, are overlapping and largely confined to the Southwestern United States, Northern Mexico, and Central America, with sporadic endemic cases also reported in Washington State [1–3]. They exist in the environment as molds with septated hyphae which contain the infectious arthroconidia. When the dry soil in which the fungus dwells is disturbed, the arthroconidia become airborne and are inhaled. Inside a host, at temperatures of 37-4°C, the mold matures to form spherules filled with endospores, which then cause local infection in 99% of cases or dissemination in <1% of the cases. It is estimated that over half of coccidioidomycosis cases are asymptomatic or minimally symptomatic and self-limited. Those who do develop pulmonary symptoms usually have complaints lasting several weeks. Respiratory symptoms include nonproductive cough, coryza, and pleuritic or dull chest pain [3]. Dissemination is most likely to occur in those of African or Filipino descent, at the extremes of age, with diabetes, pregnant, immunosuppressed, and in a newly recognized group with genetic mutations in genes related to interferon-gamma and interleukin 12 [2, 4]. The immune reaction is typically marked by caseating granulomas or pyogenic reaction, which may be misdiagnosed and mistreated as either chronic granulomatous disease or bacterial infection with abscess. Interestingly, most cases are diagnosed in winter [1]. Here, we present a rare case of coccidioidomycosis of the vocal cords in a patient complaining of chronic dysphonia or dysphagia.

2. Case Presentation

A 52-year-old male presented to the emergency department with four days of sore throat, odynophagia, and productive cough with clear-white, blood-tinged sputum. He also noted unintentional weight loss of approximately 10 pounds over the past three months but denied dyspnea, night sweats, fever, chills, or prior pulmonary complaints. Additional complaints included nausea, vomiting, polydipsia, and polyuria for the past few days after he stopped taking his long-acting insulin to adjust for decreased oral intake. He was sent to

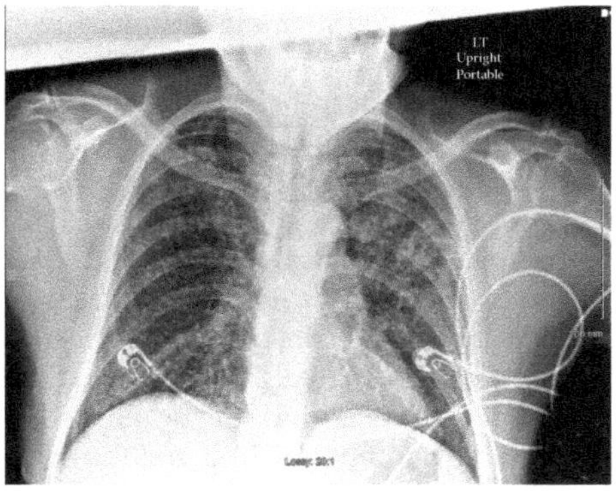

FIGURE 1: Chest radiograph upon arrival to the emergency department revealed diffuse bilateral reticulonodular opacities and airspace disease with a possible lingular cavitary lesion.

the emergency department by his primary care physician for abnormalities on chest X-ray taken the previous day, at which time he had been prescribed cephalexin empirically for suspected community acquired pneumonia.

His past medical history was significant for type 2 diabetes mellitus controlled with metformin and long-acting insulin without previous hospitalizations. He immigrated to the United States approximately 40 years ago from Central America and had never left the United States since. He works as short-distance truck driver and previously smoked heavily for a decade before quitting 20 years ago.

Upon arrival to the emergency department, his vital signs included blood pressure 123/90 mmHg, heart rate 134 beats per minute, respiratory rate 40 breaths per minute, temperature 97.8°F, and oxygen saturation 98% on room air. His physical exam revealed a cachectic man in mild distress with tachypnea, without nasal flaring or retractions, with dry mucous membranes, and hoarse voice. Lung auscultation revealed diffuse bilateral crackles. Cardiac exam revealed tachycardia with regular rhythm. Abdominal exam did not demonstrate hepatosplenomegaly or tenderness. There were no other significant physical findings on examination.

His chest X-ray revealed diffuse bilateral reticulonodular opacities and airspace disease with a possible lingular cavitary lesion (Figure 1). A thoracic CT without contrast was obtained which revealed numerous, bilateral tiny nodular densities, most prominently in the upper lobes, and confirmed the lingular cavitary lesion (Figure 2). A few scattered mediastinal lymph nodes were also noted. Serum chemistry was remarkable for an anion gap of 35, beta-hydroxybutyrate of 8.09 mmol/L, and blood glucose of 532 mg/dL. Hematology showed a white blood cell count of 13 000/μL with 0% eosinophils. Venous blood gas analysis revealed a pH of 7.13, pCO2 of 32, and lactic acid of 5.46 mmol/L. Urinalysis was positive for 4+ glucose and 3+ acetone. Later, HIV antigen testing for types 1 and 2 was negative and CD4 count was 343 cells/μL. Vancomycin 1 g and piperacillin/tazobactam 3.375 g were given intravenously in the emergency department. Intravenous insulin was started with dose adjustment according to an in-house nursing algorithm alongside vigorous hydration.

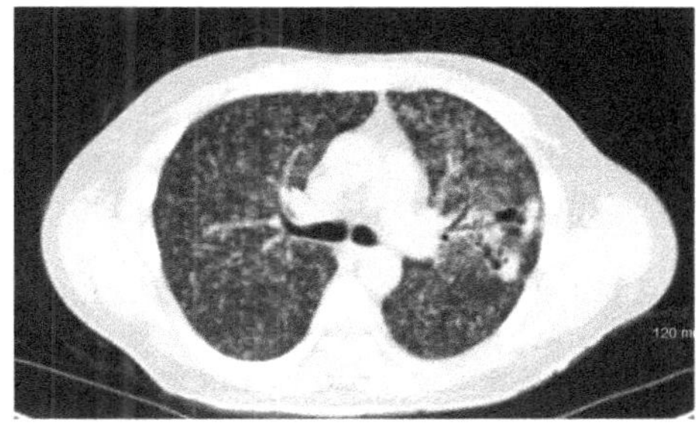

FIGURE 2: Thoracic CT scan without contrast demonstrating numerous, bilateral tiny nodular densities, most prominently in the upper lobes and confirmed a lingular cavitary lesion.

He was admitted to the ICU on airborne isolation with differential diagnoses including coccidioidomycosis, tuberculosis, and lymphangitic carcinomatosis, complicated by diabetic ketoacidosis. In the ICU, empiric antifungal therapy with fluconazole 800 mg/day was started intravenously for suspected pulmonary Coccidioides infection. Although serum anion gap and bicarbonate normalized on day two, he remained tachycardic and tachypneic and required supplemental oxygen. He also continued to have odynophagia that necessitated enteral tube feeding until hospital day five, when he was finally able to tolerate an oral diet. At this point, he developed a mild elevation of transaminases and fluconazole was changed to itraconazole 200 mg twice daily due to concern for hepatotoxicity, and abdominal ultrasound and computed tomography (CT) were obtained to rule out hepatic involvement from the suspected fungal infection. Both of these studies were negative for ascites, focal hypoattenuation within the liver, or hepatic or splenic enlargement. The CT additionally did not demonstrate abdominal adenopathy. Aminotransferases trended from their peak on hospital day three to normal on day eight.

A week after admission, he remained tachypneic, hypoxic, and hoarse. Three sputum samples were negative for acid-fast bacilli but Coccidioides antibody titer and complement fixation had not yet resulted; thus, bronchoscopy was performed, revealing irregular-appearing borders of false and true vocal cords with erythema and edema, two vocal cord polyps, inflamed upper trachea in the subglottic space, and several flesh-colored endobronchial lesions bilaterally. Forceps biopsies and brushings were performed on the endobronchial lesions, true and false cords, and posterior trachea just below the larynx. Bronchoalveolar lavage (BAL) was performed in the right middle lobe and lingula. BAL fluid cell count and differential showed a neutrophilic predominance with spherules and endospores, consistent with *Coccidioides immitis* or *Rhinosporidium seeberi*. The biopsy specimens demonstrated the same pathogen in the laryngeal tissue. The culture of the BAL fluid eventually grew *Coccidioides immitis* on the day prior to discharge (day 14), but the laryngeal tissue was not cultured.

Otolaryngology consultant recommended outpatient follow-up with consideration for laryngoscopy after resolution of his acute illness. Two days after bronchoscopy, Coccidioides antibody titer returned positive at 1 : 16. The infectious disease consultant recommended continuing itraconazole for a minimum of 12 months with serial monitoring of Coccidioides titer, transaminases, and itraconazole level every three months. He continually improved on antifungal therapy until successfully weaning from supplemental oxygen and discharge after two weeks of hospitalization.

2.1. Follow-Up. Coccidioides complement fixation returned strongly positive at 1 : 1024 nine days after discharge. Histoplasma urine antigen was positive but below the limit of quantification. At his follow-up appointments two and twelve weeks after discharge, his productive cough was present but improved and his hoarseness, dyspnea, and odynophagia had resolved. His liver enzymes remain within normal limits. At time of writing, the patient had not yet returned to have his Coccidioides titer or itraconazole level measured.

3. Discussion

It is estimated that over half of coccidioidomycosis cases are asymptomatic, minimally symptomatic, or self-limited. Those who develop pulmonary symptoms usually have complaints lasting several weeks. These include nonproductive cough, coryza, and pleuritic or dull chest pain. Common systemic symptoms include fever, headache, fatigue, and malaise. Due to the similar presentations, a majority of patients are treated with antibiotics for suspected bacterial pneumonia before eventually being correctly diagnosed [4]. There are also common extrapulmonary, immune-mediated manifestations such as mono- or oligoarthritis, especially of the knee, erythema nodosum, and erythema multiforme. These are distinct from extrapulmonary infection and give rise to the epithet, "Desert Rheumatism." The pulmonary disease can progress to cavitary pneumonia, especially of the upper lobes, and pyo- or pyopneumothorax [1]. Though rare, sepsis due to Coccidioides does occur and is associated with a mortality rate near 100% [4].

Our review of the published literature does not reveal any cases of isolated laryngeal involvement, but several cases of secondary involvement have been reported. It is unclear whether these always represent inoculation from direct contact with the infectious source or if there is a possibility of hematogenous spread to the larynx [3, 5, 6]. See Table 1 for a summary of all reported cases of laryngeal coccidioidomycosis.

Several cases of prevertebral and retropharyngeal abscesses with extension to the larynx have been reported [7–10], but very few have had vocal fold involvement without invasion from contiguous structures [5, 10–14]. Those that do not have direct extension have had concomitant involvement of another extrapulmonary site, namely, axial skeleton or skin. Laryngeal symptoms include hoarseness, sore throat, dysphagia, and odynophagia. Several of the cases previously mentioned were initially suspected to be cancerous due to their appearance on laryngoscopy before biopsy showed otherwise [5–7, 14].

Imaging of the neck in cases of laryngeal coccidioidomycosis without direct extension from another site is most often normal. In fact, only one case showed any abnormality on CT of the neck, specifically with supraglottic narrowing due to edema [5]. It should be borne in mind, however, that several of the reported cases occurred before the wide availability of CT. In cases of retropharyngeal or prevertebral abscesses, there is occasionally visible compromise of the airway by external compression.

Due to the paucity of cases of laryngeal Coccidioides, there have been large lapses in time between cases and appropriate treatment leading to substantial advances in antimicrobial therapy in the intervals. The earliest cases were treated with iodides and radiation [11] or dihydroxystilbamidine [12], followed by amphotericin B and the azole antifungals, as each agent was successively discovered over the following decades [15].

Duration of therapy for these cases has similarly evolved, with early cases treated for shorter duration than more recent cases. As several of the reported cases have been in patients with previous diagnoses of disseminated disease [5, 14], patients may end up on life-long suppressive therapy. Two cases have been reported in patients receiving immunosuppressive therapy. One of these involved a child who experienced two episodes of disseminations, once while on cyclophosphamide and prednisone for chronic granulomatous disease and again after receiving kidney transplant with further immunosuppression [16, 17]. The other case occurred in a patient taking steroids chronically for bronchiectasis [14].

The current guidelines of Infectious Disease Society of America recommend treatment of disseminated coccidioidomycosis with fluconazole 400-1200 mg/day, but do not recommend a specific duration or endpoint. The exception to this is coccidioidal meningitis, which necessitates life-long suppressive therapy regardless of symptoms. Amphotericin should be used in cases of severe or life-threatening infection or if there is treatment failure with azole therapy [2].

While any case of vocal fold coccidioidomycosis can be considered unique, there are some aspects of this case that adds to our scant literature about this subject. Firstly, this is the only reported case with concurrent diabetic ketoacidosis, despite the fact that it is known that diabetes is a risk factor for complicated pulmonary disease. Secondly, data from literature indicated that only about quarter of all sputum or BAL samples from patients with active pulmonary coccidioidomycosis culture are positive [3]. However, it is estimated that 100% of those with active pulmonary disease and sepsis or septic shock are culture positive from respiratory sources [18]. Finally, the majority of the previously reported cases had either previous pulmonary coccidioidomycosis [6, 13, 14] or other signs of disseminated disease to the skin [6, 12], meninges [5], or bone [6, 12], none of which was seen in this case.

With regard to the treatment rendered in this case, the patient was started empirically on antifungal therapy, initially with moderate-dose fluconazole 800 mg/day, which is midrange for the IDSA recommendation of 400-1200 mg/day, and transitioned to itraconazole 200 mg twice daily because of concern for developing hepatotoxicity. This change was likely premature, as the elevation in aminotransferases was mild (<2 times the upper limit of normal) and was not trended to determine if it was worsening, but the change did

TABLE 1: Reported cases of laryngeal coccidioidomycosis without contiguous spread (7, 10, 11, 12, 5, 6, 13, 14, 3).

Age/sex	Symptoms	Laryngeal diagnosis	Other sites	Treatment	Outcome
40/F [13]	Hoarseness, lymphadenopathy, fever, night sweats, dry cough, fatigue	Edematous and erythematous mucosa without focal lesions	Lymphatics, pulmonary	Fluconazole	Improvement
52/F [14]	Dysphonia, cough, weight loss, odynophagia, dysphagia	Epiglottic, aryepiglottic, and piriform fossa erythema, edema; vocal fold paralysis	Pulmonary	Fluconazole 400 mg twice daily for 6 weeks, then extended	Resolution of symptoms, left vocal fold paralysis
2.6, 14/M [14]	Not reported	Laryngeal infection on immunosuppressants, recurrence after 12 year	Not reported	"Systemic antifungal treatment"	Remission
37/M [11]	Odynophagia, dysphagia, hoarseness, night sweats, hemoptysis	Coccidioidal granuloma of the epiglottis	Lymphatic	Laryngeal irradiation and iodides for 3 months	Discharge to "full employment"
34/M [12]	Productive cough ×3 months, hoarseness, dysphagia ×1 month, weight loss	Fungating granuloma of endolarynx	Bone, pulmonary, skin	Tracheostomy, dihydroxystilbamidine 150 mg IV 4 times daily for 20 doses	None reported
45/M [6]	Productive cough, fever, malaise, hemoptysis, weight loss, dyspnea, headache, hoarseness	Aryepiglottic granuloma	Pulmonary, bone marrow	Amphotericin B 2 g, then miconazole nitrate	Laryngeal lesions cleared, disseminated infection after 3 years
34/M [5]	Not reported	Epiglottic erosion, "heaped up involvement" of entire endolarynx	Pulmonary	Tracheostomy	Not reported
20/F [5]	Not reported	Granulomatous appearance of posterior commissure, false cords, aryepiglottic folds	Meninges	Amphotericin B, parenteral and weekly intrathecal	Not reported
"Adult" age/sex not given [5]	Not reported	Granulomatous appearance of posterior commissure, false cords, aryepiglottic folds	None	Not reported	Not reported
19 mo./sex not given [5]	Not reported	Obstructive granuloma of the trachea and larynx	Pulmonary	Not reported	Not reported
4.5 mo./M [5]	Wheezing, cough	Obstructive subglottic and anterior commissure granuloma	Pulmonary	Tracheostomy, amphotericin B 0.1 mg/kg/day increasing to 1 mg/kg/day to a total of 271 mg	Improvement

not appear to impact the efficacy of the treatment. Evaluation for liver disease was performed but did not demonstrate any abnormalities. Findings that would have been consistent with the diagnosis of hepatic Coccidioides include focal hypoattenuation, ascites, hepatosplenomegaly, and abdominal adenopathy [19].

The reason for starting early treatment with antifungal therapy empirically when it was only one of three major differential diagnoses (the others being mycobacterial infection and lymphangitic carcinomatosis) was based on the acuity of his presentation. While tuberculosis was not ruled out until several days after admission, sepsis and acute respiratory failure are uncommon presentations of active TB and would be unlikely to respond quickly to antibiotics even if they were administered rapidly [20, 21]. Furthermore, the disease is endemic in our area, with 85 cases reported in our county in 2017, the most recent year for which data is available [22].

He was kept in airborne isolation until the required three negative acid-fast smears were resulted. Due to the severe presentation of his disease, he was ruled out for HIV infection but did demonstrate a low CD4+ lymphocyte count. This is likely due to the fungal infection itself rather than the cause of the infection [23]. The positivity of the Histoplasma antigen is not unexpected, as there is significant cross-reactivity between Histoplasma and Coccidioides antigens, nearly 80% in one review [24]. Another interesting point is the level of antigen titer. Previous studies have demonstrated that reactivity of greater than or equal to 1 : 16 is frequently indicative of disseminated infection, which is consistent with our patient [2].

4. Conclusion

This case highlights several important points about coccidioidomycosis, a common disease in the Southwest that appears to be on the rise. The expanding endemic region of the fungus and the increased ability to travel through endemic regions over recent decades should encourage physicians outside of the historic geographic zone to be familiar with the disease.

Due to the extreme variety of symptoms that can be caused by Coccidioides infection, clinicians should have a high index of suspicion for fungal pneumonia if the patient presents with atypical or nonresolving symptoms, especially if those symptoms are extrapulmonary. Hoarseness may be an extremely rare symptom of infection of the vocal cords in patients with pulmonary disease suspicious for coccidioidomycosis. In patients with coccidioidomycosis presenting with sepsis, early initiation of antifungal therapy may decrease mortality, contrary to previous reports.

Consent

The patient presented in this case provided informed consent for this case study.

Acknowledgments

Article processing charges were funded by the Department of Graduate Medical Education of Arrowhead Regional Medical Center, Colton, CA.

References

[1] M. A. Grippi, J. A. Elias, J. A. Fishman, R. M. Kotloff, A. I. Pack, and R. M. Senior, *Fishmans Pulmonary Diseases and Disorders*, McGraw-Hill Education, New York, 2015.

[2] J. N. Galgiani, N. M. Ampel, J. E. Blair et al., "Executive summary: 2016 Infectious Diseases Society of America (IDSA) clinical practice guideline for the treatment of coccidioidomycosis," *Clinical Infectious Diseases*, vol. 63, no. 6, pp. 717–722, 2016.

[3] N. F. Crum-Cianflone, A. A. Truett, N. Teneza-Mora et al., "Unusual presentations of coccidioidomycosis: a case series and review of the literature," *Medicine*, vol. 85, no. 5, pp. 263–277, 2006.

[4] N. F. Crum, E. R. Lederman, C. M. Stafford, J. S. Parrish, and M. R. Wallace, "Coccidioidomycosis," *Medicine*, vol. 83, no. 3, pp. 149–175, 2004.

[5] P. H. Ward, D. Morledge, G. Berci, and H. Schwartz, "Coccidioidomycosis of the larynx in infants and adults," *Annals of Otology, Rhinology & Laryngology*, vol. 86, no. 5, pp. 655–660, 1977.

[6] M. A. Platt, "Laryngeal coccidioidomycosis," *The Journal of the American Medical Association*, vol. 237, no. 12, pp. 1234-1235, 1977.

[7] J. Henley-Cohn, R. Boles, E. Weisberger, and J. Ballantyne, "Upper airway obstruction due to coccidioidomycosis," *The Laryngoscope*, vol. 89, no. 3, pp. 355–360, 1979.

[8] B. Copeland, D. White, and J. Buenting, "Coccidioidomycosis of the head and neck," *Annals of Otology, Rhinology & Laryngology*, vol. 112, no. 1, pp. 98–101, 2003.

[9] M. G. Arnold, J. C. Arnold, D. C. Bloom, D. F. Brewster, and J. K. Thiringer, "Head and neck manifestations of disseminated coccidioidomycosis," *The Laryngoscope*, vol. 114, no. 4, pp. 747–752, 2004.

[10] S. Patel and L. Snyder, "A sore throat in the southwest," *The American Journal of Medicine*, vol. 122, no. 3, pp. 233–235, 2009.

[11] C. S. Mumma, "Coccidioidomycosis of the epiglottis," *Archives of Otolaryngology-Head and Neck Surgery*, vol. 58, no. 3, pp. 306–309, 1953.

[12] H. Singh, C. J. Yast, and J. H. Gladney, "Coccidioidomycosis with endolaryngeal involvement," *Archives of Otolaryngology-Head and Neck Surgery*, vol. 63, no. 3, pp. 244–247, 1956.

[13] J. O. Boyle, S. W. Coulthard, and R. M. Mandel, "Laryngeal involvement in disseminated coccidioidomycosis," *Archives of Otolaryngology-Head and Neck Surgery*, vol. 117, no. 4, pp. 433–438, 1991.

[14] J. E. Allen and P. C. Belafsky, "Laryngeal coccidioidomycosis with vocal fold paralysis," *Ear, Nose & Throat Journal*, vol. 90, no. 5, pp. E1–E5, 2011.

[15] B. C. Walker and S. R. Walker, *Trends and changes in drug research and development: proceedings of the Society for Drug Research 20th anniversary meeting held at the Parmaceutical Society of Great Britain*, 1988, Dordrecht: Kluwer, p. 109, 1988.

[16] M. A. Keefe, E. J. Rosen, S. D. Newlands, J. Patel, A. Kalia, and N. R. Friedman, "Reactivated laryngeal Coccidioidomycosis," *Otolaryngology and Head and Neck Surgery*, vol. 125, no. 1, pp. 120-121, 2001.

[17] S. Hajare, T. A. Rakusan, A. Kalia, F. B. Gibson, and C. L. Strunk, "Laryngeal coccidioidomycosis causing airway obstruction," *The Pediatric Infectious Disease Journal*, vol. 8, no. 1, pp. 54–56, 1989.

[18] E. L. Arsura, P. L. Bellinghausen, W. B. Kilgore, J. J. Abraham, and R. H. Johnson, "Septic shock in coccidioidomycosis," *Critical Care Medicine*, vol. 26, no. 1, pp. 62–65, 1998.

[19] N. A. Gupta, M. Iv, R. P. Pandit, and M. R. Patel, "Imaging manifestations of primary and disseminated coccidioidomycosis," *Applied Radiology*, vol. 44, no. 2, pp. 9–21, 2015.

[20] Z. A. Rubin, M. K. Leonard, and G. S. Martin, "Brief report: tuberculosis sepsis and activated protein C," *The American Journal of the Medical Sciences*, vol. 332, no. 1, pp. 48–50, 2006.

[21] C. Penner, D. Roberts, D. Kunimoto, J. Manfreda, and R. Long, "Tuberculosis as a primary cause of respiratory failure requiring mechanical ventilation," *American Journal of Respiratory and Critical Care Medicine*, vol. 151, 3 part 1, pp. 867–872, 1995.

[22] Center for Infectious Diseases - Divison of Communicable Diseases - Infectious Disease Branch, A. M. Azar, and K. L. Smith, *Epidemiologic Summary of Coccidioidomycosis in California, 2017*, California Department of Public Health, 2018.

[23] U. A. Walker and K. Warnatz, "Idiopathic CD4 lymphocytopenia," *Current Opinion in Rheumatology*, vol. 18, no. 4, pp. 389–395, 2006.

[24] T. Kuberski, R. Myers, L. J. Wheat et al., "Diagnosis of coccidioidomycosis by antigen detection using cross-reaction with a Histoplasma antigen," *Clinical Infectious Diseases*, vol. 44, no. 5, pp. e50–e54, 2007.

29

Extreme Rhabdomyolysis, Acute Renal Failure and Protracted Ileus in a Case of Legionella Pneumonia

C. Laivier,[1] M.-O. Bleuze,[2] P. Hantson,[3] and J. Devos[1]

[1]Department of Intensive Care, Centre Hospitalier de Mouscron, 7700 Mouscron, Belgium
[2]Department of Pneumology, Centre Hospitalier de Mouscron, 7700 Mouscron, Belgium
[3]Department of Intensive Care, Cliniques St-Luc, Université catholique de Louvain, 1200 Brussels, Belgium

Correspondence should be addressed to J. Devos; j.devos@chmouscron.be

Academic Editor: Kurt Lenz

A 53-year-old man developed a *Legionella pneumophila* pneumonia complicated by rhabdomyolysis, acute kidney injury, and protracted ileus. Risk factors were smoking and chronic alcoholism, but the patient had no history of previous abdominal surgery. Hemodialysis was required for a period of 5 weeks with a full renal recovery. Pneumonia required respiratory support but for a limited period of 6 days. The protracted course of the ileus led to explorative laparotomy despite negative computed tomography findings. No cause of mechanical obstruction was found at surgery and common etiologies of intestinal obstruction were excluded. Parenteral nutrition was needed for a total of 4 weeks, before recovery of intestinal motility. This case illustrates the apparent discrepancy between the pulmonary symptoms and the extrapulmonary manifestations that could be seen as a consequence of an exaggerated immune response.

1. Introduction

First described in 1977, in the course of a wide community-acquired pneumonia epidemic that occurred during the American Legion's convention, Legionnaires' disease (LD) is an infectious disease caused by an aerobic gram negative bacillus [1]. *Legionella pneumophila* is the most frequently encountered species in human pathology, especially serogroup 1 (Lp-1). In over 90% of cases, transmission of LD occurs usually via the respiratory route, after inhalation of contaminated water. Interhuman transmission has never been observed [2]. Several host risk factors were described, including heavy smoking, chronic alcoholism, elderliness, diabetes, end-stage renal or pulmonary disease, and immunodeficiency (corticosteroids, cancer, hemopathy, immunosuppressive therapy, etc.) [3]. LD is a relatively rare infectious disease, with an incidence of 2 cases in Belgium per 100,000 inhabitants in 2016. The mortality rate is still high, ranging from 10% to 70% if the patient is presenting one of aforementioned risk factors [4]. A mild renal impairment is frequent in LD, while extreme rhabdomyolysis leading to acute renal failure and hemodialysis remains uncommon. The association of anuric acute renal failure and persisting ileus has not been previously reported in the setting of *L. pneumophila* pneumonia [5].

2. Case Report

A 53-year-old Caucasian man was admitted to the emergency department (ED) with complaints of diarrhea of 3 days' duration, general weakness leading to multiple falls, abdominal pain with lack of appetite, dry cough, and dyspnea on exertion since the last 6 months. His medical past history included chronic alcoholism with 28 units of alcohol per week, active tobacco smoking (22,5 pack-years), sleep apnea syndrome treated with nocturnal continuous positive airway pressure (CPAP) ventilation, high arterial blood pressure controlled by a daily dose of perindopril 5mg and bisoprolol 10 mg, and a morbid obesity with a body mass index (BMI) of 47,3 kg/m^2. There was no history of abdominal surgery. Vital signs in the ED were arterial blood pressure 106/64 mmHg, sinus tachycardia with heart rate ranging from 104

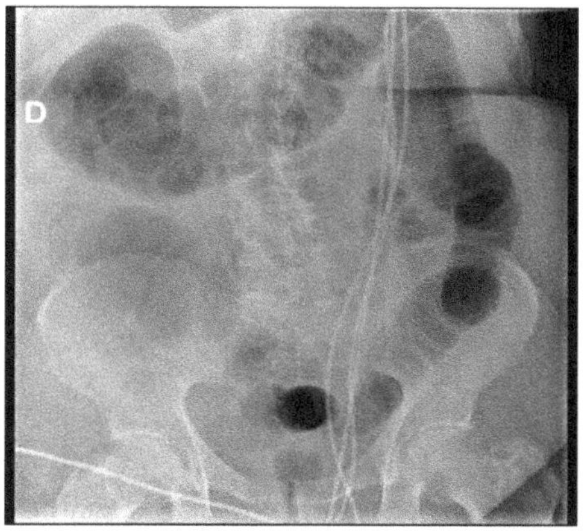

FIGURE 1: Abdomen X-ray on admission showing diffuse intestinal distension.

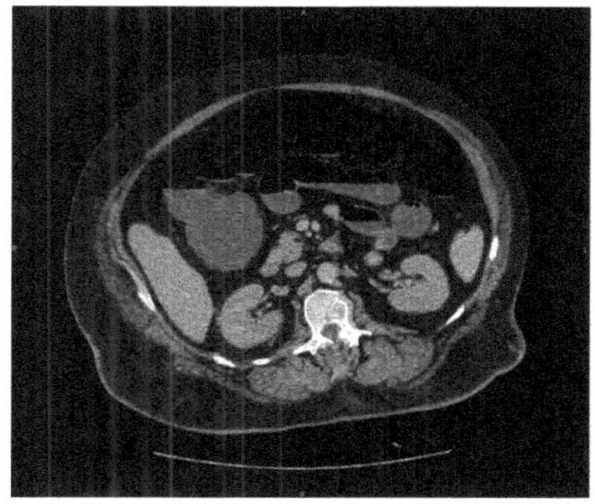

FIGURE 2: Follow-up abdomen computed tomography (CT) without evidence of mechanical obstruction, inflammatory or ischemic lesions.

to 144 bpm, respiratory rate 37/min, temperature 36.2°C, and oxygen peripheral saturation (SpO_2) 92% at room air. Initial examination revealed crackles at the basis of the right lung and abdominal distension with decreased bowel sounds. There were no clinical signs of muscular injury.

The relevant laboratory investigations were the following: CRP 192 mg/L (< 5), platelet count 115.000 /μL, serum creatinine 4.48 mg/dL, BUN 94 mg/dL, sodium 126 mmol/L, and potassium 3mmol/L. A major rhabdomyolysis was early noted: CK 96,012 IU/L (< 397), troponin-I 103.3 ng/L (< 34.2), AST 818 IU/L (< 37), and LDH 2,960 IU/L (< 214). The CK level further increased to 120,059 IU/L 4 hours after hospital admission. Arterial blood gas analysis was consistent with a compensated metabolic acidosis: pH 7.44, pCO_2 21.8 mmHg, pO_2 79.7 mmHg, bicarbonate 18.6 mmol/L, base excess -7.2 mmol/L, and lactate level 2 mmol/L (< 1.6). Urine analysis revealed moderate proteinuria (++).

The electrocardiogram showed new onset atrial fibrillation (144/min). The diagnosis of left basal pneumonia with a contralateral pleural effusion was made on chest X-ray. Small and large bowel distension was evident from abdomen X-ray with some air fluid levels (Figure 1).

The patient was transferred to the intensive care unit (ICU) for further management. He remained hypotensive (79/43 mmHg), with atrial fibrillation (166/min) and hypoxemia requiring nasal oxygen administration (5L/min). Initial therapy included fluid replacement, vasopressors, and potassium supplementation for persisting hypokalemia (2.9 mmol/L). Cefuroxime and clarithromycin were initially chosen for empirical antimicrobial therapy. No sputum was available for culture and blood cultures remained sterile. Urine *Legionella* testing returned positive for *L. pneumophila* serogroup 1 antigen and clarithromycin was continued alone.

Further clinical course was characterized by a progressive weaning of vasopressors and decrease of arterial lactate. Ileus persisted. Contrast enhanced abdominal computed tomography (CT) showed a diffuse distension of the large intestine and terminal ileum and a diffuse enhancement of the intestinal wall without evidence of bowel ischemia or stenosis (Figure 2). Renal failure worsened and the patient became anuric on day 2 with serum creatinine 7.18 mg/dl and BUN 146 mg/dl. Intermittent hemodialysis was then started. The peak level of CK (202,000 IU/L) was reached on day 2.

Mechanical ventilation was ultimately required from hospital day 4 to 10 due to the progression of hypoxemia with hypercapnia; there was also a suspicion of inhalation pneumonia secondary to persisting ileus. During the period of mechanical ventilation, the patient did not receive opioid medications that could have resulted in a decreased intestinal motility.

Despite noncontributive abdominal CT findings, an explorative laparotomy was decided on day 12 that failed to demonstrate any mechanical occlusion.

Two weeks after ICU admission, patient was transferred to the nephrology ward with persisting ileus leading to a full month of parenteral nutrition. Antimicrobial therapy was stopped after 21 days. The patient was discharged home after two months. Hemodialysis was definitely stopped after 5 weeks, and renal function returned to normal values after 6 weeks.

3. Discussion

Legionella pneumophila infection is an important cause of severe community-acquired pneumonia. The severity of pneumonia may justify ICU admission for respiratory support. In addition, extrapulmonary complications may be encountered following *Legionella* infection. The association of *Legionella* and rhabdomyolysis was first described in 1980 by Posner et al. [6]. Since that time, at least 17 additional cases have been reported in the literature [6–22]. Our patient had one of the highest ever reported CK levels [23]. The exact mechanism leading to muscular injury in case of *Legionella* infection remains unclear. The two main hypotheses are a direct invasion of the muscle by the microorganism or an indirect injury caused by endo- or exotoxin release. The role of ionic disorders may also be discussed as hyponatremia, hypokalemia, and hypophosphatemia have also been related to the occurrence of rhabdomyolysis. Our patient presented with a mild hyponatremia and hypokalemia on admission that were probably insufficient to explain the severity of rhabdomyolysis. From the literature, patients presenting with rhabdomyolysis usually require ICU admission due to the associated renal impairment. At least 13/17 patients needed intermittent hemodialysis, and among them 11 made a complete recovery [22]. The etiology of acute kidney injury (AKI) is likely related to acute tubular necrosis or acute tubule-interstitial nephritis [9]. The presence of *L. pneumophila* was exceptionally demonstrated by immunofluorescence microscopy in a renal biopsy specimen of a patient presenting acute tubulointerstitial nephritis after Legionella infection complicated with rhabdomyolysis and acute renal failure [9]. Other investigations were consistent with tubular precipitation of myoglobin casts [7]. Hypovolemia and hypotension due to gastrointestinal fluid losses may be additional factors for the development of AKI. *Legionella* pneumonia has been exceptionally complicated with Fanconi syndrome [24]. In some cases, renal anomalies can develop before the imaging demonstration of pneumonia.

To our best knowledge, there is no description of the association of rhabdomyolysis-related acute kidney injury treated with hemodialysis and bowel obstruction in the setting of *Legionella* pneumonia. There are isolated observations of segmental enteritis, ascites, or peritonitis following *L. pneumophila* infection [25–30]. Exceptionally, *L. pneumophila* has been demonstrated by direct immunofluorescent microscopic study in inflammatory colitis pieces with hemorrhagic necrosis at different stages [30]. Our patient had suffered from diarrhea during the three days preceding hospital admission. Initial hypotension was likely related to some degree of hypovolemic shock. Prichard et al. described a case of bowel obstruction in a 62-year-old woman with Legionnaires' disease. The patient had a peak CK level at 15,445 IU/L, but with a preserved renal function [5]. The abdomen CT revealed a high-grade partial small bowel obstruction. The patient was managed conservatively. The mechanism of this intestinal complication remained unknown, especially when common factors of intestinal obstruction (previous abdominal surgery, medications, ionic disorders, etc.) could be excluded. The authors hypothesized that the microorganism could activate the immune cascade by the action of lipopolysaccharide, lipid A, on the production of tumor necrosis factor alpha (TNFα); the result would be the development of diarrhea and intestinal inflammation [31–34]. A last hypothesis should be a disturbance in gut microcirculation induced by myoglobin casts. Experimental data on rats showed that severe disturbances of the small intestine blood flow may be observed when myoglobin was intravenously infused during a period of hemorrhagic hypotension [35]. Our patient did also not present usual risk factors for intestinal obstruction and gut inflammation is a potential explanation for this uncommon complication. Only one study with multivariate analysis suggested a significant statistical association between diarrhea, rhabdomyolysis, and LD [36]. The association of rhabdomyolysis and renal failure might increase the mortality rate up to 40% [9].

4. Conclusion

Among extrapulmonary complications of LD leading to ICU admission, severe rhabdomyolysis and bowel obstruction may be seen as other manifestations of the immune reaction following Legionella infection.

Consent

A written consent was obtained from the patient.

References

[1] D. Fraser, T. Tsai, W. Orenstein et al., "Legionnaires' disease," *The New England Journal of Medicine*, vol. 297, no. 22, pp. 1189–1197, 1977.

[2] J.-R. Zahar and A. Kouatchet, "Legionnaires's disease: Mise au point," *Réanimation*, vol. 17, no. 3, pp. 206–212, 2008.

[3] J. E. Stout and V. L. Yu, "Legionellosis," *The New England Journal of Medicine*, vol. 337, no. 10, pp. 682–687, 1997.

[4] N. Phin, F. Parry-Ford, T. Harrison et al., "Epidemiology and clinical management of Legionnaires' disease," *The Lancet Infectious Diseases*, vol. 14, no. 10, pp. 1011–1021, 2014.

[5] W. Prichard and L. Fick, "When diarrhea can become deadly: Legionnaires' disease complicated by bowel obstruction," *Case Reports in Gastroenterology*, vol. 10, no. 3, pp. 781–786, 2016.

[6] T. Koufakis, I. Gabranis, M. Chatzopoulou, A. Margaritis, and M. Tsiakalou, "Severe Legionnaires' Disease Complicated by Rhabdomyolysis and Clinically Resistant to Moxifloxacin in a Splenectomised Patient: Too Much of a Coincidence?" *Case Reports in Infectious Diseases*, vol. 2015, Article ID 793786, 4 pages, 2015.

[7] C. Shimura, T. Saraya, H. Wada et al., "Pathological evidence of rhabdomyolysis-induced acute tubulointerstitial nephritis accompanying Legionella pneumophila pneumonia," *Journal of Clinical Pathology*, vol. 61, no. 9, pp. 1062-1063, 2008.

[8] J. McConkey, M. Obeius, J. Valentini, and M. S. Beeson, "Legionella pneumonia presenting with rhabdomyolysis and acute renal failure: A case report," *The Journal of Emergency Medicine*, vol. 30, no. 4, pp. 389–392, 2006.

[9] A. Shah, F. Check, S. Baskin, T. Reyman, and R. Menard, "Legionnaires' disease and acute renal failure: case report and review," *Clinical Infectious Diseases*, vol. 14, no. 1, pp. 204–207, 1992.

[10] H. Erdogan, A. Yilmaz, O. Kal, A. Erdogan, and H. Arslan, "Rhabdomyolysis-induced acute renal failure associated with legionnaires' disease," *Scandinavian Journal of Urology and Nephrology*, vol. 40, no. 4, pp. 345-346, 2006.

[11] M. Abe, K. Kaizu, and K. Matsumoto, "Clinical evaluation of pneumonia-associated rhabdomyolysis with acute renal failure," *Therapeutic Apheresis and Dialysis*, vol. 12, no. 2, pp. 171–175, 2008.

[12] M. Wiegele and C. G. Krenn, "Cytosorb in a patient with legionella-pneumonia associated rhabdomyolysis," *ASAIO Journal*, vol. 61, no. 3, pp. e14–e16, 2015.

[13] K. R. Linga and D. B. Deo, "Pneumonia, rhabdomyolysis and acute renal Failure - a Deadly Cocktail!," *American Journal of Respiratory and Critical Care Medicine*, vol. 189, A1778 pages, 2014.

[14] C. Agu, M. Basunia, and D. Salhan, "Legionella pneumonia associated with severe rhabdomyolysis and acute kidney injury," *American Journal of Respiratory and Critical Care Medicine*, vol. 193, A7164 pages, 2016.

[15] S. Nakatani, H. Inariba, Y. Kumeda et al., "A case of Legionella pneumonia associated with acute renal failure," *Nihon Toseki Igakkai Zasshi*, vol. 43, no. 4, pp. 381–386, 2010.

[16] J. Li, R. Wen, H. Deng, and Q. Li, "A case of Legionella pneumonia with multiple organ failure," *Journal of Central South University (Medical Sciences)*, vol. 41, no. 6, pp. 657–660, 2016.

[17] A. Daumas, F. El-Mekaoui, S. Bataille et al., "Acute tubulointerstitial nephritis complicating Legionnaires' disease: a case report," *Journal of Medical Case Reports*, vol. 6, article 100, 2012.

[18] Y. Narita, K. Naoki, N. Horiuchi et al., "A case of legionella pneumonia associated with acute respiratory distress syndrome (ARDS) and acute renal failure treated with methylprednisolone and sivelestat," *Nihon Kokyūki Gakkai Zasshi: The Journal of the Japanese Respiratory Society*, vol. 45, no. 5, pp. 413–418, 2007.

[19] B. Sposato, S. Mariotta, A. Ricci, G. Lucantoni, and G. Schmid, "Legionnaire's pneumonia with rhabdomyolysis and acute renal failure. a case report," *Recenti Progressi in Medicina*, vol. 94, no. 9, pp. 391–394, 2003.

[20] N. Matsumoto, H. Mukae, S. Yamashita et al., "A case of severe Legionnaires' disease complicated by rhabdomyolysis, acute renal failure, liver dysfunction and encephalopathy," *Kansenshogaku Zasshi. The Journal of the Japanese Association for Infectious Diseases*, vol. 74, no. 11, pp. 989–993, 2000.

[21] H. Tokuda, N. Yahagi, S. Kasai, S. Kitamura, and Y. Otsuka, "A case of fatal pneumonia caused by Legionella pneumophila serogroup 6 developed after drowning in a public bath," *Kansenshogaku Zasshi. The Journal of the Japanese Association for Infectious Diseases*, vol. 71, no. 2, pp. 169–174, 1997.

[22] K. Seegobin, S. Maharaj, C. Baldeo, J. P. Downes, and P. Reddy, "Legionnaires' Disease Complicated with Rhabdomyolysis and Acute Kidney Injury in an AIDS Patient," *Case Reports in Infectious Diseases*, vol. 2017, Article ID 8051096, 5 pages, 2017.

[23] P. Luckoor, M. Salehi, and A. Kunadu, "Exceptionally high creatine kinase (CK) levels in multicausal and complicated rhabdomyolysis: A case report," *American Journal of Case Reports*, vol. 18, pp. 746–749, 2017.

[24] R. Koda, R. Itoh, M. Tsuchida et al., "Legionella Pneumonia Complicated with Acquired Fanconi Syndrome," *Internal Medicine*, vol. 57, no. 20, pp. 2975–2980, 2018.

[25] C. D. Roio and L. Gruner, "Légionellose et entérite," *Annales Françaises d'Anesthésie et de Réanimation*, vol. 15, no. 8, p. 1233, 1996.

[26] T. Schmidt, A. Pfeiffer, W. Ehret, E. Keiditsch, G. Ruckdeschel, and H. Kaess, "Legionella infection of the colon presenting as acute attack of ulcerative colitis," *Gastroenterology*, vol. 97, no. 3, pp. 751–755, 1989.

[27] J. P. Ozoux, L. de Calan, G. Portier, E. Legue, and J. Brizon, "Necrotizing enteritis and Legionnaires' disease," *Presse Medicale*, vol. 15, no. 2, p. 75, 1986.

[28] J. Fogliani, J. F. Domenget, N. Hohn, G. Merignargues, and N. Bornstein, "Legionnaires' disease with digestive tract lesions - One case," *Nouvelle Presse Médicale*, vol. 11, no. 36, pp. 2699–2702, 1982.

[29] E. Dournon, A. Bure, J. L. Kemeny, J. L. Pourriat, and D. Valeyre, "Legionella pneumophila peritonitis (letter)," *The Lancet*, vol. 1, no. 8285, p. 1363, 1982.

[30] V. Grangeon, L. Vincent, and Y. Pacheco, "Digestive disorders in legionnaires' disease: Accompaniment signs or infectious visceral localisation?" *Revue des Maladies Respiratoires*, vol. 17, no. 2, pp. 489–492, 2000.

[31] R. E. Bishop, "The lipid A palmitoyltransferase PagP: Molecular mechanisms and role in bacterial pathogenesis," *Molecular Microbiology*, vol. 57, no. 4, pp. 900–912, 2005.

[32] M. Cramer, "Legionnaires disease: A case study," *American Journal of Critical Care*, vol. 12, no. 3, pp. 234–238, 2003.

[33] A. Hofmann, Y. Beaulieu, F. Bernard, and P. Rico, "Fulminant Legionellosis in Two Patients Treated with Infliximab for Crohn's Disease: Case Series and Literature Review," *Canadian Journal of Gastroenterology & Hepatology*, vol. 23, no. 12, pp. 829–833, 2009.

[34] E. C. Reisinger, C. Fritzsche, R. Krause, and G. J. Krejs, "Diarrhea caused by primarily non-gastrointestinal infections," *Nature Clinical Practice Gastroenterology & Hepatology*, vol. 2, no. 5, pp. 216–222, 2005.

[35] U. Emig, G. Schmidt, G. Hellige, and F. Vetterlein, "Contribution of myoglobin-induced increases in vascular resistance to shock decompensation in experimental Crush-syndrome in anesthetized rats," *Shock*, vol. 19, no. 1, pp. 79–84, 2003.

[36] N. Sopena, M. Sabrià-Leal, M. L. Pedro-Botet et al., "Comparative study of the clinical presentation of legionella pneumonia and other community-acquired pneumonias," *Chest*, vol. 113, no. 5, pp. 1195–1200, 1998.

30

Refractory Paraneoplastic Diarrhea Secondary to Adenocarcinoma of the Lung

Lauren Howdershelt,[1] Michael J. Forte,[2] and Rahul G. Sangani[2]

[1]*Department of Family Medicine, West Virginia University, 1 Medical Center Dr., Morgantown WV 26506, USA*
[2]*Department of Medicine, Section of Pulmonary, Critical Care and Sleep Medicine, West Virginia University, 1 Medical Center Dr., Morgantown WV 26506, USA*

Correspondence should be addressed to Michael J. Forte; miforte@hsc.wvu.edu

Academic Editor: Mehmet Doganay

Paraneoplastic diarrhea is a commonly described complication of gastrointestinal tract or endocrine malignancies. It is an extremely rare complication of lung adenocarcinoma, with only one previously reported case in the literature. A 46-year-old female with newly diagnosed stage IVb lung adenocarcinoma presented to our intensive care unit in hypovolemic shock with symptoms suggestive of diabetes insipidus (DI) as well as profuse large volume watery diarrhea. Exhaustive serological and microbiological workup revealed the diarrhea to be paraneoplasitc in nature. This case represents the second known case of paraneoplastic diarrhea secondary to lung adenocarcinoma. Clinicians should be aware of this rare phenomenon.

1. Introduction

Paraneoplastic diarrhea has been seen in tumors which primarily originate in the gastrointestinal tract or endocrine system. Lung cancer, specifically lung adenocarcinoma, can develop other paraneoplastic syndromes of hypertrophic osteoarthropathy and trousseau syndrome. Only one previous case of paraneoplastic diarrhea in the setting of lung adenocarcinoma has been described. The previous report described five months of secretory diarrhea in a patient with known adenocarcinoma of the right upper lung. The patient underwent a full workup showing an elevated chromogranin-A [1]. The patient's diarrhea resolved after surgical resection. We present a second case of paraneoplastic diarrhea in the setting of lung adenocarcinoma.

2. Case Report

A 46-year-old white female with recently diagnosed, untreated stage IVb adenocarcinoma of the right lung, as well as history of bipolar disorder, previously on lithium, presented to the hospital with abdominal pain, nausea, nonbloody nonbilious vomiting, diarrhea, fevers, and chills. Workup at the outside facility showed progression of disease with new pleural and hepatic metastasis. She was treated empirically for sepsis with antimicrobials and antifungals due to suspected infected MediPort, which was removed. Microbiological workup was unremarkable. She was transferred to our facility due to ongoing circulatory shock of unknown etiology.

On arrival to our hospital, she was persistently hypotensive despite multiple fluid boluses and was noted to have a high urine output (maximum of 13 L in 24 hours) concerning for diabetes insipidus (DI) along with profuse, high output of watery diarrhea. She was diagnosed with DI given her urine osmolarity of 202 mOsm/kg, urine specific gravity of 1.005, and urine sodium of 47 mOsm/kg in conjunction with a serum osmolarity of 298 mOsm/kg. Based on nephrology recommendations, she was continually treated with desmopressin, hydrochlorothiazide

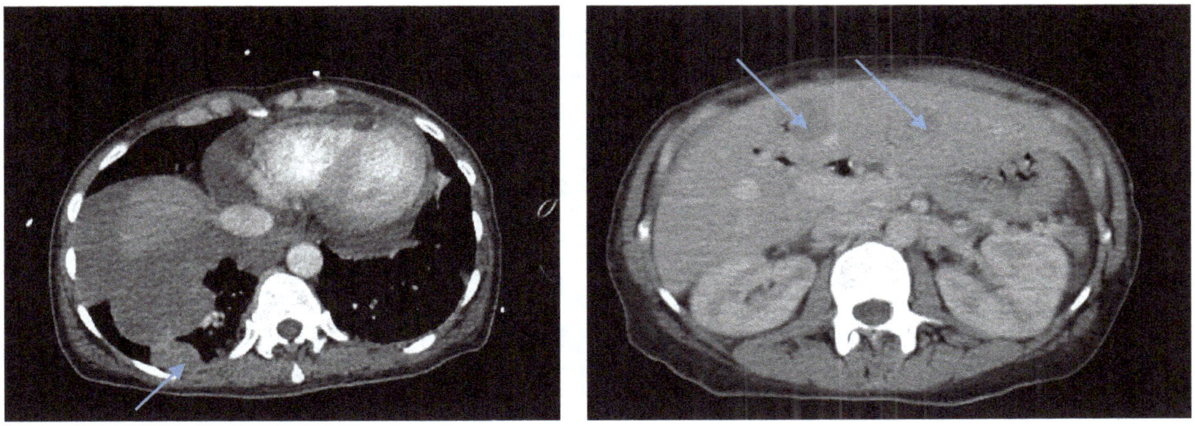

(a) (b)

FIGURE 1: (a) New pleural based metastasis (blue arrow) with known large right lung mass and (a) 2 new metastatic liver lesions (blue arrows).

(HCTZ), and triamterene for mixed central and nephrogenic DI process.

Despite her urine output decreasing, her stool output remained high, averaging 2700 mL per day. Clostridium difficile toxin and stool cultures were negative. New pleural and liver metastasis were visible on a repeat CT abdomen and pelvis as part of the workup with no other abnormalities seen in the GI tract (Figures 1(a) and 1(b)). Despite trials of loperamide, stool bulking agents, and later diphenoxylate/atropine, her diarrhea persisted. In addition, our gastroenterology colleagues deemed her too unstable for any endoscopic evaluation including colonoscopy. Given her history, the possibility of a paraneoplastic phenomenon was explored. A complete serological workup revealed only significantly elevated levels of chromogranin A and calcitonin (Table 1). Her overall conditioned continued to deteriorate and she developed multiorgan failure, refractory pain symptoms, and continued high stool output. Given her overall illness, she was deemed not a candidate for treatment of malignancy and opted for hospice care.

TABLE 1

Patient's stool studies	Normal values in parenthesis
Infectious disease	
Stool leukocytes	No PMNs
Stool culture	Vibrio-negative Salmonella-negative Campylobacter-negative Shigella-negative
Clostridium difficile toxin PCR assay	Negative
Parasitic studies	
Ova and parasites screen	Negative
Cryptosporidium/Giardia	Negative
Endocrine studies	
5-HIAA, 24-hour urine	4.7 (<8 mg/24 hours)
ACTH	18.8 (6.0-59 pg/mL)
Cortisol (p.m.)	9.3 (2.0-14.0 ug/dL)
Calcitonin	229 (<7.6 pg/mL)
Chromogranin-A	152 (<92 ng/mL)
Gastrin	52 (0-180 pg/mL)
Serotonin	131 (<230 ng/mL)
Somatostatin	9 (up to 25 pg/mL)
VIP, plasma	Undetectable

Key: HIAA = 5-hydroxyindoleacetic acid, VIP = vasoactive intestinal peptide.

3. Discussion

Given the significant elevation in Chromogranin A and calcitonin in the setting of otherwise normal hormonal markers and negative infectious workup, we believe that the profuse, watery diarrhea experienced by our patient was a paraneoplastic phenomenon incited by her lung adenocarcinoma.

Typically, lung adenocarcinoma is associated with hypertrophic osteoarthropathy and not diarrhea. Of the three main types of lung cancer, small cell lung cancer has the highest rate of developing a paraneoplastic syndrome via the release of an endogenous substance and at times may result in free water retention or GI dysmotility [1]. However, secretory diarrhea defined as diarrhea that generates excessive amounts of stool with no osmotic gap and persists with fasting, secondary to a neoplasm is rarely reported in the literature [2].

Secretory diarrheas are more commonly associated with pancreatic neuroendocrine tumors such as gastrinomas, vasoactive intestinal peptide- (VIP-) omas, somatostatinomas, and carcinoid tumors. Our patient had normal or undetectable levels of these three pancreatic hormones essentially ruling these out. We additionally ruled out carcinoid tumor via normal levels of serotonin and urine metanephrines and the liver metastasis was known to be of lung origin.

With similar manifestations of diarrhea and cutaneous flushing, medullary thyroid cancer originates in the parafollicular C cells of the thyroid that produce calcitonin. This paraneoplastic phenomenon is often found in advanced medullary thyroid carcinoma and is due to elevated systemic calcitonin [3]. Calcitonin levels of >10 pg/mL often manifests in secretory diarrhea [4]. Our patient was found to have a calcitonin level of 229 pg/mL; however, no tumors were detected within her thyroid on imaging and had normal thyroid function panel.

Even though lung cancer has the largest association with paraneoplastic syndromes secretory diarrhea has rarely been found and few case reports exist within the literature. Tischer et al. [5] proposed secretory diarrhea as an atypical paraneoplastic syndrome in a patient with chronic diarrhea for three months who found relief from diarrhea after the resection of a solitary pulmonary nodule found to be small cell lung cancer. The endogenous molecule was not discovered. Later, adrenocorticotropic hormone (ACTH) and calcitonin causing diarrhea and metabolic abnormalities was found in the setting of small cell lung cancer [6]. Diarrhea associated with large cell carcinoma has been described in the literature twice; once in the setting of elevated VIP and calcitonin [7] and another in the case of elevated gastrin levels [8]. A similar scenario of paraneoplastic diarrhea in the setting of adenocarcinoma with elevated chromogranin-A to our case has been described. The authors reported that profuse diarrhea, once requiring up to doses of 12 mg of loperamide daily to control, completely resolved following surgical resection of the tumor [1].

In our case, the disease was too far advanced to consider surgical treatment; however, she demonstrated elevated chromogranin-A similar to the previous report with adenocarcinoma. Thus, we postulate that our patient's secretory diarrhea was due to the elevated chromogranin-A and calcitonin. We also hypothesize that the patient might have exhibited concomitant neuroendocrine features on her predominant histopathology of adenocarcinoma, but unfortunately, her pathology slides were not able to be transferred to our facility for further assessment. This case emphasizes the need for increased awareness among the clinicians regarding uncommon phenomenon of paraneoplastic diarrhea leading to critical illness. Early surgical management likely is key for resolution, as medical management alone carries a high risk of failure.

References

[1] A. D. Nguyen, M. A. Valasek, and E. Burstein, "Paraneoplastic diarrhea in a patient with lung adenocarcinoma," *Clinical Journal of Gastroenterology*, vol. 6, no. 5, pp. 357–360, 2013.

[2] A. I. Vinik and C. Chaya, "Clinical presentation and diagnosis of neuroendocrine tumors," *Hematology/Oncology Clinics of North America*, vol. 30, no. 1, pp. 21–48, 2016.

[3] M. W. Zafereo, "Thyroid cancer," in *Conns Current Therapy*, R. Kellerman, Ed., pp. 369–373, Elsevier, Philidelphia, NY, USA, 1st edition, 2019.

[4] J. Robbins, M. J. Merino, J. D. Boice Jr. et al., "Thyroid cancer: a lethal endocrine neoplasm," *Annals of Internal Medicine*, vol. 115, no. 2, pp. 133–147, 1991.

[5] T. Tischer, W. Sienel, O. Thetter, and B. Passlick, "Chronic diarrhea as a first manifestation of small cell lung cancer. A case report," *Zentralblatt für Chirurgie*, vol. 126, no. 11, pp. 926–928, 2001.

[6] K. Coners, S. E. Woods, and M. Webb, "Dual paraneoplastic syndromes in a patient with small cell lung cancer: a case report," *Journal of Medical Case Reports*, vol. 5, no. 1, p. 318, 2011.

[7] K. W. Pratz, C. Ma, M. C. Aubry, T. J. Vrtiska, and C. Erlichman, "Large cell carcinoma with calcitonin and vasoactive intestinal polypeptide-associated Verner-Morrison syndrome," *Mayo Clinic Proceedings*, vol. 80, no. 1, pp. 116–120, 2005.

[8] A. Abou-Saif, J. Lei, T. J. McDonald et al., "A new cause of Zollinger–Ellison syndrome: Non–Small cell lung cancer," *Gastroenterology*, vol. 120, no. 5, pp. 1271–1278, 2001.

31

Considerations in Neuromuscular Blockade in the ICU

Jessica D. Workum,[1,2] Stephanie H.V. Janssen,[1,3] and Hugo R.W. Touw[1]

[1]*Department of Intensive Care, Radboud University Medical Center, Geert Grooteplein Zuid 10, 6525 GA, Nijmegen, Netherlands*
[2]*Department of Clinical Pharmacology, Radboud University Medical Center, Geert Grooteplein Zuid 10, 6525 GA, Nijmegen, Netherlands*
[3]*Department of Anaesthesiology, Radboud University Medical Center, Geert Grooteplein Zuid 10, 6525 GA, Nijmegen, Netherlands*

Correspondence should be addressed to Jessica D. Workum; jessica.workum@radboudumc.nl

Academic Editor: Kenneth S. Waxman

Neuromuscular blocking agents are regularly used in the intensive care unit (ICU) to facilitate mechanical ventilation in patients with acute respiratory distress syndrome and patient-ventilator dyssynchronies. However, prolonged neuromuscular blockade is associated with adverse effects like ICU-acquired weakness. Residual neuromuscular blockade is, however, not routinely monitored in the intensive care unit, and as such, this phenomenon might be unrecognized and underreported. We report a case in which an unusual prolonged effect of neuromuscular blockade was seen after cessation of the drug, which illustrates the complexity of neuromuscular blockade in the ICU. We advocate for the use of train-of-four measurements in the ICU, recommend to choose cisatracurium over rocuronium in critically ill patients due to their pharmacokinetics when continuous neuromuscular blockade is considered, and propose a subsequent strategy once the choice has been made to start neuromuscular blockade.

1. Introduction

Neuromuscular blocking agents (NMBAs) are used in the intensive care unit (ICU) for various indications, for instance, to facilitate intubation in the treatment of status asthmaticus and to facilitate mechanical ventilation in patients with acute respiratory distress syndrome (ARDS). The ACURASYS trial by Papazian et al. [1] found a beneficial effect of continuous neuromuscular blockade on the mortality of ARDS patients. This has led to an increase in the use of continuous NMBAs in the ICU, as the current guideline for sustained neuromuscular blockade in the adult critically ill patient now recommends starting continuous NMBAs early in ARDS [2]. In contrary to the ACURASYS trial, the recently published ROSE trial found no reduction in mortality with early continuous neuromuscular blockade in ARDS [3]. Furthermore, it was associated with an increase in ICU-acquired weakness and serious adverse cardiovascular events. Neuromuscular blockade should, therefore, be used cautiously and only in selected individuals in which other strategies have failed.

Neuromuscular blockade can have residual effects. Residual neuromuscular blockade can cause postoperative pulmonary complications [4], ranging from a reduced ability to swallow by a loss of coordination of tongue and throat musculature, which carries a higher risk of aspiration [5, 6], to general muscle weakness, loss of ventilatory hypoxic drive, atelectasis, and airway obstruction. An additional important complication is awareness. These complications can lead to an increased length of hospital stay with a threefold higher chance to be admitted to the ICU [7]. In the critically ill patients, the consequences of residual neuromuscular blockade have not been investigated; however, it is reasonable to assume a risk similar to prolonged infusion.

The degree of (residual) neuromuscular blockade can be determined by measuring the neuromuscular response on peripheral nerve stimulation, for instance, with a train-of-four (TOF) measurement. During TOF stimulation, four stimuli are delivered at 0.5 second intervals, and the response of the innervated muscle is assessed. With an increasing depth of neuromuscular blockade, this response (twitches) decreases in force. When there is no response on TOF stimulation, a deep neuromuscular blockade may be present, the intensity of which can be measured using the posttetanic count (PTC). During a PTC measurement, a 5-second tetanic stimulus of 50 Hz is administered, followed by a series of single twitch stimuli delivered at 1 Hz for 20 seconds. A response to this stimulation will be seen in the early stages of recovery [8]. Despite the frequent use of NMBAs in the ICU, it is not yet common practice to measure TOF or PTC in the critically ill and as such, residual neuromuscular blockade might be unrecognized and underreported.

We present a case that illustrates the complexity of continuous neuromuscular blockade in a critically ill patient. Furthermore, we review the literature and pharmacokinetics of neuromuscular blockade in the ICU and propose a subsequent strategy, once the choice has been made to start neuromuscular blockade.

2. Case Report

A 76-year-old woman was admitted to our ICU with pyogenic spondylodiscitis, due to *Staphylococcus aureus* bacteremia with unknown focus, complicated by an epidural abscess for which she received a laminectomy with subsequent drainage of the abscess. Her medical history consisted of a coronary artery bypass graft and hypertension. In the days following surgery, she developed ventilator-acquired pneumonia (VAP) with difficult mechanical ventilation, as expressed by patient-ventilator dyssynchronies like reverse triggering. As deep sedation with midazolam, sufentanyl, and propofol showed no improvement, it was decided to start continuous neuromuscular blockade with rocuronium. Though this did improve the quality of ventilation, we did find extensive residual effect of the neuromuscular blockade.

After 48 hours of continuous infusion, rocuronium was ceased. To rule out any form of residual neuromuscular blockade, TOF and PTC measurements were performed 5 hours after cessation of the rocuronium by stimulating the ulnar nerve. TOF response was zero, and no motor response could be provoked from the PTC stimulation either. It was concluded that there was still residual neuromuscular blockade, and therefore sedation was continued.

The next day, 22 hours after cessation of the rocuronium, both measurements were performed again under unchanged conditions. The results were similar: TOF response remained zero, and there was no response on PTC stimulation.

Approximately 60 hours after cessation of the continuous rocuronium infusion, the TOF remained immeasurably low, but this time, PTC stimulation gave a clear motor response that consisted of a few twitches with visible fading. We, therefore, administered 500 mg sugammadex intravenously split into two doses to antagonize rocuronium, after which the TOF ratio subsequently rose to 94 percent.

The following morning, the TOF ratio has fallen to 4 percent again without intervention due to recurarization. The measurement was repeated 5 hours later, and it had risen to 92 percent without intervention, upon which sedation was stopped successfully.

3. Discussion

3.1. Nondepolarizing Neuromuscular Blocking Agents. Nondepolarizing NMBAs bind to the alpha-subunit of the skeletal muscle postsynaptic nicotinic receptor, preventing acetylcholine from binding to the receptor and depolarizing the cell and thus inhibiting muscular contraction. They can be divided into two classes: the benzylisoquinolinium (e.g., atracurium and cisatracurium) and the aminosteroid compounds (e.g., rocuronium, vecuronium, and pancuronium). In the ICU, aminosteroid compounds are more commonly used than their benzylisoquinolinium counterparts, based on familiarity of the physician with the drug [9]. Unlike benzylisoquinolium NMBAs, aminosteroid NMBAs can be antagonized with sugammadex, a selective binding agent with high affinity. Sugammadex encapsulates the aminosteroid NMBA, negating its effect [10].

3.2. Pharmacokinetics of Rocuronium. Like all neuromuscular blockers, rocuronium is administered intravenously, as it is not effective orally. It is an aminosteroid compound which rapidly distributes throughout the body, following a three compartment model. The rapid distribution half-life is 1 to 2 minutes, whereas the slower distribution half-life is 14–18 minutes. It has a volume of distribution of 0.21–0.27 l/kg in the adult population, which decreases slightly in the elderly population. Protein binding is approximately 30%. Rocuronium is partially metabolized to the active metabolite 17-desacetyl-rocuronium, which is approximately 20 times less potent than rocuronium itself. Elimination half-life varies between 60 and 90 minutes. The primary route for excretion is biliary, whereas 33–47% of rocuronium is excreted unchanged in urine.

3.3. Pharmacokinetics of Cisatracurium. Cisatracurium is a benzylisoquinolinium compound. It is an isomer of atracurium with more favorable characteristics: it is four times more potent, does not cause histamine release, and has no direct cardiovascular effects. It has a shorter onset, with its peak within 1-2 minutes. It has a volume of distribution of 0.145 l/kg, and it is mainly metabolized through Hofmann elimination, with a plasma elimination half-life of 22 minutes. Renal and hepatic metabolism is negligible; however, the inactive metabolites are excreted renally. With 40–90 minutes, its duration of action is slightly longer than atracurium.

3.4. Train-of-Four in the Critically Ill. Currently, the guideline for sustained neuromuscular blockade in the adult critically ill patient recommends against monitoring the depth of neuromuscular blockade using TOF alone, but it suggests to use it in conjunction with clinical assessment [2]. Clinical assessment proves, however, to be an unreliable method for assessing the depth of neuromuscular blockade when compared to TOF, even in the critically ill [11].

It is not clear yet if the depth of neuromuscular blockade in patients with ICU-acquired weakness can be adequately measured with peripheral nerve stimulation [12]. TOF measurements are lower in patients with ICUAW than in those without. Results should, therefore, be interpreted with great care in this group of patients.

3.5. Neuromuscular Blockade in the Critically Ill. Though several sources have indicated that renal insufficiency does not impair rocuronium clearance [13, 14], clinical studies have shown prolonged neuromuscular effects of rocuronium in patients with renal failure [15, 16], though none come close to our patient. Liver disease affects rocuronium volume of distribution and clearance, increasing the duration of its effect [17, 18].

A study performed by Circeo et al. [19] showed a profound prolonged effect of rocuronium after continuous infusion in critically ill patients with multiple organ failure (MOF) compared to single organ failure. Mean time to recovery, as measured with the train-of-four, was 599 minutes for the MOF group versus 230 minutes in the non-MOF group. Furthermore, the MOF group required only 40% of the amount of rocuronium used non-MOF group (0.2 mg/kg/hour versus 0.5 mg/kg/hour).

It is, therefore, postulated that the prolonged effect of rocuronium in our patient is multifactorial. She had received a continuous dose of 0.3 mg/kg/hour twice the recommended maintenance dose of 0.1–0.15 mg/kg/hour. Her volume of distribution would have been increased as a result of excessive fluid administration due to prior shock as well as profound hypoalbuminemia (13 g/L, normal range 35–45 g/L), causing a prolonged distribution half-life. She showed signs of hepatic injury, with slight increases in transaminase levels (ALT 49 U/L and AST 184 U/L), elevated yGT (417 U/L), AF (319 U/L) and bilirubin levels (direct 43 umol/L, total 44 umol/L), attributed to high dose flucloxacillin as liver and biliary pathology was excluded on ultrasound, but no signs of liver failure as her glucose levels, platelet count, and coagulation panel were normal. And she had profound renal impairment (GFR <10 ml/min) for which continuous renal replacement therapy was started. Both could contribute to a decrease in rocuronium clearance, causing a prolonged clinical effect.

The administration of sugammadex and its subsequent reversal of neuromuscular blockade confirmed our suspicion of residual neuromuscular blockade. As sugammadex is predominantly renally cleared, its half-life is increased in renal dysfunction, possibly causing rocuronium-sugammadex complexes to circulate longer in the system. However, these complexes have a very low dissociation rate, so there is little to no concern of recurarization. In addition, the reversal rate is as rapid and effective as in patients with normal renal function. [20].

4. Conclusion

This case illustrates the complex pharmacokinetics of rocuronium in the critically ill, especially when administered as a continuous infusion, with an unexpectedly prolonged clinical effect. Combined with the recent findings of the ROSE trial, we strongly advise to exercise restrained use of continuous neuromuscular blockade in the ICU in general and advise to consider using intermittent boluses instead. If, however, the choice has been made to start continuous neuromuscular blockade, we strongly advise to monitor TOF levels during continuous infusion and after cessation of the drug. We furthermore advise to choose cisatracurium over a steroid-based NMBA like rocuronium in these situations, due to their more favorable pharmacokinetics in critically ill patients.

4.1. Proposed Strategy and Recommendations. For rapid sequence induction, we recommend a steroid-based NMBA like rocuronium, due to its rapid onset and the possibility to antagonize its effects with sugammadex.

If continuous neuromuscular blockade is considered, then

(1) Consider other strategies
  (a) Deeper sedation
  (b) Optimizing patient-ventilator synchrony
  (c) Others

(2) Consider intermittent boluses instead

(3) Consider your patient: if multiple organ failure, then
  (a) Monitor the effect with TOF
  (b) Choose cisatracurium over an aminosteroid NMBA

(4) Consider monitoring TOF levels in all patients

(5) If prolonged effects are observed after cessation of the drug, consider antagonizing with sugammadex if an aminosteroid (rocuronium, vecuronium, or pancuronium) was chosen. Mind that due to their distribution, this may need to be repeated.

References

[1] L. Papazian, J.-M. Forel, A. Gacouin et al., "Neuromuscular blockers in early acute respiratory distress syndrome," *New England Journal of Medicine*, vol. 363, no. 12, pp. 1107–1116, 2010.

[2] M. J. Murray, H. DeBlock, B. Erstad et al., "Clinical practice guidelines for sustained neuromuscular blockade in the adult critically ill patient," *Critical Care Medicine*, vol. 44, no. 11, pp. 2079–2103, 2016.

[3] M. Moss, D. T. Huang, R. G. Brower et al., "Early neuromuscular blockade in the acute respiratory distress syndrome," *The New England Journal of Medicine*, vol. 380, no. 21, pp. 1997–2008, 2019.

[4] E. Kirmeier, L. I Eriksson, H Lewald et al., "Post-anaesthesia pulmonary complications after use of muscle relaxants (POPULAR): a multicentre, prospective observational study," *The Lancet. Respiratory Medicine*, vol. 7, no. 7, pp. 129–140, 2019.
[5] F. Donati, "Residual paralysis: a real problem or did we invent a new disease?," *Canadian Journal of Anesthesia/Journal Canadien D'anesthésie*, vol. 60, no. 7, pp. 714–729, 2013.
[6] T. Fuchs-Buder, R. Nemes, and D. Schmartz, "Residual neuromuscular blockade," *Current Opinion in Anaesthesiology*, vol. 29, no. 6, pp. 662–667, 2016.
[7] S. D. Grabitz, N. Rajaratnam, K. Chhagani et al., "The effects of postoperative residual neuromuscular blockade on hospital costs and intensive care unit admission," *Anesthesia & Analgesia*, vol. 128, no. 6, pp. 1129–1136, 2019.
[8] M. Naguib, S. J. Brull, and K. B. Johnson, "Conceptual and technical insights into the basis of neuromuscular monitoring," *Anaesthesia*, vol. 72, no. 1, pp. 16–37, 2017.
[9] D. H. Rhoney and K. R. Murry, "National survey of the use of sedating drugs, neuromuscular blocking agents, and reversal agents in the intensive care unit," *Journal of Intensive Care Medicine*, vol. 18, no. 3, pp. 139–145, 2003.
[10] A. Srivastava and J. M. Hunter, "Reversal of neuromuscular block," *British Journal of Anaesthesia*, vol. 103, no. 1, pp. 115–129, 2009.
[11] P. Bouju, J. M. Tadie, N. Barbarot et al., "Clinical assessment and train-of-four measurements in critically ill patients treated with recommended doses of cisatracurium or atracurium for neuromuscular blockade: a prospective descriptive study," *Ann Intensive Care*, vol. 7, no. 1, p. 10, 2017.
[12] S. Deem, "Intensive-care-unit-acquired muscle weakness," *Respiratory Care*, vol. 51, no. 51, pp. 1042-1043, 2006.
[13] R. D. R. U. G. D. E. X. Evaluations. 2019, Micromedex.
[14] Rocuronium. 2019, DrugBank.ca.
[15] H. J. Sparr, J. M. Wierda, J. H. Proost, C. Keller, and K. S. Khuenl-Brady, "Pharmacodynamics and pharmacokinetics of rocuronium in intensive care patients," *British Journal of Anaesthesia*, vol. 78, no. 3, pp. 267–273, 1997.
[16] S. Kocabas, D. Yedicocuklu, and F. Z. Askar, "The neuromuscular effects of 0.6 mg kg-1 rocuronium in elderly and young adults with or without renal failure," *European Journal of Anaesthesiology*, vol. 25, no. 11, pp. 940–946, 2008.
[17] M. Khalil, G. D'Honneur, P. Duvaldestin, V. Slavov, C. D. Hys, and R. Gomeni, "Pharmacokinetics and pharmacodynamics of rocuronium in patients with cirrhosis," *Anesthesiology*, vol. 80, no. 6, pp. 1241–1247, 1994.
[18] M. M. van Miert, N. B. Eastwood, A. H. Boyd, C. J. R. Parker, and J. M. Hunter, "The pharmacokinetics and pharmacodynamics of rocuronium in patients with hepatic cirrhosis," *British Journal of Clinical Pharmacology*, vol. 44, no. 2, pp. 139–144, 1997.
[19] L. E. Circeo and S. T. Reeves, "Multicenter trial of prolonged infusions of rocuronium bromide in critically ill patients," *Southern Medical Journal*, vol. 94, no. 1, pp. 36–42, 2001.
[20] L. M. Staals, M. M. J. Snoeck, J. J. Driessen et al., "Reduced clearance of rocuronium and sugammadex in patients with severe to end-stage renal failure: a pharmacokinetic study," *British Journal of Anaesthesia*, vol. 104, no. 1, pp. 31–39, 2010.

A Curious Case of MRSA Bacteremia and Septic Pulmonary Embolism Secondary to Peripheral Venous Catheter

Joshua Twito, Syeda Sahra, Abdullah Jahangir, and Neville Mobarakai

Staten Island University Hospital, Staten Island, NY 10305, USA

Correspondence should be addressed to Syeda Sahra; ssahra@northwell.edu

Academic Editor: Mabrouk Bahloul

Background. Central venous catheters (CVCs) have been frequently associated with septic thrombophlebitis, bacteremia, and septic emboli. Right-sided infective endocarditis is seen concurrently in patients with septic pulmonary emboli. A case of methicillin-resistant Staphylococcus aureus (MRSA) bacteremia and septic pulmonary emboli secondary to infected peripheral venous catheter (PVC) is reported. Transesophageal echocardiogram (TEE) showed no evidence of infective endocarditis. *Case Presentation.* A 44-year-old female presented to E.R. with left upper extremity pain and swelling at the previously inserted peripheral 18-gauge intravenous catheter site. She also had chest pain, which worsened with inspiration. The patient was found to be in septic shock. Her clinical condition deteriorated acutely. Right upper extremity deep venous thrombosis (DVT) and pulmonary emboli were seen on imaging. Blood cultures grew MRSA. Transthoracic and transesophageal echocardiograms showed no vegetations. The patient responded well to appropriate antibiotics and anticoagulation. *Conclusion.* Peripherally inserted catheters are an important portal for pathogen entry and need periodic site assessment and frequent evaluation of their need for insertion. Septic pulmonary emboli can also be seen without any evidence of right-sided infective endocarditis.

1. Introduction

Catheter-associated infections are common in hospitalized patients, particularly with central venous catheters in critically ill patients. These infections include but are not limited to soft tissue abscesses, cellulitis, septic phlebitis, pneumonia, and bacteremia. Upper extremity DVTs formed secondary to central venous catheters have been associated with pulmonary emboli [1–4]. Staphylococcus aureus is usually the incriminated organism in catheter-associated infections, and Staphylococcus bacteremia outcomes, if overlooked, can be life-threatening. Right-sided infective endocarditis is a common precedent with septic emboli [5]. The hospital stay and clinical course in these patients are complicated by the need for prolonged antibiotics and anticoagulation [6]. Rare and infrequently, Staphylococcus bacteremia is also seen with peripherally inserted catheters [7]. We present a case of thrombophlebitis from a peripherally inserted catheter leading to Staphylococcus bacteremia and pulmonary embolism without any evidence of infective endocarditis on transthoracic and transesophageal echocardiogram. The patient received appropriate antibiotics and anticoagulation. Physicians should keep the likelihood of staphylococcal bacteremia and showering of septic emboli in mind even with peripherally inserted catheters. Right-sided infective endocarditis is not necessarily always present with septic pulmonary emboli. Observation of hygienic measures while insertion, periodic site assessment, and prompt discontinuation of the catheter when not indicated should be performed to prevent the catheter-associated infections [8].

2. Case

A 44-year-old female presented to our emergency department with pain, swelling, and weakness in the left upper extremity. She also complained of pain in her chest, which worsened with inspiration. The patient had noticed having trouble typing on her computer keyboard and an episodic bilateral leg numbness for the past few days. She had a past medical history of recently diagnosed multiple sclerosis, chronic migraines, and seizure disorder (on antiepileptic drug (AED) therapy). The patient was seen two weeks earlier

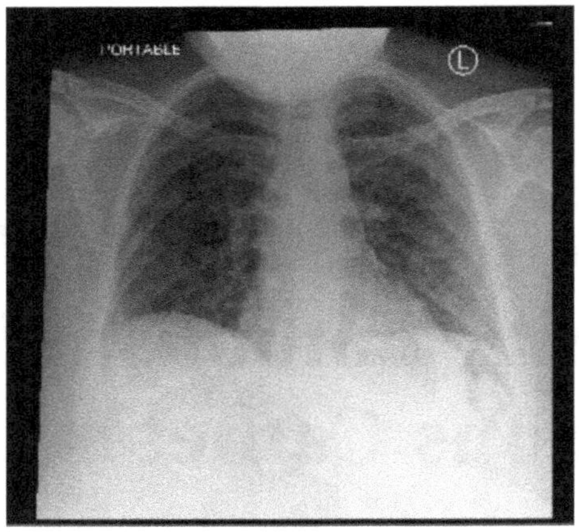

FIGURE 1: Chest X-ray on arrival showing diffuse bilateral opacities.

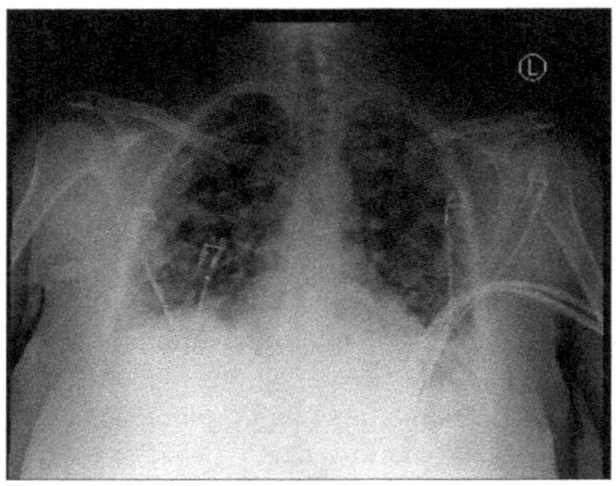

FIGURE 2: Chest X-ray showing worsening bilateral nodular opacities on hospital day 1.

in the Emergency Room with generalized weakness, left arm numbness, and headache. Stroke workup was unremarkable, and the patient was subsequently discharged to follow-up with neurology outpatient.

She denied any other complaints in the time preceding her admission. The patient reported an active lifestyle and denied any tobacco usage, alcohol, or intravenous drug abuse.

On physical examination, the patient displayed a worsening tachycardia, hypotension with a blood pressure of 75/40 mmHg, and a drop in oxygen saturation to 88% at room air. Supplemental oxygen therapy via nasal cannula at a rate of 5 liters per minute improved her oxygen saturation to 99%. A low-dose norepinephrine infusion was started for the hypotension.

The left upper extremity showed tenderness to palpation and swelling where an intravenous catheter was inserted on her last visit to the E.R. two weeks ago. The 18-gauge PVC was inserted by the nursing department in the Emergency Room and was removed 12 hours after the insertion. The patient noticed some redness and tenderness, which had started few days after being discharged and progressively worsened.

The patient received Cefazolin and Vancomycin. Blood work was significant for leukocytosis, mildly elevated blood urea (30 mg/dL), serum glucose of 164 mg/dL, serum lactate 2.5 mg/dL, erythrocyte sedimentation rate (ESR) 49 mm/hr, and a quantitative D-dimer of 3624 ng/mL. Coagulation studies showed activated partial thromboplastin time (aPTT) 25.4 s, and an INR (international normalized ratio) elevated to 1.42 s.

Chest radiograph revealed worsening diffuse nodular opacities bilaterally in the lung fields (Figures 1 and 2). C.T. angiography of the chest with IV contrast revealed changes consistent with septic pulmonary emboli (Figure 3). Left upper extremity duplex ultrasonography revealed acute deep vein thrombosis of the left axillary and brachial veins, thrombosis of the cephalic vein, and a patent basilic vein.

The patient was admitted to the ICU for management of septic shock. Antimicrobial therapy was adjusted to Cefepime and Azithromycin, and therapeutic anticoagulation was started.

On hospital day 2, the left antecubital fossa was erythematous and painful, with purulent fluid expression. Nafcillin and Vancomycin were started based on preliminary cultures growing gram-positive bacteria. Final cultures revealed MRSA bacteremia, and Nafcillin was discontinued. The patient continued to experience chest pain, shortness of breath, and left arm pain with worsening leukocytosis. Transthoracic echocardiogram (TTE) showed no evidence of endocarditis. The patient was found to have septic thrombophlebitis of the brachiocephalic vein on surgical exploration and required excisional debridement and resection of a portion of the brachiocephalic vein. Fungitell, Aspergillus galactomannan assay, and HIV ½ testing were negative.

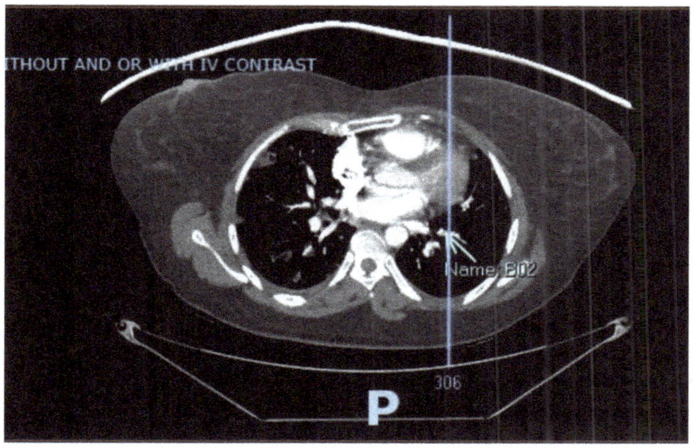

FIGURE 3: C.T. chest angiogram showing diffuse, multifocal nodular opacities throughout the bilateral lungs, some of which appeared cavitary, with the largest measuring approximately 1.8 cm located in the lower right lobe.

Vancomycin, Ceftaroline, and Clindamycin were started on the basis of final cultures. Transesophageal echocardiogram (TEE) on hospital day eight did not show any evidence of right-sided endocarditis. Blood cultures were cleared from MRSA on hospital day ten, and we transitioned the anticoagulation to low molecular weight heparin (LMWH). Blood pressure support was weaned off. She got discharged home on intravenous Vancomycin for 6-8 weeks and was reported doing well on follow-up.

3. Discussion and Conclusion

Septic pulmonary emboli are characterized by fever, tachycardia, shortness of breath along with nodular opacities, and cavitation on imaging [9]. Septic systemic emboli are seen secondary to left-sided infective endocarditis, and pulmonary emboli are generated secondary to right-sided infective endocarditis [10].

CVC catheter placement is a risk factor for upper extremity DVT [2]. Septic pulmonary embolism follows as its natural consequence. Ultrasonography and color flow doppler are diagnostic modalities for DVTs.

The catheter site serves as a portal for infection. Seeding of community-based and nosocomial pathogens (most commonly Staphylococcus) from the skin has been established to cause bacteremia and right-sided infective endocarditis [5, 11, 12].

There is a substantial emphasis on periodic assessment of centrally placed catheters in critical care units and their prompt removal once they are no longer needed. All emergently placed nonsterile accesses are recommended to be replaced by a sterile catheter as soon as the patient is clinically stable [13]. These ICU protocols have been created and followed after the deadly consequences of catheter-associated infections became well established.

This case is unusual as the patient developed MRSA bacteremia and septic pulmonary emboli from a peripheral venous catheter despite being immunocompetent and having no history of intravenous drug abuse. Another interesting finding was the absence of any right-sided infective endocarditis in this patient confirmed on the transesophageal echocardiogram. Infected PVCs are mostly accompanied by fever, erythema, and tenderness, which resolve with warm compressions and limb elevation. There have been very few bacteremia cases and showering of septic emboli from a peripherally placed venous catheter owing to suppurative thrombophlebitis [14].

A similar case has been reported in the literature recently, but the pathogen was ESBL Klebsiella pneumonia [15]. The authors conclude that peripherally inserted intravenous catheter infections can cause bacteremia and septic emboli. The septic pulmonary emboli are possible without cardiac vegetations as well. Regular assessment of catheter site for erythema and swelling, hygienic measures during insertion, choosing an anatomically favored location for lesser chances of infection (antecubital fossa), and early removal of the catheter can help minimize catheter-associated thrombophlebitis and its complications [8].

Abbreviations

AEDs: Antiepileptic drugs
CVC: Central venous catheter
DVT: Deep venous thrombosis
ER: Emergency Room
ICU: Intensive care unit
LMWH: Low molecular weight heparin
MSSA: Methicillin-sensitive Staphylococcus aureus
MRSA: Methicillin-resistant Staphylococcus aureus
PVC: Peripheral venous catheter
PTT: Partial thromboplastin time
TTE: Transthoracic echocardiogram
TEE: Transesophageal echocardiogram.

Consent

The patient and family were contacted during the hospital stay and after discharge. Consent was obtained over the telephone for use of patient data, images, and blood work for the publication of case for purely educational and research purposes to which the family agreed. No identifying information usage was explained.

Authors' Contributions

The manuscript was written by J.T. and S.S. The literature review was done by A.J. Supervision and proofreading were done by N.M.

References

[1] G. S. Hyman and D. D. Cardenas, "Upper-extremity deep vein thrombosis associated with peripherally inserted central catheters in acute spinal cord injury: a report of 2 cases," *Archives of Physical Medicine and Rehabilitation*, vol. 83, no. 9, pp. 1313–1316, 2002.

[2] P. Prandoni, P. Polistena, E. Bernardi et al., "Upper-extremity deep vein thrombosis. Risk factors, diagnosis, and complications," *Archives of Internal Medicine*, vol. 157, no. 1, pp. 57–62, 1997.

[3] M. Monreal, A. Raventos, R. Lerma et al., "Pulmonary embolism in patients with upper extremity DVT associated to venous central lines–a prospective study," *Thrombosis and Haemostasis*, vol. 72, no. 4, pp. 548–550, 1994.

[4] M. D. Black, G. J. French, P. Rasuli, and A. C. Bouchard, "Upper extremity deep venous thrombosis. Underdiagnosed and potentially lethal," *Chest*, vol. 103, no. 6, pp. 1887–1890, 1993.

[5] A. S. Beláustegui, S. Flagel, E. A. Soraide, G. Guzmán, B. Perazzi, and A. Famiglietti, "Septic pulmonary embolism of cutaneous origin," *Medicina (B Aires)*, vol. 72, no. 4, pp. 325–328, 2012.

[6] R. W. Dib, A.-M. Chaftari, R. Y. Hachem, Y. Yuan, D. Dandachi, and I. I. Raad, "Catheter-related Staphylococcus aureus bacteremia and septic thrombosis: the role of anticoagulation therapy and duration of intravenous antibiotic therapy," *Open Forum Infectious Diseases*, vol. 5, no. 10, 2018.

[7] E. D. Austin, S. B. Sullivan, S. Whittier, F. D. Lowy, and A.-C. Uhlemann, "Peripheral intravenous catheter placement is an underrecognized source of Staphylococcus aureus bloodstream infection," *Open forum infectious diseases*, vol. 3, no. 2, 2016.

[8] M. Blauw, B. Foxman, J. Wu, J. Rey, N. Kothari, and A. N. Malani, "Risk factors and outcomes associated with hospital-onset peripheral intravenous Catheter–AssociatedStaphylococcus aureusBacteremia," *Open forum infectious diseases*, vol. 6, no. 4, 2019.

[9] R. Ye, L. Zhao, C. Wang, X. Wu, and H. Yan, "Clinical characteristics of septic pulmonary embolism in adults: a systematic review," *Respiratory Medicine*, vol. 108, no. 1, pp. 1–8, 2014.

[10] R. Patti, S. S. Gupta, and Y. Kupfer, "Right sided infective endocarditis and systemic emboli," *QJM*, vol. 112, no. 1, pp. 57-58, 2019.

[11] M. Grewal, S. Gupta, M. Muranjan, and S. Karande, "Managing pulmonary embolism secondary to suppurative deep vein thrombophlebitis due to community-acquired Staphylococcus aureus in a resource-poor setting," *Journal of Postgraduate Medicine*, vol. 64, no. 3, pp. 164–169, 2018.

[12] J. G. Bartlett, "Methicillin-resistant Staphylococcus aureus infections," *Topics in HIV Medicine*, vol. 16, no. 5, 2008.

[13] P. K. Patel, A. Gupta, V. M. Vaughn, J. D. Mann, J. M. Ameling, and J. Meddings, "Review of strategies to reduce central line-associated bloodstream infection (CLABSI) and catheter-associated urinary tract infection (CAUTI) in adult ICUs," *Journal of Hospital Medicine*, vol. 13, no. 2, pp. 105–116, 2018.

[14] D. N. Lipe, L. A. Foris, and K. C. King, *Septic Thrombophlebitis in StatPearls*, StatPearls Publishing Copyright © 2020, StatPearls Publishing LLC, Treasure Island (F.L.), 2020.

[15] A. Baidya, V. Ganakumar, R. S. Jadon, P. Ranjan, S. Manchanda, and R. Sood, "Septic pulmonary emboli as a complication of peripheral venous cannula insertion," *Drug Discoveries & Therapeutics*, vol. 12, no. 2, pp. 111–113, 2018.

33

Super-Refractory Status Epilepticus Treated with High Dose Perampanel: Case Series and Review of the Literature

Christopher R. Newey,[1,2] **Naresh Mullaguri**,[1] **Stephen Hantus**,[1,2] **Vineet Punia**,[2] **and Pravin George**[1]

[1]*Cerebrovascular Center, Neurological Institute, Cleveland Clinic, 9500 Euclid Avenue, Cleveland, OH 44195, USA*
[2]*Epilepsy Center, Neurological Institute, Cleveland Clinic, 9500 Euclid Avenue, Cleveland, OH 44195, USA*

Correspondence should be addressed to Christopher R. Newey; neweyc@ccf.org

Academic Editor: Chiara Lazzeri

Introduction. Acute symptomatic seizures are frequent in the critically ill patient and can be difficult to treat. The novel anticonvulsant perampanel may be effective in the treatment of status epilepticus considering its mechanism of action of being an AMPA antagonist. We present four cases of super refractory status epilepticus treated with high dose perampanel. *Method.* Case report. *Cases.* Four patients were treated with perampanel for their refractory status epilepticus. One patient had new onset refractory status epilepticus of unknown etiology. Three other patients had status epilepticus as a result of their cardiac arrest. Two of the cardiac arrest patients had myoclonus. In all patients, the additional of perampanel resulted in a reduction of seizure burden without affecting hemodynamics or hepatic or renal function. *Conclusion.* Perampanel may be effective in the treatment of super-refractory status epilepticus of varying etiologies. A larger, prospective study is needed to further assess this therapy.

1. Introduction

Acute symptomatic seizures—convulsive or nonconvulsive—are frequent in the critically ill patient [1]. As seizures persist, the efficacy of GABAergic agents is reduced by the internalization of postsynaptic GABA-A receptors allowing for glutamate to promote ictal activity by binding to AMPA receptors [2]. Stepwise algorithms have been created to guide medical management with little to poor evidence behind them outside of administering benzodiazepine early [3–5]. Unfortunately, the treatment of status epilepticus can be difficult and is often associated with high morbidity [6–8]. Newer anticonvulsants, such as perampanel, may be effective and well-tolerated in the treatment of status epilepticus [9]. We present four cases of super refractory status epilepticus, in very different clinical settings, treated with high dose perampanel.

2. Cases

2.1. Case 1. A 28-year-old male with history of smoking and autism presented with acute altered mental status, increased combativeness, and an upper respiratory viral illness. He had no prior history of seizures or head trauma. Urine drug screen was positive for the tetrahydrocannabinol. His initial physical and neurological examinations were unremarkable. Labs were remarkable for leukocytosis (13040 cells/mm^3) and mild transaminitis (alanine transaminase 102 U/mL and aspartate transaminase 75 U/mL). Hepatitis panel and human immunodeficiency virus serologies were unremarkable. Computerized tomography of the brain was unremarkable.

While in the emergency department (ED), he complained of severe thirst and suddenly suffered a generalized tonic-clonic seizure with urinary incontinence lasting approximately one-minute. He was treated with intravenous lorazepam and levetiracetam. He was admitted to the neurological intensive care unit. A lumbar puncture was performed which revealed a mildly elevated protein (84 mg/dL), lymphocytic predominant pleocytosis (16 cells/mm^3), and normal glucose. He was started on broad-spectrum antibiotics including vancomycin, ceftriaxone, and acyclovir. VZV-PCR, and HSV-PCR returned negative; thus, antibiotics and anti-virals were de-escalated. Magnetic resonance imaging (MRI) of the brain with and without contrast was unremarkable. He was monitored on continuous electroencephalography (CEEG). Two days into his hospitalization, he had worsening exam and required intubation for airway protection. CEEG showed nonconvulsive seizures from bilateral frontotemporal regions. His levetiracetam dose was increased and he was given fosphenytoin. Despite these changes, his seizures progressed to convulsive and nonconvulsive status epilepticus. Autoimmune and paraneoplastic encephalitis panels were negative except for elevated anti-thyroid peroxidase antibodies (>1548 IU/mL (range 0–60 IU/mL)) and anti-thyroglobulin antibodies (128 IU/mL (range 0–60 IU/mL)). He was started on intravenous high dose methylprednisolone (1 g/day). Repeat lumbar puncture showed improving pleocytosis (13 cells/mm^3) and protein (54 mg/dL). He continued to have nonconvulsive seizures on CEEG. He was started on continuous infusion of midazolam along with the propofol to achieve burst suppression. He was also loaded with phenobarbital. He continued to have breakthrough seizures and required pentobarbital. He was subsequently loaded with lacosamide and valproic acid and was eventually started on a ketamine infusion. Given lack of response to high dose steroids, plasma exchange was started on day ten of his hospitalization. He received 4 total doses of plasma exchange. His CEEG showed predominantly a burst suppression pattern but prolonged bursts (>30 s) had evolving seizures (Figure 1(a)). Thus, in an effort to break his continuous seizures, he was loaded with 32 mg of oral perampanel. A few hours after his perampanel dose, his continuous seizures broke, and he was able to be maintained in burst suppression to complete suppression for 48 h with no clinical or electrographic seizures (Figures 1(b) and 1(c)). He was started on a maintenance perampanel dose of 8 mg daily. There were no hemodynamic or organ dysfunction from the perampanel load (Table 1).

Unfortunately, he developed an ileus with severe lactic acidosis and multiorgan failure. Family decided to pursue comfort measures. He passed away on day seventeen.

2.2. Case 2. A 69-year-old man with no past medical history called emergency medical service (EMS) from home for new onset shortness of breath. On arrival to the house, there was no answer at the door. Forced entry was required. Patient was found on floor unresponsive in pulseless electrical activity (PEA). Advanced cardiac life support (ACLS) measures were started. He only required two rounds of chest compressions and epinephrine before return of spontaneous circulation (ROSC). He was taken to the ED where he was emergently intubated. CT of the head was negative for acute intracranial process. He was subsequently started on hypothermia protocol. He was admitted to the medical intensive care unit (MICU). On examination, he was noted to have myoclonic jerks particularly with stimulation. He was loaded with levetiracetam, valproic acid, and started on a propofol infusion. CEEG was placed which showed a burst-suppression pattern with 5–8 bursts per minute (Figure 2(a)). Each burst corresponded with myoclonus. His levetiracetam was adjusted without improvement. He was then loaded with 32 mg of oral perampanel through nasogastric tube. After 30 minutes, his CEEG showed 1-2 bursts per minute (Figure 2(b)). His bursts

Table 1: Hemodynamic and laboratory values for patients treated with high dose perampenal.

	Patient 1	Patient 2	Patient 3	Patient 4
Systolic blood pressure (mmHg)				
Baseline	109	144	111	98
2 h post	106	142	101	101
24 h post	102	135	129	91
48 h post	105	106	133	92
Creatinine (mg/dL)				
Baseline	0.77	0.79	1.13	1.58
24 h post	0.8	0.57	1.19	1.62
48 h post	0.79	0.93	1.17	1.6
Alanine aminotransferase (ALT) (U/L)				
Baseline	137	41	77	85
24 h post	53	44	47	79
48 h post	56	26	26	68
Aspartate aminotransferase (AST) (U/L)				
Baseline	58	178	52	77
24 h post	18	166	33	73
48 h post	23	186	30	67

Abbreviations: mmHg, millimeters of Mercury; mg, milligrams; dL, deciliter; U, Units; L, liter.

maintained this rate for next 8 h. He had a mild transaminitis of 44 U/L ALT (alanine aminotransferase; normal 12–78 U/L) and 126 U/L AST (aspartate aminotransferase; normal 9–37 U/L) prior to anticonvulsants. Post anticonvulsants, his liver function tests and creatinine remained relatively unchanged (Table 1). His myoclonus improved and was not appreciated further after 36 h from perampanel load. Two weeks after his admission, his neurological examination had no improved further. The family proceeded with comfort care measures.

2.3. Case 3. A 67-year-old man was admitted to an outside hospital (OSH) after being found unresponsive and in PEA. He received ACLS in the field. ROSC was obtained after 20 minutes. He was intubated and received induced hypothermia for 24 h. He was rewarmed. His examination remained poor. On examination his pupils were sluggishly reactive. He had no motor response to noxious stimulation. His family requested transfer to our facility for second opinion. MRI of the brain was obtained which fluid attenuated inversion recovery changes in the bilateral basal ganglia. Somatosensory evoked potentials showed present N20 response bilaterally. CEEG showed generalized slowing as well as lateralized slowing in the left hemisphere with periodic discharges in the left parieto-occipital region (Figure 3(a)). He was started on levetiracetam. His CEEG then showed frequent non-convulsive seizures arising from the left parieto-occipital region (Figure 3(b)). He was started on lacosamide and then valproic acid with no improvement. Midazolam infusion was started along with load of perampanel 32 mg (Figures 3(c) and 3(d)). There was no change in his hepatic or renal panel, and his hemodynamics remained stable (Table 1). His maintenance dose was 12 mg for 5 days and then reduced to 6 mg. CEEG continued to be negative for seizures. His levetiracetam and lacosamide were

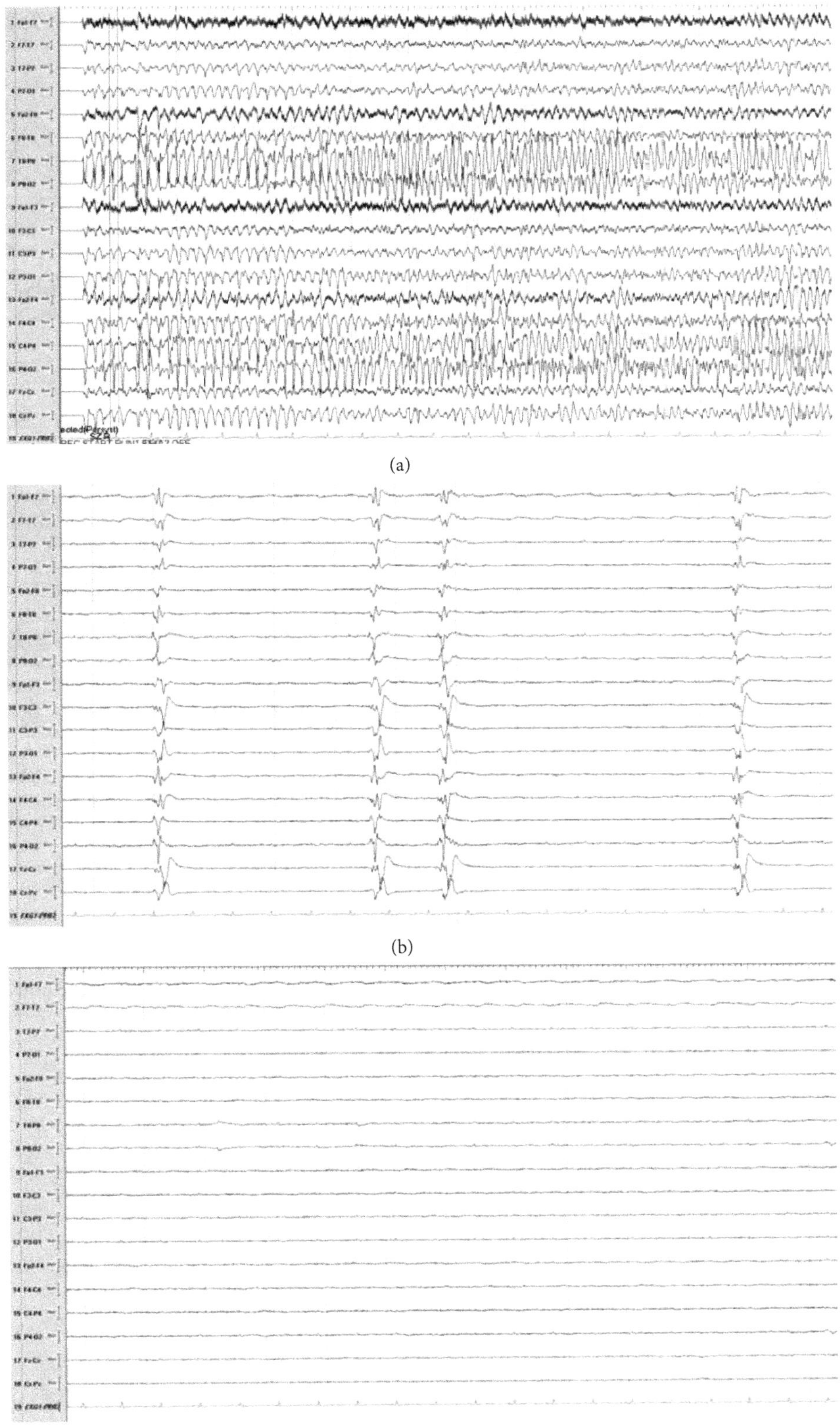

(a)

(b)

(c)

Figure 1: Electroencephalography (EEG): (a) EEG seizure arising from the right hemisphere, maximum temporo-parietal region. Seizures were seen occurring at a rate of 6–10 per hour lasting up to 3 minutes in duration without clinical signs. Seizures were frequent despite levetiracetam, lacosamide, phenobarbital, valproic acid, phenytoin, ketamine, midazolam, and pentobarbital. Sharply contoured generalized periodic discharges were seen interictally (b). Two hours after perampanel load (32 mg), the EEG transitioned to background suppression, and no further seizures were observed for the next 72 hours (c). Bitemporal montage, sens 7 uV, Lf 1.6 Hz, HF 70 Hz, 15 s epoch.

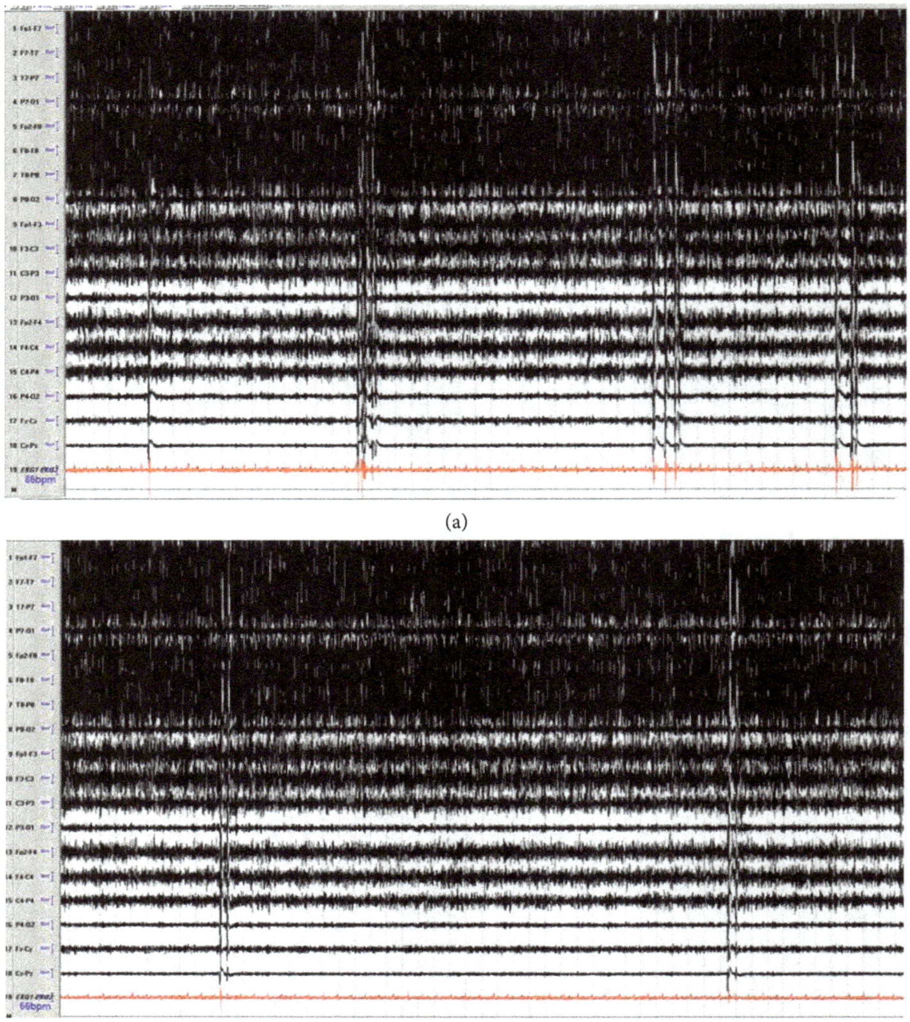

(a)

(b)

FIGURE 2: Electroencephalography (EEG): (a) Generalized burst suppression was seen occurring at a rate of 5–8 bursts per minute. Each burst was associated with generalized myoclonus despite the use of levetiracetam, valproic acid, and propofol. (b) Following 32 mg of perampanel, the bursts reduced to about 1-2 times per minute. Bitemporal montage, sens 7 uV, Lf 1.6 Hz, HF 70 Hz, 60 s epoch.

eweaned off. He was eventually discharged to long-term acute care hospital on valproic acid and perampanel 6 mg.

2.4. Case 4. A 53-year-old woman with a history of congestive heart failure was admitted in PEA arrest post left heart catheterization. ROSC was obtained after 30 minutes. CT head was negative for any acute intracranial process. She underwent hypothermia (32C) for 24 h followed by rewarming and normothermia. Her exam post rewarming showed intact brainstem reflexes and withdrawing in the extremities. Over the course of a week, she developed generalized myoclonic jerks, particularly of the axial muscles and face. It was unclear if these myogenic jerks had underlying CEEG correlate. She was subsequently given a sedative and a paralytic, which showed an underlying generalized periodic discharge (Figures 4(a) and 4(b)). She was loaded with levetiracetam (2000 g) without improvement in CEEG (Figure 4(c)). She was then loaded with 32 mg of perampanel. Two hours post perampanel load, her myogenic activity subsided, and her CEEG showed a generalized periodic pattern. She was maintained on 12 mg of perampanel daily for next three days. This was then reduced to 4 mg per day. Her myoclonus remained improved. There were no changes with her hepatic function panel or hemodynamics following the load of perampanel (Table 1). She eventually had a tracheostomy and PEG placed and transferred to a long-term acute care facility.

3. Discussion

These four cases highlight the effectiveness and tolerability of high dose perampanel in the management of patients with super refractory status epilepticus. Patient 1 had super refractory status epilepticus likely from an underlying autoimmune disorder. Patients 2, 3, and 4 had super refractory status epilepticus from varying degrees of anoxic injury. Patients 3 and 4 had generalized status epilepticus whereas patients 1 and 2 had focal seizures. In all cases, perampanel was effective in

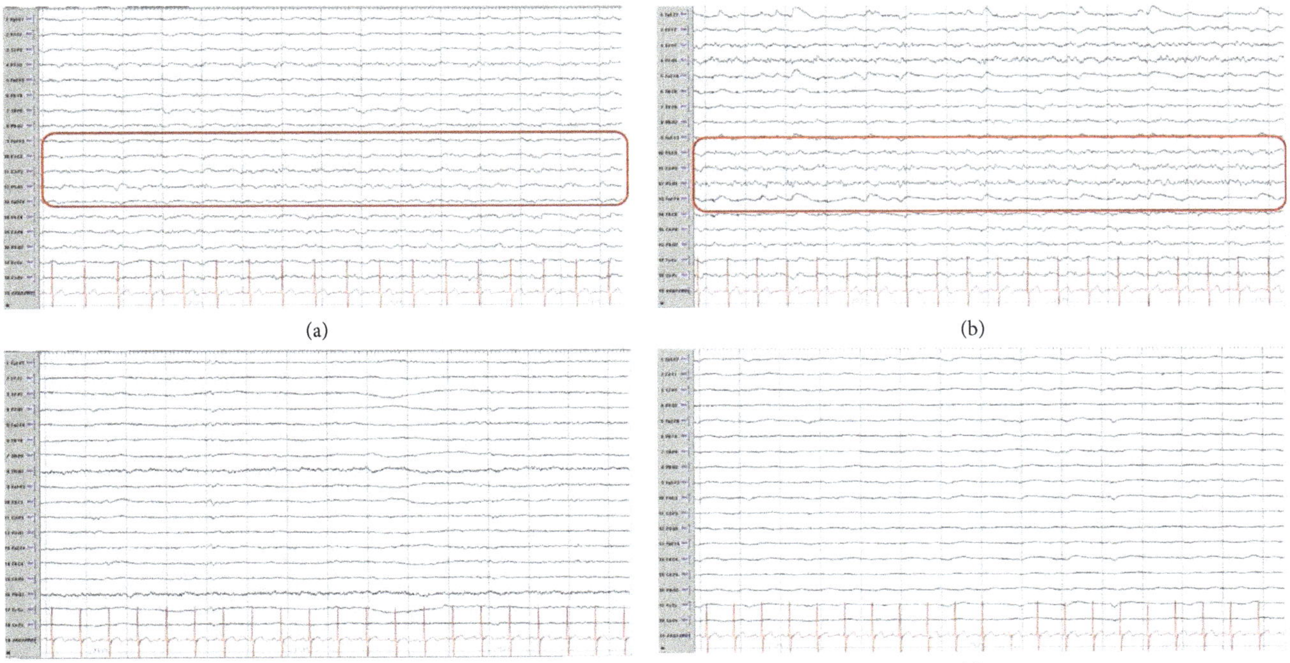

(a) (b) (c) (d)

FIGURE 3: Electroencephalography (EEG): (a) Generalized slowing is seen with lateralized slowing in the left hemisphere. Periodic lateralized epileptiform discharges are seen in the left parieto-occipital region (red box). (b) Frequent seizures without clinical signs were seen arising from the left parieto-occipital region (red box). (c) Immediately before perampanel. At this time, the patient was receiving levetiracetam, lacosamide, valproic acid, and midazolam infusion. (d) 2 h after perampanel, there is diffuse slowing. No further seizures occurred. Midazolam was stopped. He was eventually weaned off the levetiracetam and lacosamide and discharged on perampanel and valproic acid. Bitemporal montage, sens 7 uV, Lf 1.6 Hz, HF 70 Hz, 15 s epoch.

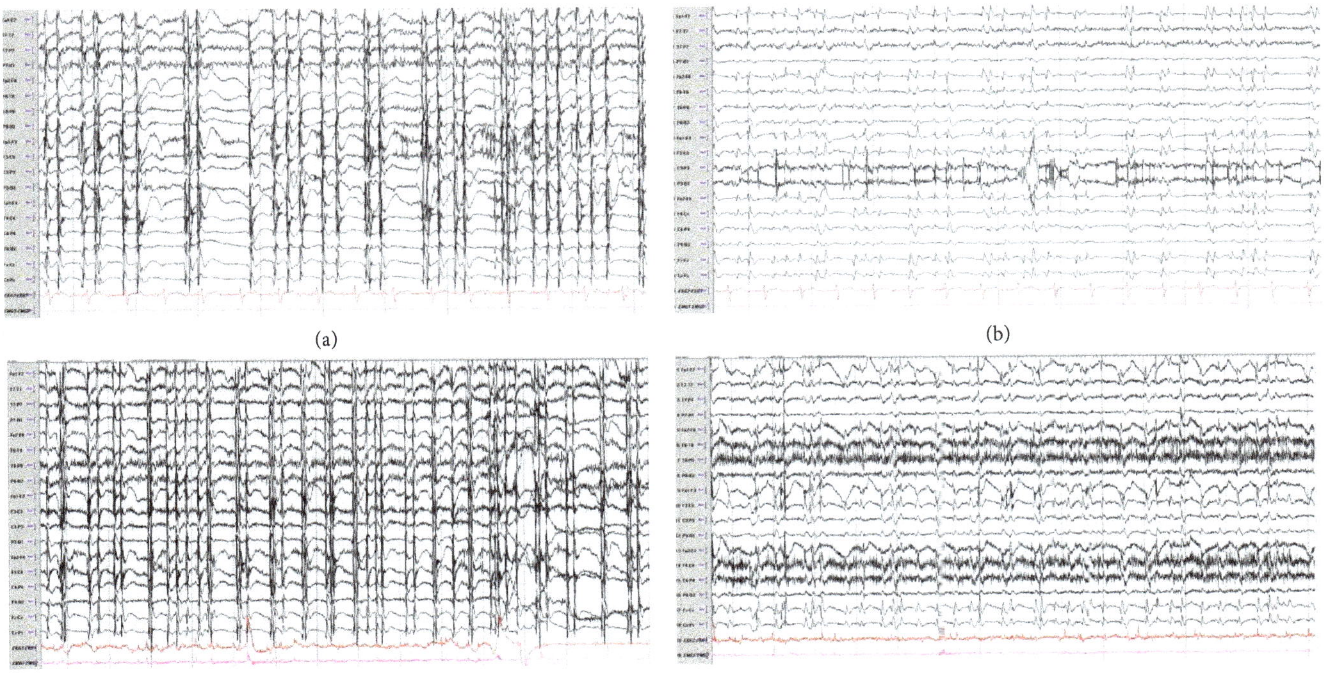

(a) (b) (c) (d)

FIGURE 4: Electroencephalography (EEG): (a) Generalized myogenic artifact is seen throughout the record. (b) Following sedation and paralytic, generalized periodic discharges were seen. She was loaded with levetiracetam without improvement in the CEEG. (c) She was subsequently loaded with 32 mg of perampanel. (d) Two hours post load, her myoclonus had improved. CEEG, however, continued to show the generalized periodic discharge. Bitemporal montage, sens 7 uV, Lf 1.6 Hz, HF 70 Hz, 15 s epoch.

either stopping or reducing the seizure burden with no adverse effects.

Perampanel is a noncompetitive glutamate alpha-amino-3-hydroxy-5-methyl-4-isoxazolepropionic acid (AMPA) receptor antagonist [10]. It has a terminal half-life of ~105 h and reaches steady state in 10–19 days [11]. It has a time to peak of 0.5 (fasting) to 2.5 h (nonfasting) with 100% bioavailability and is extensively (>90%) metabolized by CYP450 3A4 [11]. Thus, a loading dose (such as 32 mg) may be necessary to achieve a therapeutic plasma level [2]. Additionally, a higher maintenance dose may be necessary to maintain the appropriate therapeutic serum concentration. Perampanel has been previously shown to be effective for treatment of status epilepticus after failure of benzodiazepines [2, 12, 13]. This favorable profile is likely explained by the glutamate and gamma-aminobutyric acid (GABA) receptor composition in ongoing seizures [14, 15]. In a single-center study of 30 patients with refractory status epilepticus, the addition of perampanel was given following administration of standard treatment algorithm (median of 4 IV drugs, range 2–7 before perampanel) [13]. Perampanel was given as an initial higher dose (median 32 mg, range 16–32 mg) in 14 patients and a median of 4 mg (range 2–12 mg) in 16 patients [13]. Clinical response was observed by a median of 24 h (range 8–48 h) and EEG response by median of 60 h (range 12–72 h) with a shorter time to treatment response in those with high dose loading (16 vs 18 h for clinical response; 24 vs 72 h for EEG response) [13]. In ~23–63% of patients, a mild hepatic/cholestatic injury was observed following perampanel [10, 13]. No patient had changes in cardiorespiratory parameters following loading dose of perampanel [10, 13]. One patient developed multi-organ failure from the use of high doses of pentobarbital. We have previously reported on the observed surgical and medical complications that accompany high dose pentobarbital [6]. With the development of the new AEDs, the goal should be to stop seizures prior to having to use a barbiturate given the complications directly and indirectly associated with this therapeutic option.

Perampanel may also have a role in the treatment of post-anoxic status epilepticus. In a small pilot study of 8 post-anoxic patients with super-refractory, nonconvulsive status epilepticus (NCSE) and favorable prognostic indicators, the addition of perampanel (median dose of 6 mg; range 6–12 mg) after a median time of 9.5 days (range 4–35 days) from cardiac arrest to the standard of care [median number of 3 AEDs (range 2–5) and 3 anesthetics (range 1–4)] resulted in cessation of NCSE in six (75%) patients by 72 h [10]. For those patients with postanoxic myoclonic seizures, perampanel has been shown to cause clinically meaningful improvement in myoclonus despite the use of other commonly administered antiepileptic medications [16]. These findings highlight the effectiveness of perampanel in refractory cases of status epilepticus.

These cases highlight the use of the novel anticonvulsant perampanel in the treatment of super-refractory status epilepticus. Perampanel was effective in treatment of status epilepticus in these cases with varying etiologies and was well tolerated. A larger, prospective study is needed to test this treatment option.

Disclosure

Pravin George serves on the medical advisory board of Lifebanc. Christopher R. Newey serves on the medical advisory board of Lifebanc and has served as a speaker for BARD medical. Stephen Hantus has served on the speaker's bureau for UCB Pharma.

References

[1] C. R. Newey, T. G. Kinzy, V. Punia, and S. Hantus, "Continuous electroencephalography in the critically ill: clinical and continuous electroencephalography markers for targeted monitoring," *Journal Clinical Neurophysiology*, vol. 35, pp. 325–331, 2018.

[2] F. Brigo, S. Lattanzi, A. Rohracher et al., " Perampanel in the treatment of status epilepticus: a systematic review of the literature," *Epilepsy & Behavior*, vol. 86, pp. 179–186, 2018.

[3] D. M. Treiman, P. D. Meyers, N. Y. Walton et al., "A comparison of four treatments for generalized convulsive status epilepticus," *New England Journal of Medicine*, vol. 339, no. 12, pp. 792–798, 1998.

[4] R. Silbergleit, V. Durkalski, D. Lowenstein et al., "Intramuscular versus intravenous therapy for prehospital status epilepticus," *New England Journal of Medicine*, vol. 366, no. 7, pp. 591–600, 2012.

[5] A. M. Hussain, J. W. Lee, B. J. Kolls et al., "Randomized trial of lacosamide versus fosphenytoin for nonconvulsive seizures," *Annals of Neurology*, vol. 83, no. 6, pp. 1174–1185, 2018.

[6] C. R. Newey, D. Wisco, P. Nattanmai, and A. Sarwal, "Observed medical and surgical complications of prolonged barbiturate coma for refractory status epilepticus," *Therapeutic Advances in Drug Safety*, vol. 7, no. 5, pp. 195–203, 2016.

[7] C. R. Newey, P. George, P. Nattanmai, C. Ahrens, S. Hantus, and A. Sarwal, "Evolution of cerebral atrophy in a patient with super refractory status epilepticus treated with barbiturate coma," *Case Reports in Neurological Medicine*, vol. 2017, 4 pages, 2017.

[8] N. Mullaguri, N. Katyal, A. Sarwal et al., "Pitfall in pupillometry: exaggerated ciliospinal reflex in a patient in a barbiturate coma mimicking a nonreactive pupil," *Cureus*, vol. 30, p. e2004, 2017.

[9] A. Strzelcyk, S. Knake, R. Kalviainen et al., "Perampanel for treatment of status epilepticus in Austria, Finland, Germany, and Spain," *Acta Neurologica Scandinavica*, vol. 139, no. 4, pp. 369–376, 2019.

[10] S. Beretta, G. Padovano, A. Stabile et al., "Efficacy and safety of perampanel oral loading in postanoxic super-refractory status epilepticus: a pilot study," *Epilepsia*, vol. 59, pp. 243–248, 2018.

[11] P. N. Patsalos, "The clinical pharmacology profile of the new antiepileptic drug perampanel: a novel noncompetitive AMPA receptor antagonist," *Epilepsia*, vol. 56, no. 1, pp. 12–27, 2015.

[12] T. Hanada, K. Ido, and T. Kosasa, "Effect of perampanel, a novel AMPA antagonist, on benzodiazepine-resistant status epilepticus in a lithium-pilocarpine rat model," *Pharmacology Research &Perspectives*, vol. 2, no. 5, p. e00063, 2014.

[13] A. Rohracher, G. Kalss, C. Neuray et al., "Perampanel in patients with refractory and super-refractory status epilepticus in a neurological intensive care unit: a single center audit of 30 patients," *Epilepsia*, vol. 59, pp. 234–242, 2018.

[14] T. Loddenkemper, D. M. Talos, R. T. Cleary et al., "Subunit composition of glutamate and gamma-aminobutyric acid receptors in status epilepticus," *Epilepsy Research*, vol. 108, no. 4, pp. 605–615, 2014.

[15] E. Santamarina, M. Sueiras, R. M. Lidon et al., "Use of perampanel in one case of super-refractory hypoxic myoclonic status: case report," *Epilepsy Behav*, vol. 4, pp. 56–59, 2015.

[16] B. J. Steinhoff, M. Bacher, C. Kurth, M. Anke, and R. Kornmeier, "Add-on perampanel in Lance-Adams syndrome," *Epilepsy & Behavior Case Reports*, vol. 6, pp. 28–29, 2016.

Right Sided Intracardiac Thrombosis during Veno-Arterial Extracorporeal Membrane Oxygenation

Anusha Ganapati Bhat,[1] **Armand Golchin**,[2]
Deepak Kumar Pasupula,[3] **and Jaime A. Hernandez-Montfort**[4]

[1] *Department of Internal Medicine, Baystate Medical Center, University of Massachusetts Medical School, Springfield, MA, USA*
[2] *Division of Critical Care Medicine, Baystate Medical Center, University of Massachusetts Medical School, Springfield, MA, USA*
[3] *Department of Internal Medicine, University of Pittsburgh Medical Center, Pittsburgh, PA, USA*
[4] *Division of Cardiology, The University of Texas Medical Branch, Galveston, TX, USA*

Correspondence should be addressed to Anusha Ganapati Bhat; anusha.bhatmd@baystatehealth.org

Academic Editor: Chiara Lazzeri

Veno-Arterial Extracorporeal Membrane Oxygenation is a common technology of the modern era used as a bridge in severe refractory cardiac and respiratory failure until definitive management is planned. However, early recognition and management of one of the most challenging complications, intracardiac thrombus, continue to remain a conundrum. The incidence of the clinical scenario is very rare. Therefore, due to the lack of literature, there are no guidelines for risk stratification, prevention, or management of intracardiac thrombus. We describe a case of massive pulmonary embolism, who developed a sudden right sided intra-cardiac thrombosis while being optimally anticoagulated on VA ECMO. We also review the literature to describe the pathophysiology, risk stratification, prevention, and management of this rare entity.

1. Introduction

Veno-Arterial Extracorporeal Membrane Oxygenation is a technology of the modern era that has progressed quickly and continues to evolve in the world of critical care. Since its initial use in 1970s for postcardiotomy cardiogenic shock, its indications have broadened to involve temporary management of severe refractory cardiac and respiratory failure until a definitive management is planned. But there have been complications associated with them. Based on Extracorporeal Life Support (ECLS) registry report 2017, intracardiac thrombus (ICT) accounts for 5-6% of all the complications of VA ECMO. To our knowledge, most of the ICT is developing while on VA ECMO involved left side or all the chambers of the heart simultaneously. We describe a case of massive pulmonary embolism, who developed a sudden right sided intra-cardiac thrombosis (ICT) while being optimally anticoagulated on VA ECMO. The incidence of the clinical scenario is very rare and reduced even more with the advancement in the ECMO technology. Therefore, due to the lack of sufficient reporting of this clinical entity, there are no guidelines for risk stratification, prevention, or management of ICT. This paper describes the risk factors and pathophysiology for development of intra-cardiac thrombus in a patient treated with VA-ECMO. We will also review the literature describing this rare entity.

2. Case Report

A 63-year-old gentleman with a past medical history of alcoholic cirrhosis presented with acute dyspnea, tachycardia, and hypotension to an outside hospital. He was found to have a massive pulmonary embolism bilaterally on Computed Tomography Angiography (CTA) chest. Additionally, there was a sizable thrombus in the right atrium partially extending through patent foramen ovale. Ultrasound Doppler of

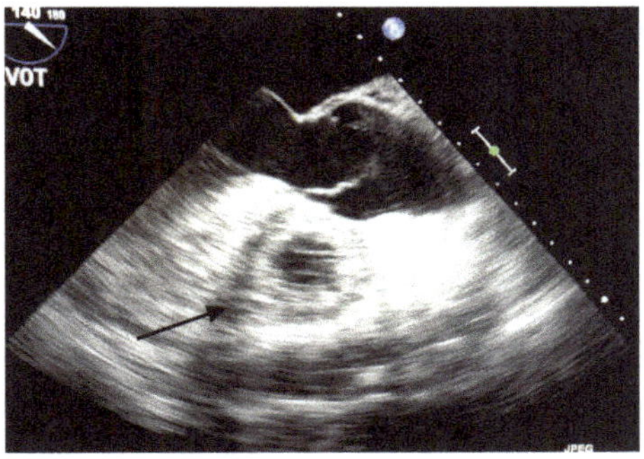

Figure 1: Transesophageal echocardiogram with ME AV LAX view showing extensive thrombus formation in the right ventricle.

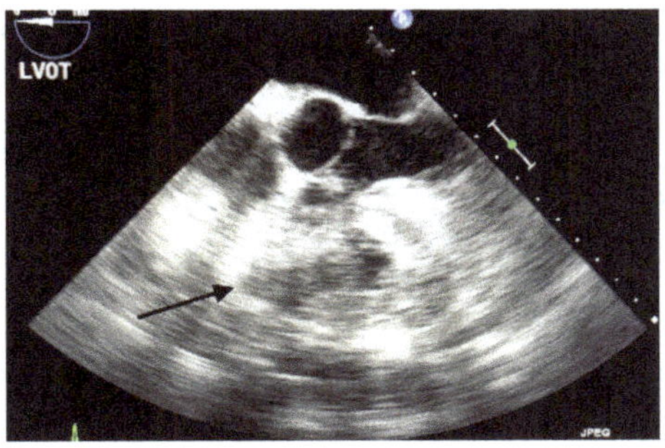

Figure 2: Transesophageal echocardiogram with ME 4CH view showing poor endocardial definition of the right ventricle and the thrombus.

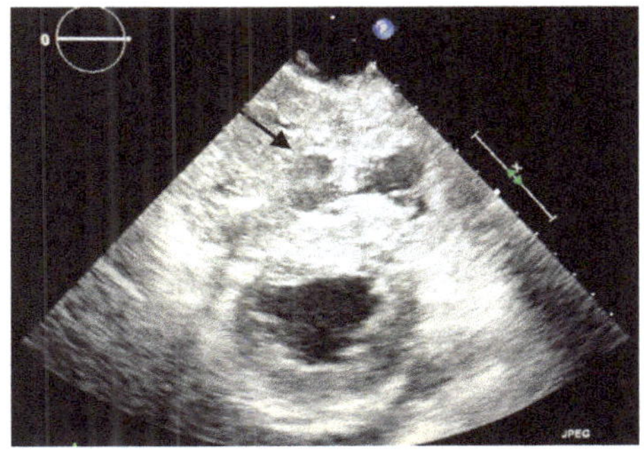

Figure 3: Transesophageal echocardiogram with TG SAX view showing extensive thrombus formation in the right ventricle.

lower extremities was negative for deep venous thrombosis. The massive PE was managed surgically for immediate stabilization with complete embolectomy followed by patent foramen ovale closure. There was no residual thrombus noted; however, CTA scan was not repeated to evaluate peripheral pulmonary artery thrombosis. Unfortunately, the procedure was complicated by postcardiotomy shock. He failed to be wean from the cardiopulmonary bypass machine and vasopressors (vasopressin, norepinephrine, and epinephrine), thus requiring central Venous-Arterial Extracorporeal Membrane Oxygenation (VA ECMO) support until recovery. Anticoagulation provided perioperatively kept his activated clotting time (ACT) greater than 300s for a few hours. Once ACT was within therapeutic range, he was reinitiated on anticoagulation with a heparin bolus of 50units/kg, followed by continuous infusion at 7.5 units/kg thereafter per ECMO management protocol of the hospital. VA ECMO settings were maintained with a flow of 4.6-4.8 L/min and sweep gas flow rate of 3-4 L/min. His mean arterial pressure was above 65 mmHg and pulmonary arterial pressure was elevated at 29-65 mmHg systolic and 7-25 mmHg diastolic.

On postoperative day 1 (POD 1) he continued to have high flow on VA ECMO, but was noted to have increasing bleed from his nasogastric tube. His hemoglobin dropped from 13.9 gm/dL to 7.5 gm/dL with a hematocrit of 21.6%. His workup was also significant for chronic unchanged thrombocytopenia of 40-50 k/mm3. At this time, systemic anticoagulation was transiently discontinued due to continued bleeding. He was managed with a transfusion of packed red blood cell, platelets, cryoprecipitate, and fresh frozen plasma over a span of 12 hours. In the meantime, he also underwent upper endoscopy, which revealed erosive esophagitis and gastric mucosal erythema, for which he received high dose intravenous proton pump inhibitors. After the completion of the blood products transfusion, his bleeding stopped. Thereafter, he was started on heparin drip at the rate of 10 units/kg/hour and managed with an activated clotting time over 200s, activated partial thromboplastin time 35-75s, and anti-Xa level 0.30-0.70 IU/ml.

His settings and flow on VA ECMO remained unchanged and he seemed to improve hemodynamically with less requirement of vasopressors in the next 24 hours. He was weaned off epinephrine. His point of care echocardiogram also revealed good cardiac activity without any visible clots. However, towards the end of POD 3, he was noted to develop worsening tachycardia, reduction in ECMO flow to 3.6L/min, and thrombosis of the mediastinal tube. Serotonin release assay for assessment of heparin induced thrombocytopenia (HIT) was negative. A bedside transesophageal echocardiogram revealed global hypokinesis and severe LV dysfunction. Additionally, there was a notably large in situ right ventricular thrombus with a posterior circumferential pericardial clot extending from 3 to 9 o'clock position surrounding the left and right ventricles. He was re-operated immediately with the removal of 1.5L blood and thrombus from the pericardium and mediastinum. There was no obvious site of bleeding noted; however repeat transesophageal echocardiogram suggested reformation of a total right ventricular thrombus, which was confirmed by a transthoracic echocardiogram. The thrombus extended to the main pulmonary artery and its branches. At this point, the family decided to pursue palliative care due to his poor prognosis and the patient expired within the next few minutes (Figures 1, 2, and 3).

3. Discussion

ECMO has been used for approximately four decades in intensive care units around the world. Over the years, there have been significant advancements in the technology resulting in improved outcomes and survival rates. Currently, VA ECMO is used for the management of cardiac arrest, cardiomyopathy, myocarditis, and congenital defect and in cardiogenic shock that are difficult to wean from cardiopulmonary bypass (CPB). However, early recognition and management of one of the most challenging complications, intracardiac thrombus, remain a conundrum.

The first case series that introduced ICT as a complication of ECMO was in 1995, where, out of 30 patients on ECMO, 6 developed ICT accounting for 20% incidence rate [1]. Mechanical clots accounted for 15.6% of all the complications and the mortality rate of thromboembolic events while on ECMO has been predicted to be 8.7% [2].

ECMO circuit is a prothrombotic stimulus since it is sensed as a foreign body physiologically. VA ECMO in particular has additional sites of thrombus formation in the heart unlike Veno-Venous ECMO (VV ECMO). Cardiac surgery causes high tissue injury, which may be worsened by further tissue injury during cannulation for vascular access. In addition, blood upon contact with the negatively charged plastic linings connecting ECMO circuit further augments Virchow's triad and sets off the coagulation cascade. In our case, the patient also had a history of alcoholic cirrhosis, which may have hindered coagulation system in the patient with subsequent massive PE in the first place. During the hospital course, his pulmonary arterial pressure (PAP) was high, indicative of evolving pulmonary hypertension as a result of PE, although we cannot ascertain if he already had developed microthrombi in his pulmonary vasculature. Thromboembolism into the blood vessels of the lungs leads to inflammation and interstitial edema subsequently leading to PH, which elevates afterload for the right heart.

Impaired right cardiac output leads to systolic dysfunction, cardiac hypokinesis, and blood stasis, ultimately resulting in ICT, which may be the most likely explanation in our case. In the setting of high prothrombotic risk factors such as coagulopathy from liver disease, additional hypercoagulability induced from multiple blood products transfusion has also been associated with increased odds of thrombosis. A systemic review by Williams et al. established risk factors for the development of ICT following CPB, where patients with surgery for over 2 hours and preexisting congestive heart failure and those undergoing blood products transfusion and antifibrinolytic administration were at a major risk. Of all the blood products, 37.5% of patients developed ICT after platelet transfusion and 27% following plasma transfusion [3].

To prevent ICT, patients are systemically anticoagulated mostly with unfractionated heparin, less frequently low molecular weight heparin, direct thrombin inhibitors, or novel anticoagulation agents, unless heparin is contraindicated. Some instances where thrombus developed while on therapeutic heparin were related to resistance to heparin, which have been partially evidenced to improve with supplemental antithrombin, but definitive evidences are scarce. Although we did not check endogenous antithrombin III level, this intervention is optional in patients undergoing cardiac surgery with CPB, the elderly, and diabetics [4–8]. Also, several advances have been made to the ECMO circuit to minimize hypercoagulability. Use of hollow microfibers to prevent direct blood-gas interactions, preventing artificial surface-blood interactions to reduce hypercoagulability, reducing turbulent flow with low-resistance oxygenators, shorter connections, and minimum circulatory volume are other interventions [9]. These changes in the technology may have reduced incidence of ECMO circuit related thrombosis, but cardiac chambers would still be at risk of forming clots due to low pressure when on VA ECMO. Therefore, systemic anticoagulation is of utmost importance, even though it is challenging as in our case due to increased bleeding potential.

Current protocol for anticoagulation is by combined measurement and assessment of activated clotting time, partial thromboplastin time, and anti-factor Xa levels to adjust anticoagulation therapy to prevent bleeding and clotting imbalance, although in our case they had poor clinical correlatability, which may indicate inappropriate estimation of anticoagulation level.

With anticoagulation, the unfortunate drawback is the risk of bleeding. Disseminated intravascular coagulation, mechanical hemolysis, gastrointestinal hemorrhage, and surgical site bleeds are accountable for up to 50.1% of all the complications from ECMO [10]. But, systemic anticoagulation is one of the key factors to ensure prevention of ICT and requires close monitoring to strike a balance between clotting and bleeding potential. Furthermore, observing pressure gradient changes in the system, timely echocardiograms, and watching for hemodynamic instability will ensure early recognition even when ICT forms.

Once ICT has developed, management options are not evidence based, but based on clinical experience and small studies. Systemic thrombolytic therapy may be fatal due to ongoing bleeds, as in our case, whereas local instillation of thrombolytics may not be helpful due to poor reachability of the medication to the site of ICT due to poor blood flow. Furthermore, inactivation of plasminogen by use of antifibrinolytics during surgery as well as dilutional drop in their levels from volume supplementation for hemodynamic stability may lead to ineffectiveness of tissue plasminogen activator [11].

Current modality used for management of ICT includes surgical thrombectomy, local thrombolysis, or usage of ventricular assist device to ensure adequate forward flow of blood to prevent new thrombus formation from stasis [12, 13]. With ICT on VA ECMO, most patients assume palliative care due to poor outcomes [14]. There is scarce data in the literature to make final conclusion about guidelines for management. But, we can try to improve risk factor predictions and manage patients based on their individual risk stratification. Future research should concentrate on conducting large scale studies for patients on VA ECMO to recognize risk factors and possible successful management of ICT to improve overall mortality outcomes.

References

[1] D. D. Muehrcke, P. M. McCarthy, R. W. Stewart et al., "Complications of extracorporeal life support systems using heparin-bound surfaces: The risk of intracardiac clot formation," *The Journal of Thoracic and Cardiovascular Surgery*, vol. 110, no. 3, pp. 843–851, 1995.

[2] A. Beiras-Fernandez, M.-A. Deutsch, S. Kainzinger et al., "Extracorporeal membrane oxygenation in 108 patients with low cardiac output-A single-center experience," *The International Journal of Artificial Organs*, vol. 34, no. 4, pp. 365–373, 2011.

[3] B. Williams, B. Wehman, M. A. Mazzeffi et al., "Acute Intracardiac Thrombosis and Pulmonary Thromboembolism After Cardiopulmonary Bypass," *Anesthesia & Analgesia*, vol. 126, no. 2, pp. 425–434, 2018.

[4] J. W. Byrnes, C. J. Swearingen, P. Prodhan, R. Fiser, and U. Dyamenahalli, "Antithrombin III supplementation on extracorporeal membrane oxygenation: Impact on heparin dose and circuit life," *ASAIO Journal*, vol. 60, no. 1, pp. 57–62, 2014.

[5] M. E. Carr, "Diabetes mellitus: a hypercoagulable state," *Journal of Diabetes and its Complications*, vol. 15, no. 1, pp. 44–54, 2001.

[6] M. G. Conlan, A. R. Folsom, A. Finch et al., "Associations of factor VIII and von Willebrand factor with age, race, sex, and risk factors for atherosclerosis. The Atherosclerosis Risk in Communities (ARIC) study," *Thrombosis and Haemostasis*, vol. 70, no. 3, pp. 380–385, 1993.

[7] V. Muedra, D. Barettino, P. D'Ocón, A. Zuñiga, and L. Moreno, "Antithrombin activity and outcomes in patients undergoing cardiac surgery with cardiopulmonary bypass," *Blood Coagulation & Fibrinolysis*, vol. 24, no. 4, pp. 454–457, 2013.

[8] M. Ranucci, A. Ditta, A. Boncilli et al., "Determinants of antithrombin consumption in cardiac operations requiring cardiopulmonary bypass," *Perfusion*, vol. 19, no. 1, pp. 47–52, 2004.

[9] D. A. Murphy, L. E. Hockings, R. K. Andrews et al., "Extracorporeal membrane oxygenation-hemostatic complications," *Transfusion Medicine Reviews*, vol. 29, no. 2, pp. 90–101, 2015.

[10] R. R. Thiagarajan, R. P. Barbaro, P. T. Rycus et al., "Extracorporeal Life Support Organization Registry International Report 2016," *ASAIO Journal*, vol. 63, no. 1, pp. 60–67, 2017.

[11] S. L. Diamond and S. Anand, "Inner clot diffusion and permeation during fibrinolysis," *Biophysical Journal*, vol. 65, no. 6, pp. 2622–2643, 1993.

[12] A. Salsano, E. Sportelli, G. M. Olivieri, N. Di Lorenzo, S. Borile, and F. Santini, "RVAD support in the setting of submassive pulmonary embolism," *Journal of Extra-Corporeal Technology*, vol. 49, no. 4, pp. 304–306, 2017.

[13] F. Sangalli, G. Greco, L. Galbiati, F. Formica, S. Calcinati, and L. Avalli, "Regional Thrombolysis with Tenecteplase During Extracorporeal Membrane Oxygenation: A New Approach for Left Ventricular Thrombosis," *Journal of Cardiac Surgery*, vol. 30, no. 6, pp. 541–543, 2015.

[14] M. Alhussein, Y. Moayedi, J. D. Posada et al., "Ventricular Thrombosis Post-Venoarterial Extracorporeal Membrane Oxygenation," *Circulation: Heart Failure*, vol. 10, no. 2, 2017.

Circulatory Collapse due to Hyperinflation in a Patient with Tracheobronchomalacia: A Case Report and Brief Review

Niclas Lundström,[1] Gert Henriksson,[2] Ola Börjesson,[3] Malin Jonsson Fagerlund,[1] and Johan Petersson[1]

[1] *Function Perioperative Medicine and Intensive Care (PMI), Karolinska University Hospital, Sweden*
[2] *Department of ENT Surgery, Karolinska University Hospital, Sweden*
[3] *Department of Rheumatology, Karolinska University Hospital, Sweden*

Correspondence should be addressed to Niclas Lundström; niclas.lundstrom@sll.se

Academic Editor: Kenneth S. Waxman

We present a case of repeated cardiac arrests derived from dynamic hyperinflation in a patient with severe tracheobronchomalacia. Mechanical ventilation led to auto-PEEP with hemodynamic impairment and pulseless electric activity. Adjusted ventilation settings, deep sedation, and muscle paralysis followed by acute stenting of the affected collapsing airways restored ventilation and prevented recurrent circulatory collapse. We briefly review the pathophysiology and treatment options in patients with dynamic hyperinflation.

1. Introduction

Patients with expiratory flow limitation are at risk of developing dynamic hyperinflation and auto-PEEP, which in extreme cases can cause circulatory collapse [1]. Aggravated by overzealous positive pressure ventilation, it is crucial that the cause of collapse is immediately recognized in order to relieve intrathoracic pressure and adapt ventilator treatment [2]. Previously described in patients with severe asthma and COPD [3–5], this case also demonstrates the risk of hyperinflation causing cardiac arrest in patients with tracheobronchomalacia. In such a case, rapid stenting of the collapsing airways can be a lifesaving procedure. Patient informed consent was obtained.

2. Case

A 66-year-old man arrived at the emergency room after a cardiac arrest with successful prehospital resuscitation.

He had a medical history of hypertension, diabetes, and obstructive sleep apnea. Recently he had also been diagnosed with granulomatosis polyangiitis (GPA) with positive C-ANCA and respiratory tract involvement. Severe tracheobronchial inflammation had led to stenosis and secondary tracheobronchomalacia, with the distal trachea and main bronchi most affected on previous CT scans. At the time of the reported events, he received treatment with azathioprine 100 mg per day and prednisolone 10 mg per day. Noninvasive mask ventilation with positive airway pressure was used at night because of worsened symptoms when recumbent. There was a plan to consult ENT surgeons regarding the possibility of placing airway stents to treat the condition.

Pulmonary function test done the month before showed marked nonreversible expiratory flow limitation with forced expiratory volume in 1 second (0.6 L, 18% of expected) and hyperinflation with a reduced forced vital capacity (2.7L, 58% of expected), an increased residual volume (3.0L, 139% of expected), and functional residual capacity (4.3L, 131% of expected). Total lung capacity and diffusion capacity were normal.

The patient had undergone bronchoscopy under general anesthesia the previous year which was complicated by severe bronchospasm, hypoventilation, and subsequent hypercapnia requiring unplanned delayed extubation and ICU admission.

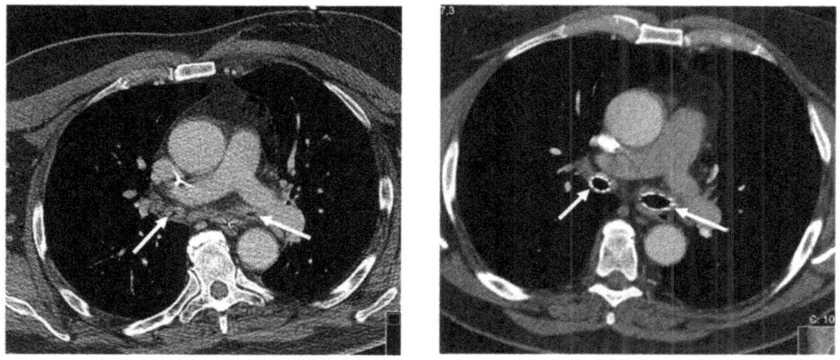

(a) (b)

FIGURE 1: CT imaging before (a) and after (b) stenting. Arrows pointing at main bronchi.

The cardiac arrest took place during a visit at an out-of-hospital urology clinic. It was preceded by obstructive breathing and coughing leading up to respiratory arrest, and he became pulseless before the arrival of paramedics. Cardiopulmonary resuscitation (CPR) was started. When paramedics arrived, they found pulseless electrical activity, CPR was continued including administration of adrenaline, and after 10 minutes there was return of spontaneous circulation and breathing.

At the hospital emergency room he was unresponsive but with stable pulse and blood pressure. After intubation he was taken to the ICU. Arterial blood gas showed respiratory acidosis with pH at 6.88, $PaCO_2$ 16.6 kPa. Ventilating the patient sufficiently to normalize $PaCO_2$ was difficult. Regardless of ventilation mode, high inspiratory and end-expiratory pressures were needed for acceptable tidal volumes and gas exchange. PEEP at 14-16 cmH2O was considered optimal. Remaining air flow at end-expiration indicated auto-PEEP; therefore, the expiratory phase was prolonged with I:E ratio 1:4. Bronchoscopy showed very narrow bronchi and inflammation. CT scan confirmed narrow conditions in the proximal airways, especially in the main bronchi (Figure 1(a)). No signs of pulmonary embolism were seen.

The second day at the ICU, the situation quickly deteriorated, with increasing respiratory acidosis. The patient seemed stressed and hypertensive and triggered the ventilator. Suddenly the blood pressure dropped to immeasurable. CRP was started, the ventilator was disconnected, and bag ventilation was attempted. Adrenaline was administered and after about 2-3 minutes of CPR circulation returned. During the CPR, muscle relaxant with rocuronium (Esmeron®) was also administered to ease continued ventilation after return of circulation. The assessment at this point was that hyperinflation and auto-PEEP due to the expiratory flow obstruction likely had caused the circulatory collapse. Increasing sedation and muscle paralysis stabilized the situation and the patient was therefore kept deeply sedated.

The ENT surgeons were consulted to discuss urgent stenting of the collapsing airways. Stenting of each main bronchus using two stents was conducted a few hours later in the operating theater. The procedure was done with aid of rigid bronchoscopy with ongoing jet ventilation during general anesthesia. The diameter of the right main bronchus was approximately 2-3 mm wide and in the left main bronchus hardly any lumen was seen.

With the stents in place (Figure 1(b)), respiratory compliance improved immediately, and peak pressure and PEEP could be reduced with maintained minute volume. The patient was extubated in the operation room. He was neurologically intact and the continued care was uneventful. The following years though, he has needed treatment at hospital several times, due to recurrent respiratory problems with mucus stagnation, infections and granulation tissue in proximity to the stents, well-known complications to long term stent treatment. However, he has experienced no further episode of circulatory collapse.

3. Discussion

This case illustrates the risk of dynamic hyperinflation and circulatory collapse in patients with severe expiratory flow limitation and the potentially lifesaving effects of timely airway stenting in patients with obstruction of the central airways as in tracheobronchomalacia. In the following, we briefly discuss lung hyperinflation, auto-PEEP and circulatory compromise and lastly tracheobronchomalacia.

Lung hyperinflation essentially means that the lung volume at the end of expiration is above normal [6, 7]. Static hyperinflation refers to a consistent increase in the functional residual capacity (FRC). Dynamic hyperinflation refers to a variable increase in end-expiratory lung volume (EELV), often caused by expiratory flow limitation that prevents the lung from emptying to its resting volume before inspiration. Dynamic hyperinflation varies with changes in flow limitation, minute ventilation, and breathing pattern. In this situation of incomplete expiration, alveolar pressure at end-expiration remains higher than proximal airway pressure at the start of next inspiration. This is called intrinsic PEEP or auto-PEEP [1]. Physiologically, auto-PEEP differs from externally applied PEEP set on a ventilator, as auto-PEEP is present only distal to airways with flow limitation and not equally distributed in the lungs [2, 8]. During invasive ventilation auto-PEEP leads to decreased lung compliance, resulting in reduced tidal volumes during pressure controlled ventilation

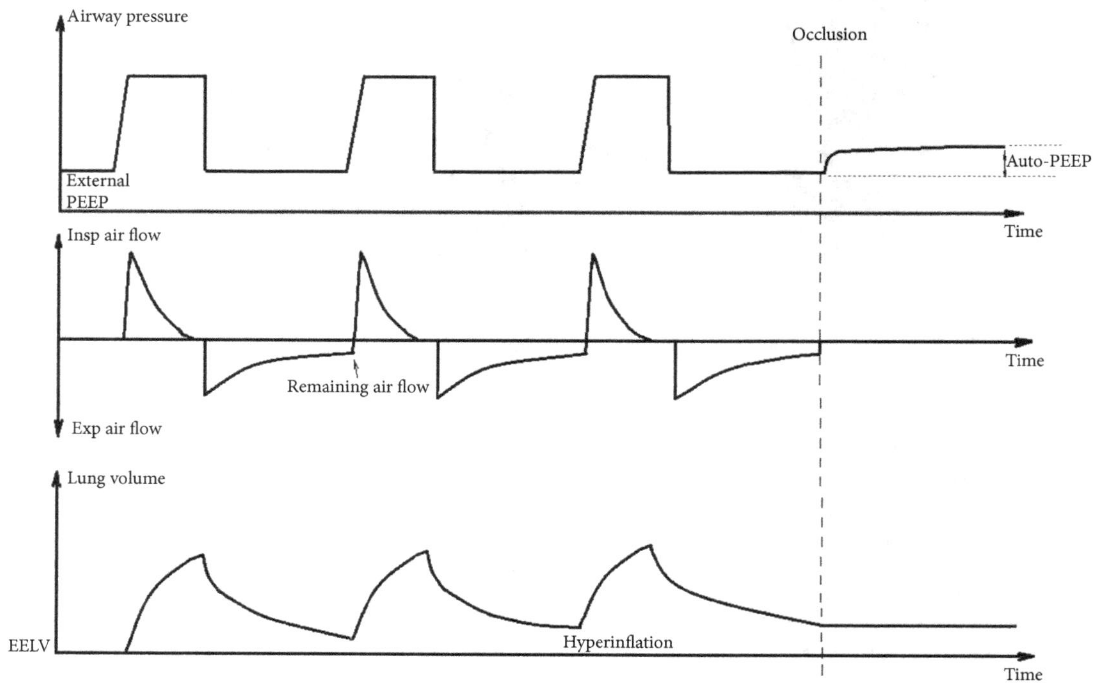

FIGURE 2: Ventilatory curves for three consecutive breaths during pressure controlled ventilation in a patient with dynamic hyperinflation and auto-PEEP, measurement of static auto-PEEP after occlusion.

and increased peak pressures in volume controlled modes [9]. Auto-PEEP can be measured in most ventilators from the airway pressure during prolonged expiration with a closed expiration valve (Figure 2). This requires a passive patient.

Auto-PEEP can generate the same hemodynamic effects as externally added PEEP. The resulting elevated intrathoracic pressure reduces venous return and thus cardiac output [10–13]. Hyperinflation may also reduce cardiac output through increased pulmonary vascular resistance, impairing right ventricular function leading to reduction of left ventricular preload. Bradycardia and vasodilation via autonomic reflexes are also possible adverse effects of hyperinflation [14].

As described, our patient suffered two episodes of cardiac arrest, and our discussion centers around the second occasion during invasive ventilation. However, in patients with obstructive lung disease, a worsening of expiratory flow limitation and increased breathing frequency can cause significant dynamic hyperinflation and auto-PEEP also during spontaneous breathing. This can both increase work of breathing further and impair cardiac output [6]. As the primary cardiac arrest was preceded by obstructive respiratory distress with forced and rapid breathing, we believe increasing dynamic hyperinflation and auto-PEEP played a key role in the rapid development of respiratory failure and circulatory compromise with hypoxemia and hypotension leading to cardiac arrest.

The second cardiac arrest during invasive ventilation was preceded by acceptable oxygenation but ventilation difficulties with reduced tidal volumes and hypercapnia. After a brief period of hypertension, blood pressure dropped quickly before onset of the cardiac arrest (Figure 3). The circulatory collapse can in this case be considered caused directly by dynamic hyperinflation and deleterious auto-PEEP levels generated during positive pressure ventilation.

The sudden collapse could have been related to swelling of the airways with further lumen reduction, and stress from light sedation with patient triggered breaths and forced expiration likely worsened airway collapse and flow limitation further. With diminishing expiration, auto-PEEP approaches the inspiratory pressure delivered by the ventilator. Progressively increasing respiratory acidosis and respiratory efforts sets the stage for a vicious circle culminating in extreme intrathoracic pressures and circulatory collapse. Attempting to increase the minute ventilation with the ventilator in this situation could aggravate the situation even more by further increasing auto-PEEP. Instead tidal volume or respiratory rate needs to be reduced, with permissive hypercapnia if necessary, to allow lung emptying and reduce auto-PEEP. This might require heavy sedation to suppress the patient's ventilatory drive. If sedation is insufficient to achieve patient-ventilator synchrony or is poorly tolerated due to hemodynamic instability, muscle paralysis might be necessary [2, 8, 9].

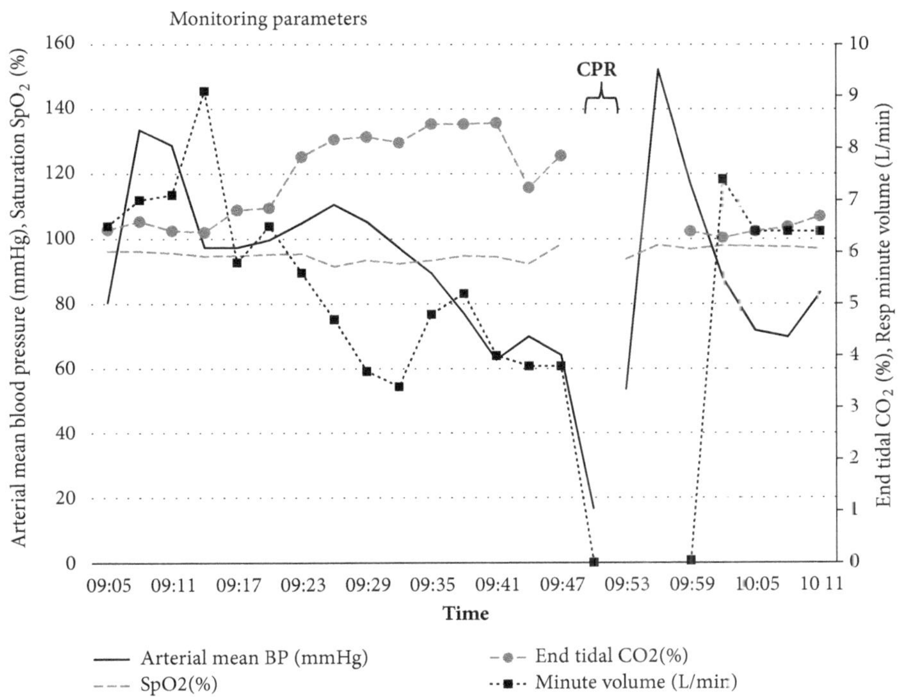

FIGURE 3: Vital parameters. Preceding the second cardiac arrest, expired minute volume is reduced, resulting in elevated end tidal carbon dioxide concentration. Blood pressure is initially elevated, probably secondary to stress, before it suddenly drops. Saturation is maintained through increased oxygen fraction in inspired air.

If the situation progresses to cardiac arrest, decreasing intrathoracic pressure by disconnecting the patient from the ventilator might restore venous return. Switching to manual bag ventilation is crucial to allow sufficient expiration time as rapid bag ventilation may also generate high auto-PEEP which could impair CPR outcome [2, 15]. Hyperinflation and auto-PEEP have been suggested as underestimated cause of persistent pulseless electrical activity during CPR in patients with obstructive airway diseases [5, 16].

Any action that might reduce flow limitation, e.g., bronchodilating therapy or exchange of an obstructed endotracheal tube, should be taken as rapidly as possible. The placement of stents to improve airway patency of the most affected bronchi solved the most severe expiratory air flow limitation in our case, preventing further episodes of dynamic hyperinflation and circulatory compromise which we believe confirms the pathophysiology outlined above.

Applying external PEEP may be useful in patients with flow limitation and dynamic hyperinflation, especially in cases with expiratory airway collapse such as COPD or tracheobronchomalacia. It may improve the airway patency, equalize PEEP between lung regions, and improve gas exchange. As long as applied PEEP is lower than auto-PEEP, it should exert little effect on peak pressure. In pressure support mode or noninvasive ventilation, external PEEP can ease triggering and reduce work of breathing. With applied PEEP balancing auto-PEEP, the relative negative pressure change needed for inspiration is reduced. Some literature recommended applying external PEEP at 75-85% of estimated auto-PEEP [8–10].

4. Tracheobronchomalacia

Our patient was diagnosed with GPA, a disease commonly involving the lower respiratory tract, e.g., causing subglottic stenosis, alveolar bleeding, pulmonary granulomas, tracheobronchial inflammation, and tracheobronchomalacia [17, 18].

Tracheobronchomalacia is a condition with weakened tracheal or bronchial cartilage. It can be secondary to trauma, surgery, intrathoracic processes, chronic inflammation, and necrosis in the bronchial tissues. Obstruction of air flow primarily occurs at active expiration, when the intrathoracic pressure exceeds the intrabronchial pressure, leading to collapse of the weakened parts [19, 20].

If medical treatment is insufficient, further treatment include laser treatment, surgery, and stenting with silicone or metal stents (Figure 4) in order to prevent airway collapse [18, 19]. Stents are ideally inserted for a shorter time, but sometimes long term treatment is necessary, which can cause problems with mucus stagnation, infections, and granulation tissue forming at the ends of the stent. Surgical tracheobronchoplasty is done at some centra, a procedure that aims to stabilize the airway by suturing a mesh to the posterior membrane of the trachea and bronchi. [20–22].

Additional Points

Key Points. This case highlights potentially life-threatening effects of dynamic hyperinflation and auto-PEEP caused by flow limitation in patients with tracheobronchomalacia and the difficulties with mechanical ventilation in these patients.

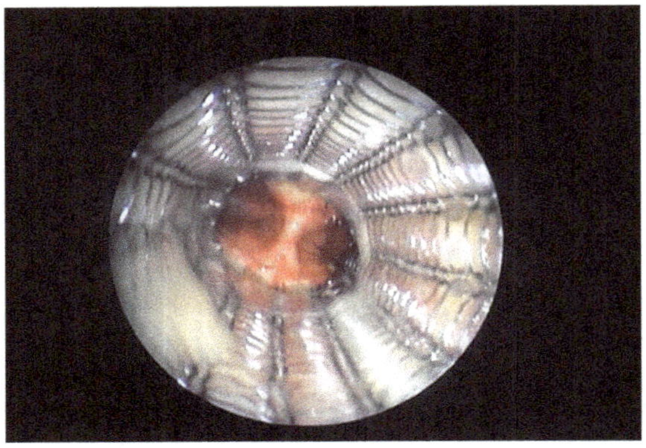

Figure 4: A metal stent in the trachea. This nitinol stent is covered except at the ends. The image is from another patient.

Acute stenting of the affected airways is an important treatment option.

Acknowledgments

No funding has been received, except for the article processing fee, financed through the Karolinska Institute.

References

[1] P. E. Pepe and J. J. Marini, "Occult positive end-expiratory pressure in mechanically ventilated patients with airflow obstruction: the auto-PEEP effect," *The American Review of Respiratory Disease*, vol. 126, no. 1, pp. 166–170, 1982.

[2] L. Blanch, F. Bernabe, and U. Lucangelo, "Measurement of air trapping, intrinsic positive end-expiratory pressure, and dynamic hyperinflation in mechanically ventilated patients," *Respiratory Care*, vol. 50, no. 1, pp. 110–123, 2005.

[3] P. S. Myles, H. Madder, and E. B. Morgan, "Intraoperative cardiac arrest after unrecognized dynamic hyperinflation," *British Journal of Anaesthesia*, vol. 74, no. 3, pp. 340–342, 1995.

[4] J. Sprung, K. Hunter, G. M. Barnas, and D. L. Bourke, "Abdominal distention is not always a sign of esophageal intubation: Cardiac arrest due to 'auto-PEEP'," *Anesthesia & Analgesia*, vol. 78, no. 4, pp. 801–804, 1994.

[5] P. L. Rogers, R. Schlichtig, A. Miro, and M. Pinsky, "Auto-PEEP during CPR: An 'occult' cause of electromechanical dissociation?" *CHEST*, vol. 99, no. 2, pp. 492-493, 1991.

[6] D. E. O'Donnell, K. A. Webb, and J. A. Neder, "Lung hyperinflation in COPD: Applying physiology to clinical practice," *COPD Research and Practice*, vol. 1, p. 4, 2015.

[7] A. Rossi, Z. Aisanov, S. Avdeev et al., "Mechanisms, assessment and therapeutic implications of lung hyperinflation in COPD," *Respiratory Medicine*, vol. 109, no. 7, pp. 785–802, 2015.

[8] J. J. Marini, "Dynamic hyperinflation and auto-positive end-expiratory pressure lessons learned over 30 years," *American Journal of Respiratory and Critical Care Medicine*, vol. 184, no. 7, pp. 756–762, 2011.

[9] M. Oddo, F. Feihl, M.-D. Schaller, and C. Perret, "Management of mechanical ventilation in acute severe asthma: practical aspects," *Intensive Care Medicine*, vol. 32, no. 4, pp. 501–510, 2006.

[10] D. Berlin, "Hemodynamic consequences of auto-PEEP," *Journal of Intensive Care Medicine*, vol. 29, no. 2, pp. 81–86, 2014.

[11] M. Dambrosio, G. Cinnella, N. Brienza et al., "Effects of positive end-expiratory pressure on right ventricular function in COPD patients during acute ventilatory failure," *Intensive Care Medicine*, vol. 22, no. 9, pp. 923–932, 1996.

[12] V. M. Ranieri, M. Dambrosio, and N. Brienza, "Intrinsic PEEP and cardiopulmonary interaction in patients with COPD and acute ventilatory failure," *European Respiratory Journal*, vol. 9, no. 6, pp. 1283–1292, 1996.

[13] F. Baigorri, A. De Monte, L. Blanch et al., "Hemodynamic responses to external counterbalancing of auto-positive end-expiratory pressure in mechanically ventilated patients with chronic obstructive pulmonary disease," *Critical Care Medicine*, vol. 22, no. 11, pp. 1782–1791, 1994.

[14] M. R. Pinsky, "Cardiovascular issues in respiratory care," *CHEST*, vol. 128, suppl 2, no. 5, pp. 592S–597S, 2005.

[15] T. P. Aufderheide, G. Sigurdsson, R. G. Pirrallo et al., "Hyperventilation-induced hypotension during cardiopulmonary resuscitation," *Circulation*, vol. 109, no. 16, pp. 1960–1965, 2004.

[16] S. E. Lapinsky and R. S. Leung, "Auto-PEEP and electromechanical dissociation," *The New England Journal of Medicine*, vol. 335, no. 9, p. 674, 1996.

[17] C. A. Langford and G. S. Hoffman, "Wegener's granulomatosis," *Thorax*, vol. 54, no. 7, pp. 629–637, 1999.

[18] T. E. Daum, U. Specks, T. V. Colby et al., "Tracheobronchial involvement in Wegener's granulomatosis," *American Journal of Respiratory and Critical Care Medicine*, vol. 151, no. 2 Pt 1, pp. 522–526, 1995.

[19] K. A. Carden, P. M. Boiselle, D. A. Waltz, and A. Ernst, "Tracheomalacia and tracheobronchomalacia in children and adults: an in-depth review," *CHEST*, vol. 127, no. 3, pp. 984–1005, 2005.

[20] S. Murgu and H. Colt, "Tracheobronchomalacia and excessive dynamic airway collapse," *Clinics in Chest Medicine*, vol. 34, no. 3, pp. 527–555, 2013.

[21] A. Majid, J. Guerrero, S. Gangadharan et al., "Tracheobronchoplasty for severe tracheobronchomalacia: a prospective outcome analysis," *CHEST*, vol. 134, no. 4, pp. 801–807, 2008.

[22] S. P. Gangadharan, C. T. Bakhos, A. Majid et al., "Technical aspects and outcomes of tracheobronchoplasty for severe tracheobronchomalacia," *The Annals of Thoracic Surgery*, vol. 91, no. 5, pp. 1574–1580, 2011.

Successful Use of Octreotide Therapy for Refractory Levofloxacin-Induced Hypoglycemia: A Case Report and Literature Review

Matthew R. Watson,[1] **Ceressa T. Ward**,[1] **Amit Prabhakar**,[2] **Babar Fiza**,[2] **and Vanessa Moll**[2]

[1]*Pharmaceutical Services, Emory University Hospital Midtown, Atlanta, Georgia, USA*
[2]*Department of Anesthesiology, Emory Center of Critical Care, Emory School of Medicine, Atlanta, Georgia, USA*

Correspondence should be addressed to Vanessa Moll; vanessa.moll@emory.edu

Academic Editor: Gil Klinger

Fluoroquinolones are commonly prescribed antimicrobials that have been implicated in alterations of glucose metabolism. We report a case of refractory fluoroquinolone-induced hypoglycemia in a patient with type-2 diabetes mellitus on glipizide that was successfully treated with octreotide. A patient was admitted with hypoglycemia after having been initiated on levofloxacin therapy. Despite treating the hypoglycemia supportively with multiple boluses of 25 g of dextrose, a continuous dextrose infusion, and glucagon, the patient experienced repeated episodes of rebound hypoglycemia. The persistent hypoglycemia was eventually reversed with the administration of subcutaneous octreotide. Clinicians should be cognizant of this adverse effect of fluoroquinolones, as well as predisposing risk factors, and consider octreotide as an adjunctive therapy for refractory hypoglycemia cases.

1. Introduction

Fluoroquinolones are a commonly prescribed class of broad-spectrum antimicrobials used for a variety of bacterial infections given their excellent degree of tissue penetration and high oral bioavailability [1]. Although appropriate for select indications, routine use of fluoroquinolones has been questioned due to associated risks. Serious adverse effects have been linked to fluoroquinolones prompting recent updates to the safety labeling which now includes potential risk for significant hypoglycemia resulting in coma [2]. The mechanism of fluoroquinolone-induced hypoglycemia is poorly understood. However, it is postulated that fluoroquinolones interact with insulin producing pancreatic β-cells. Currently, there are no targeted therapeutic options for treating this adverse effect. Given the hypothesized mechanism, octreotide may represent a novel treatment for reversal of fluoroquinolone-induced hypoglycemia. We report a case of severe life-threatening and refractory hypoglycemia from levofloxacin successfully treated with octreotide.

2. Case Report

A 73-year-old Caucasian male with a past medical history of coronary artery disease, heart failure, atrial fibrillation, chronic obstructive pulmonary disease, and type-2 diabetes mellitus was admitted after having a witnessed seizure at his nursing rehabilitation facility. When emergency medical services arrived, the patient was found to be hypoglycemic with blood glucose (BG) of 21 mg/dL. He was administered 25 g of dextrose 50% (D50) resulting in some improvement in his mental status. He was then transferred to our emergency department (ED).

In the ED, the patient was minimally responsive to both verbal and physical cues. The initial laboratory results were significant for hypokalemia with potassium of 2.9 mmol/L (normal 3.6-5.1 mmol/L), acute kidney injury with serum creatinine at 2.52 mg/dL (normal 0.7-1.3 mg/dL; baseline approximately 1.5 mg/dL), albumin of 2 g/dL (normal 3.5-5.7 g/dL), and hypoglycemia with a BG of 34 mg/dL (normal 70-105 mg/dL). Liver function tests (LFTs) were all within

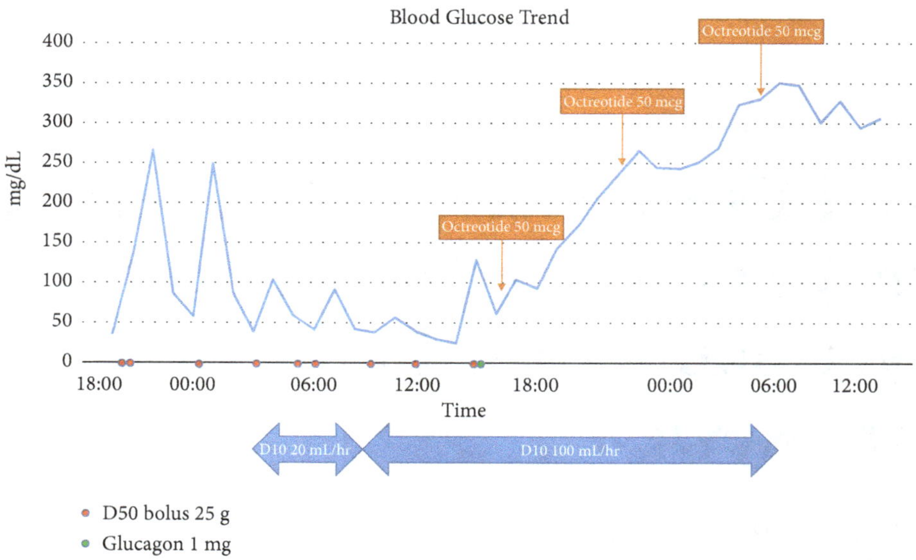

FIGURE 1: Blood glucose values in response to D10 infusion, D50 boluses, glucagon, and octreotide. D10, dextrose 10%; D50, dextrose 50%.

normal limits. The patient was immediately given 50 g of D50 resulting in a repeat BG of 134 mg/dL. Review of the patient's home medication list identified that the patient was prescribed levofloxacin 750 mg daily for pneumonia on discharge from a hospitalization three days prior with no other medication changes. Chronic medications were inclusive of aspirin 81 mg daily, atorvastatin 80 mg daily, glipizide 10 mg daily, losartan 25 mg daily, mometasone 220 mcg/inhalation three times daily, spironolactone 25 mg daily, torsemide 100 mg daily, and warfarin. The patient required four additional boluses of D50 and a continuous dextrose 10% (D10) infusion to maintain euglycemia before transfer to the intensive care unit (ICU).

In the ICU, the patient continued to experience multiple episodes of severe rebound hypoglycemia despite an additional four boluses of D50, increasing the D10 infusion rate to 100 mL/hr (see Figure 1) and withholding home medications. Glucagon 1 mg intramuscularly only led to a transient increase in BG. Given the patient's refractory hypoglycemia to standard supportive care therapies, octreotide 50 mcg subcutaneously was administered every six hours for a total of three doses. Within three hours of administration of the first dose of octreotide, there was a significant increase in BG levels (ranging from 170 to 237 mg/dL) and no further D50 boluses were required. Due to persistent hyperglycemia (BG >250 mg/dL), the D10 infusion was discontinued 5.5 hours after the second dose of octreotide. The patient eventually required an insulin infusion the following day and was transferred to the floor. The patient was ultimately discharged to his nursing rehabilitation facility in stable condition.

3. Discussion

Hypoglycemia is a rare but a known potential adverse effect of fluoroquinolone therapy. Several published case reports have specifically implicated levofloxacin as the causative agent of hypoglycemia with some resulting in fatal outcomes [3–13]. This case report adds to the emerging data documenting fluoroquinolone-induced hypoglycemia. The exact incidence of this adverse effect is not known. However, a total of 67 cases of fluoroquinolone-associated hypoglycemia have been identified through review of the FDA Adverse Event Reporting System (FAERS) and published literature from 1987 to 2017 [14]. This figure is likely conservative due to probable underrecognition and thus underreporting. Due to hypoglycemia having the potential to lead to serious morbidity and mortality, it is important for clinicians to recognize risk factors associated with this adverse event and increase monitoring or choose alternative therapy when appropriate [15].

Several risk factors may predispose patients to hypoglycemia while being treated with fluoroquinolones including diabetes, concomitant use of sulfonylureas or insulin, renal insufficiency, and elderly which is conventionally defined as greater than 65 years old [2, 16, 17]. Although levofloxacin was dosed appropriately for renal function at the time of prescription for pneumonia, our patient did have multiple risk factors (i.e., elderly with diabetes on glipizide) that could have prompted discussion regarding alternative treatment. If a fluoroquinolone is determined to be the most optimal antibiotic based on indication, there is data to support that differences in risk of hypoglycemia exist among this class that could assist in guiding therapy.

In a large population-based cohort study of over 78,000 diabetic patients newly prescribed a fluoroquinolone, the absolute risk of hypoglycemia per 1,000 people for moxifloxacin, levofloxacin, and ciprofloxacin was found to be 10.0, 9.3, and 7.9, respectively. This is in comparison to 3.7 for macrolides and 3.2 for cephalosporins [18]. In contrast to this study, the FAERS found moxifloxacin to be the least associated with hypoglycemia. Moxifloxacin, ciprofloxacin, and levofloxacin accounted for 9, 12, and 44 of the 67 cases of hypoglycemia reported, respectively. This data is consistent with published work from the Veteran Affairs system where levofloxacin was noted to confer a higher risk of hypoglycemia in comparison to ciprofloxacin. Moxifloxacin was not studied in that publication due to low usage at the time of the study [19]. The interpretation of this data may be limited by reporting/publication bias. Nonetheless, the differences can likely be explained by variations in molecular structure which have been seen with other toxicities associated with fluoroquinolones [20].

The mechanisms by which fluoroquinolones induce hypoglycemia have not yet been fully elucidated. However, in vitro and animal model studies have provided evidence on proposed pharmacodynamic pathways that modulate insulin secretion. These studies in addition to the known pharmacokinetic profile of levofloxacin provide potential explanations for this clinical scenario.

Adenosine triphosphate-sensitive potassium (KATP) channels located in pancreatic β-cells play a key role in sensing plasma glucose levels and triggering the release of insulin to maintain euglycemia [21, 22]. In vitro studies suggest that fluoroquinolones block this channel resulting in membrane depolarization leading to an influx of calcium through voltage-gated calcium channels and subsequent increase in insulin release [23, 24]. These similar molecular mechanisms occur when sulfonylureas bind to the sulfonylurea receptor 1 subunit on the KATP channels. This results in the same downstream signaling resulting in exocytosis of insulin secretory granules via calcium signaling [25]. Due to the varying risks of hypoglycemia reported in the literature among the fluoroquinolones, further research is needed to understand possible unidentified biochemical triggering factors [26].

In addition to pharmacodynamics, a pharmacokinetic mechanism in our case should be explored. On admission, our patient was noted to be on concomitant therapy with glipizide for type-2 diabetes. Hence, the possibility of a combined drug-drug interaction between levofloxacin and glipizide should be considered as another mechanism to explain the refractory hypoglycemia. Glipizide is primarily metabolized by the cytochrome P-450 (CYP) system, specifically isoenzyme CYP2C9 [27]. It has been shown in an in vitro model of human liver microsomes that levofloxacin weakly inhibits CYP2C9 [28]. Due to the existence of genetic polymorphisms of CYP2C9, patients may exhibit different baseline metabolism rates that variably change by the addition of a CYP2C9 inhibitor. This could possibly explain the differences in clinical outcomes and/or adverse events between patients on these two medications. Moreover, levofloxacin and glipizide are approximately 24-38% and 98-99% protein bound primarily to albumin, respectively [29, 30]. Given these ratios, albumin binding affinities, and different primary albumin binding sites, the probability of levofloxacin causing a significant displacement of glipizide to increase its free drug fraction, thus its therapeutic/adverse effects, is unlikely [31, 32].

Although supportive care therapies such as glucose and glucagon administration remain the cornerstone of treatment for hypoglycemia, complications have been reported. In this therapeutic approach, transient beneficial increases in serum glucose are offset by rebound hypoglycemia that can especially occur in patients taking medications affecting pancreatic KATP β-cell channels such as sulfonylureas. This is caused by the additional glucose further stimulating insulin release in patients with intact pancreatic function (e.g., nondiabetics or patient with type-2 noninsulin dependent diabetes) [33, 34]. Given the similarities in biological mechanism to sulfonylureas, it is reasonable to propose that this phenomenon of rebound hypoglycemia may occur with fluoroquinolones as well. Although there are no specific therapies to reverse fluoroquinolone-induced hypoglycemia, octreotide may represent a novel adjunctive treatment given its well-documented success in sulfonylurea toxicity [35, 36].

Octreotide is a potent and long-acting synthetic analog of the inhibitory peptide hormone somatostatin [33]. Voltage-gated calcium channels on the pancreatic β-cell membrane are coupled to G-protein somatostatin-2 receptors. When these receptors are bound by octreotide, the voltage-gated calcium channels remain closed preventing calcium influx into the cell, therefore, inhibiting insulin release. This mechanism occurs downstream of the KATP channel thus inhibiting the cascade of molecular signaling induced by sulfonylureas and fluoroquinolones. Following the initial administration of octreotide to our patient, there was a significant increase in the ability to maintain euglycemia within 3 hours which was previously unable to be achieved with other supportive care therapies. Octreotide therapy also assisted in limiting the amount of infused fluids as the D10 infusion was discontinued 5.5 hours after the second dose. This benefit is important to consider when caring for patients with cardiac or renal failure where fluid overload can further complicate care.

The dosage and interval of octreotide therapy were based on published literature for insulin and sulfonylurea overdoses. In adults, doses of 50-100 mcg subcutaneously or intravenously every 6 to 12 hours have been reported [35]. Octreotide with its relatively benign adverse effect profile is well tolerated by most adult and pediatric patients [34, 36, 37]. The most common side effects are pain at the injection site and gastrointestinal disturbances. Given the anticipated short-term use of octreotide, the risks of this off-label therapy are minimal.

To our knowledge, this is the second case report to describe the successful use of octreotide for treating life-threatening hypoglycemia caused by levofloxacin in combination with glipizide. The first case by Kelesidis and Canseco was similar to ours in that an elderly woman with type-2 diabetes mellitus treated with glipizide and chronic kidney disease experienced refractory hypoglycemia to supportive measures complicated by seizures after one dose of ciprofloxacin [6]. After the administration of a single dose of 50 mcg octreotide intravenously, the patient's glucose normalized in approximately 2 hours. The time course for the ability to maintain euglycemia after the first subcutaneous octreotide administration was similar in our case at 3 hours. The difference in time to therapeutic effect could be explained by the different routes of administration. Conversely, the time to hypoglycemic event took 4 days to develop in our case in comparison to after a single dose. This highlights the importance of frequent monitoring for this adverse effect early and often after fluoroquinolone initiation.

This case is limited by the fact that causation cannot unequivocally establish levofloxacin as the sole cause of hypoglycemia given other potential contributing factors, including the use of sulfonylureas where both pharmacodynamic and pharmacokinetic mechanisms may have contributed. Based on the Naranjo score of 4, it is possible the hypoglycemia was attributed to levofloxacin [38]. Though appropriately dosed at the time of initiation days prior, our patient presented with acute renal insufficiency as evidenced by a greater than twofold increase in serum creatinine. This likely caused an accumulation of levofloxacin secondary to delayed renal clearance and a more pronounced dose-dependent pharmacodynamic effect. While all sulfonylureas independently increase the risk for hypoglycemia, it is unlikely that glipizide was the predominant driver of this adverse effect in this case. The patient had been on a stable dose of immediate release glipizide 10 mg daily for several years and there was no reason to suspect intentional overdose given that the patient came from a nursing rehabilitation facility. Moreover, glipizide is metabolized extensively by the liver yielding inactive metabolites with data to support its use in patients with chronic kidney disease or on dialysis. Given that our patient presented with normal LFTs, there is low suspicion there was a metabolism deficiency. Furthermore, the clearance of levofloxacin is three times longer than that of glipizide in patients with acute renal impairment [29, 30] Additionally, this patient had chronic low albumin suggesting the free drug fraction of glipizide has been steadily maintained and is an unlikely explanation for the acute effect seen in this case.

It should also be noted that the patient was initiated on high calorie, high fiber enteral nutrition (EN) at 50 mL/hr at the time octreotide was initiated. However, the carbohydrates provided by EN in addition to that provided by the D10 infusion at 100 mL/hr only supplied the patient with 20.8 g of carbohydrates per hour. This amount of carbohydrates is less than that provided by each bolus of D50 (25 g) and thus, unlikely to account for the sudden maintenance of euglycemia.

Our case and review of the literature highlight the safety concern of potential hypoglycemia with the use of levofloxacin in patients with identified risk factors and support the use of octreotide to reverse this phenomenon. Early recognition of this potential complication and subsequent treatment are necessary to prevent increased morbidity and mortality. Clinicians should exercise caution when prescribing fluoroquinolones by evaluating patients for known risk factors for hypoglycemia especially when unavoidable drug-drug interactions are possible. In patients unresponsive to standard supportive care therapies, the early adjunctive use of octreotide appears to be a reasonable off-label treatment option for fluoroquinolone-induced hypoglycemia.

4. Conclusion

Severe hypoglycemia is a known adverse effect of fluoroquinolones. However, until the recent updates in safety labeling, general awareness of this adverse effect was lacking. Clinicians should be aware of the risk factors and increase monitoring or choose alternative therapy when appropriate. It is essential clinicians are cognizant of these lesser-known adverse effects and drug-drug interactions to ensure prompt recognition and treatment using appropriate adjuncts. Octreotide may represent a novel reversal agent in addition to supportive care therapies for patients presenting with refractory, fluoroquinolone-induced hypoglycemia. To the best of the authors' knowledge, this is the second case report to describe the successful use of octreotide to treat severe and refractory hypoglycemia caused by levofloxacin in a patient with type-2 diabetes mellitus receiving glipizide.

Disclosure

Abstract was presented at the Society of Critical Care Medicine Annual Congress meeting in San Diego, February 17th, 2019.

Authors' Contributions

Watson and Ward were responsible for drafting of the manuscript. Watson, Ward, Prabhakar, Fiza, and Moll were responsible for critical revision of the manuscript for important intellectual content. Moll was responsible for study supervision.

References

[1] M. K. Bolon, "The newer fluoroquinolones," *Medical Clinics of North America*, vol. 95, no. 4, pp. 793–817, 2011.

[2] "Safety alerts for human medical products - fluoroquinolone antibiotics: FDA requires labeling changes due to low blood sugar levels and mental health side effects," 2019, https://www.fda.gov/Safety/MedWatch/SafetyInformation/SafetyAlertsforHumanMedicalProducts/ucm612979.htm.

[3] S. Fusco, F. Reitano, N. Gambadoro et al., "Severe hypoglycemia associated with levofloxacin in a healthy older woman," *Journal of the American Geriatrics Society*, vol. 61, no. 9, pp. 1637-1638, 2013.

[4] N. Bansal, D. Manocha, and B. Madhira, "Life-threatening metabolic coma caused by levofloxacin," *American Journal of Therapeutics*, vol. 22, no. 2, pp. e48–e51, 2015.

[5] H. Parra-Riffo and J. Lemus-Peñaloza, "Severe levofloxacin-induced hypoglycaemia: a case report and literature review," *Nefrologia*, vol. 32, no. 4, pp. 546-547, 2012.

[6] T. Kelesidis and E. Canseco, "Quinolone-induced hypoglycemia: a life-threatening but potentially reversible side effect," *American Journal of Medicine*, vol. 123, no. 2, pp. e5–e6, 2010.

[7] T. Kelesidis and E. Canseco, "Levofloxacin-induced hypoglycemia: a rare but life-threatening side effect of a widely used antibiotic," *American Journal of Medicine*, vol. 122, no. 3, pp. e3–e4, 2009.

[8] K. R. Lawrence, M. Adra, and C. Keir, "Hypoglycemia-induced anoxic brain injury possibly associated with levofloxacin," *Infection*, vol. 52, no. 6, pp. e177–e180, 2006.

[9] L. V. Friedrich and R. Dougherty, "Fatal hypoglycemia associated with levofloxacin," *Pharmacotherapy*, vol. 24, no. 12, pp. 1807–1812, 2004.

[10] L. Micheli, M. Sbrilli, and C. Nencini, "Severe hypoglycemia associated with levofloxacin in Type 2 diabetic patients receiving polytherapy: two case reports," *International Journal of Clinical Pharmacology and Therapeutics*, vol. 50, no. 4, pp. 302–306, 2012.

[11] A. E. Gibert and F. S. Porta, "Hypoglycemia and levofloxacin: a case report," *Clinical Infectious Diseases*, vol. 46, no. 7, pp. 1126-1127, 2008.

[12] S. M. Garber, M. W. Pound, and S. M. Miller, "Hypoglycemia associated with the use of levofloxacin," *American Journal of Health-System Pharmacy*, vol. 66, no. 11, pp. 1014–1019, 2009.

[13] M. Kanbay, T. Aydogan, R. Bozalan et al., "A rare but serious side effect of levofloxacin: hypoglycemia in a geriatric patient," *Diabetes Care*, vol. 29, no. 7, pp. 1716-1717, 2006.

[14] FDA Drug Safety Communication, https://www.fda.gov/downloads/Drugs/DrugSafety/UCM612834.pdf.

[15] J. Morales and D. Schneider, "Hypoglycemia," *American Journal of Medicine*, vol. 127, no. 10, pp. S17–S24, 2014.

[16] T. M. Parekh, M. Raji, Y.-L. Lin, A. Tan, Y.-F. Kuo, and J. S. Goodwin, "Hypoglycemia after antimicrobial drug prescription for older patients using sulfonylureas," *JAMA Internal Medicine*, vol. 174, no. 10, pp. 1605–1612, 2014.

[17] K. L. LaPlante, T. L. Mersfelder, K. E. Ward, and B. J. Quilliam, "Prevalence of and risk factors for dysglycemia in patients receiving gatifloxacin and levofloxacin in an outpatient setting," *Pharmacotherapy*, vol. 28, no. 1, pp. 82–89, 2008.

[18] H.-W. Chou, J.-L. Wang, C.-H. Chang, J.-J. Lee, W.-Y. Shau, and M.-S. Lai, "Risk of severe dysglycemia among diabetic patients receiving levofloxacin, ciprofloxacin, or moxifloxacin in Taiwan," *Clinical Infectious Diseases*, vol. 57, no. 7, pp. 971–980, 2013.

[19] S. L. Aspinall, C. B. Good, R. Jiang, M. McCarren, D. Dong, and F. E. Cunningham, "Severe dysglycemia with the fluoroquinolones: a class effect?" *Clinical Infectious Diseases*, vol. 49, no. 3, pp. 402–408, 2009.

[20] R. C. Owens and P. G. Ambrose, "Antimicrobial safety: focus on fluoroquinolones," *Clinical Infectious Diseases*, vol. 41, Suppl 2, pp. S144–S157, 2005.

[21] J. C. Koster, M. A. Permutt, and C. G. Nichols, "Diabetes and insulin secretion: the ATP-sensitive K+ channel (K ATP) connection," *Diabetes*, vol. 54, no. 11, pp. 3065–3072, 2005.

[22] A. L. Gloyn, E. R. Pearson, J. F. Antcliff et al., "Activating mutations in the gene encoding the ATP-sensitive potassium-channel subunit Kir6.2 and permanent neonatal diabetes," *The New England Journal of Medicine*, vol. 350, no. 18, pp. 1838–1849, 2004.

[23] N. Maeda, T. Tamagawa, I. Niki et al., "Increase in insulin release from rat pancreatic islets by quinolone antibiotics," *British Journal of Pharmacology*, vol. 117, no. 2, pp. 372–376, 1996.

[24] A. Saraya, M. Yokokura, T. Gonoi, and S. Seino, "Effects of fluoroquinolones on insulin secretion and beta-cell ATP-sensitive K+ channels," *European Journal of Pharmacology*, vol. 497, no. 1, pp. 111–117, 2004.

[25] D. Sola, L. Rossi, G. P. C. Schianca, P. Maffioli, M. Bigliocca, R. Mella et al., "Sulfonylureas and their use in clinical practice," *Archives of Medical Science*, vol. 11, no. 4, pp. 840–848, 2015.

[26] H. Ghaly, C. Kriete, S. Sahin et al., "The insulinotropic effect of fluoroquinolones," *Biochemical Pharmacology*, vol. 77, no. 6, pp. 1040–1052, 2009.

[27] D. Van Booven, S. Marsh, H. McLeod et al., "Cytochrome P450 2C9-CYP2C9," *Pharmacogenetics and Genomics*, vol. 20, no. 4, pp. 277–281, 2010.

[28] L. Zhang, M. Wei, C. Zhao, and H. Qi, "Determination of the inhibitory potential of 6 fluoroquinolones on CYP1A2 and CYP2C9 in human liver microsomes," *Acta Pharmacologica Sinica*, vol. 29, no. 12, pp. 1507–1514, 2008.

[29] "Levofloxacin, Lexi-Drugs, Lexicomp [Internet]," 2019, http://online.lexi.com.

[30] "Glipizide, Lexi-Drugs, Lexicomp [Internet]," http://online.lexi.com.

[31] N. Seedher and P. Agarwal, "Competitive binding of fluoroquinolone antibiotics and some other drugs to human serum albumin: a luminescence spectroscopic study," *Luminescence*, vol. 28, no. 4, pp. 562–568, 2013.

[32] N. Seedher and M. Kanojia, "Mechanism of interaction of hypoglycemic agents glimepiride and glipizide with human serum albumin," *Central European Journal of Chemistry*, vol. 7, no. 1, pp. 96–104, 2009.

[33] P. E. R. Lheureux, S. Zahir, A. Penaloza, and M. Gris, "Bench-to-bedside review: antidotal treatment of sulfonylurea-induced hypoglycaemia with octreotide," *Critical Care*, vol. 9, no. 6, pp. 543–549, 2005.

[34] P. P. Dougherty and W. Klein-Schwartz, "Octreotide's role in the management of sulfonylurea-induced hypoglycemia," *Journal of Medical Toxicology*, vol. 6, no. 2, pp. 199–206, 2010.

[35] W. Klein-Schwartz, G. L. Stassinos, and G. K. Isbister, "Treatment of sulfonylurea and insulin overdose," *British Journal of Clinical Pharmacology*, vol. 81, no. 3, pp. 496–504, 2016.

[36] M. Glatstein, D. Scolnik, and Y. Bentur, "Octreotide for the treatment of sulfonylurea poisoning," *Clinical Toxicology*, vol. 50, no. 9, pp. 795–804, 2012.

[37] C. J. Fasano, G. O'Malley, P. Dominici, E. Aguilera, and D. R. Latta, "Comparison of octreotide and standard therapy versus standard therapy alone for the treatment of sulfonylurea-induced hypoglycemia," *Annals of Emergency Medicine*, vol. 51, no. 4, pp. 400–406, 2008.

[38] C. A. Naranjo, U. Busto, E. M. Sellers et al., "A method for estimating the probability of adverse drug reactions," *Clinical Pharmacology & Therapeutics*, vol. 30, no. 2, pp. 239–245, 1981.

Does Dexmedetomidine Improve or Worsen Restless Leg Syndrome under Sedation: A Case Report and Extensive Review

Sandra Iskandar,[1] **Marina Souto Martins**,[2] **Andrew Hudson**,[3] **Jason G. Hirsch**,[3] **and Jonathan S. Jahr**[3]

[1]*University of California-Riverside Medical Student, Riverside, CA, USA*
[2]*School of Medicine, University of Fortaleza, Brazil SA*
[3]*David Geffen School of Medicine at UCLA, USA*

Correspondence should be addressed to Jonathan S. Jahr; j.s.jahr@ucla.edu

Academic Editor: Kenneth S. Waxman

Background. Restless leg syndrome (RLS) is a common neurological condition that manifests as creeping, nonpainful urges to move lower extremities and is relieved with movements of the legs. RLS is associated with comorbidities such as gastric surgery, diabetes mellitus, uremia, and iron deficiency anemia, and it is misdiagnosed in many cases. Drugs like levodopa, ropinirole, pramipexole, cabergoline, and pergolide that target the dopaminergic system have been traditionally used to treat symptoms of RLS. α2-adrenoceptor (α2-AR) agonists, like clonidine and dexmedetomidine, have also been reported to show improvement of RLS symptoms during sedation. *Specific Aim.* This case report suggests that dexmedetomidine may have worsened RLS during sedation in a 71-year-old male with no prior diagnosis of RLS or reported symptoms. The patient had a procedure for right first metatarsophalangeal joint (MTPJ) fusion, with second digit proximal interphalangeal joint (PIPJ) arthrodesis, and flexor tendon transfer due to pain on walking and failing conservative therapy. He underwent intravenous sedation/monitored anesthesia care (MAC) with propofol, dexmedetomidine, and a peripheral regional block for intraoperative anesthesia and postoperative analgesia. During the surgery, the patient experienced continuous bilateral leg movement, unpredictable, and unrelated to surgical stimulation or level of consciousness within 5 minutes of administration of dexmedetomidine. The patient tolerated the procedure, and the unpredicted leg movement was managed by the surgeons intraoperatively. *Conclusion.* Although no previous literature exists and mechanisms are unclear, this case report hypothesizes that dexmedetomidine may contribute to worsening RLS symptoms.

1. Introduction

Restless leg syndrome (RLS) [1] is a relatively common condition affecting from 1% to 15% of the general population [2] and may be challenging to treat if present during moderate to deep sedation [3]. Dexmedetomidine has been reported to improve RLS during sedation [3]. We report a case where dexmedetomidine may have worsened RLS associated lower extremity movement during sedation and then present the current literature on RLS, and the case report is describing dexmedetomidine actions improving RLS during sedation. We comment that dexmedetomidine may exacerbate RLS under sedation and discuss mechanisms whereby this may occur.

2. Case Presentation

A 71-year-old man was scheduled for right first metatarsophalangeal joint (MTPJ) fusion, with second digit proximal interphalangeal joint (PIPJ) arthrodesis, and flexor tendon transfer due to pain on walking and failing conservative therapy. His extensive past medical history included hypertension (HTN), hypersensitivity lung disease (HLD), and chronic chest pain under investigation. He was also diagnosed with asthma and depression. He had a history of previous surgeries, without any reported problems related to anesthesia. His medications included metoprolol, atorvastatin, budesonide/formoterol, ipratropium, venlafaxine, albuterol, and clonidine. He had a smoking history for 3 years, which he quit during his twenties. Alcohol drinking habits were described as rare, and the patient denied cannabis or other substance use.

He did not have any finding during physical exam on preoperative anesthesia assessment, and for his preoperative laboratory work up, the only finding was an electrocardiogram (EKG) with sinus rhythm (SR) and a right bundle branch block (RBBB). The patient remained a candidate for intravenous sedation/monitored anesthesia care (MAC), with a peripheral regional block for intraoperative anesthesia and postoperative analgesia.

His baseline blood pressure (BP) and HR during the procedure were 156/92 mmHg and 91/min, respectively. His oxygen saturation (SpO2) was 96% while breathing room air. The patient received 20 milligram (mg) perineural infusion of mepivacaine 1.5%/mL during preoperative care. Additionally, after intravenous access was obtained, the patient received 20 micrograms (mcg) of dexmedetomidine and was placed on propofol infusion. He also received 30 mg of ketamine for multimodal anesthesia throughout the procedure.

His intraoperative course was complicated by the unanticipated event of almost continuous bilateral leg movement, unpredictable and unrelated to surgical stimulation or level of consciousness within 5 minutes of administration of dexmedetomidine. His depth of sedation was varied to deep sedation all the way to light sedation, with no improvement in symptoms of leg movements. The surgical team was able to continue surgery by placing the anesthetized foot in a padded restraint.

However, the nonoperative leg continued to move and caused challenges for both anesthesia and surgical teams. Discussion as to whether to convert to a general anesthetic occurred, but the surgeons believed they could complete the surgery safely and successfully, despite suboptimal conditions. The anesthesia team was concerned that a general anesthetic, with the patient's significant comorbidities, might prolong his postoperative course and even require a hospitalization.

The procedure was managed with varying the depth of sedation with the propofol infusion and later, addition of ketamine, in an attempt to provide additional sedation, improve the surgical operating conditions, and decrease leg movement. In the end, the patient tolerated the procedure under sedation and the surgeons managed to deal with the unpredictable leg movements, and no noticeable improvements occurred with either propofol at varying depths of sedation, dexmedetomidine, or later the case, ketamine. The patient did not receive any ondansetron or metoclopramide as antiemetics.

The surgery lasted three hours and seventeen minutes. The patient was transferred to the postoperative anesthetic care unit (PACU) for further observation. His postoperative course was uneventful and was discharged to a 23-hour observation unit and discharged home the next day without untoward events, unaware of his RLS history.

3. Discussion

Restless leg syndrome (RLS) or Willis-Ekbom disease is a chronic movement disorder that manifests as creeping, nonpainful urges to move lower extremities and is relieved with movements of the legs. The disorder has diurnal patterns, and it manifests during sleep or at rest. In the United States, there are more than three million cases per year [1]. Diagnosis of RLS is often missed, and patients endure their symptoms for years without treatment [2]. Therefore, taking a detailed patient history along with polysomnography studies is key to diagnosing the syndrome. Another related movement disorder is periodic limb movement disorder (PLMD) which manifests in repetitive and jerking movements during sleep. Even though RLS is a sensory phenomenon, PLMD is often associated with RLS.

3.1. Etiology. RLS can be broken down into two types: primary and secondary. Primary can be further subcategorized as being either idiopathic or familial in origin. Familial restless leg syndrome tends to occur at younger than 45 years of age [1]. The inheritance pattern of familial cases follows an autosomal dominant pattern with multiple loci [4, 5]. Years of research into the genetics behind RLS have revealed the genetic heterogeneity of the condition leading RLS to be considered a complex genetic disease [6]. Secondary disease is associated with comorbidities such as gastric surgery, diabetes mellitus, uremia, and iron deficiency anemia [4, 7]. Varied responses to treatment have been seen depending on the etiology of the disease, making it imperative to distinguish the cause of patients' symptoms [4]. Some studies suggest increasing prevalence with age [8], and others show that the cardiovascular and metabolic changes that occur with age are related to RLS [9].

RLS is associated with reduced intracortical inhibition rather than a specific lesion in the central nervous system (CNS) [4]. RLS symptoms seem to result from abnormal spinal sensorimotor integration at the spinal cord level and abnormal central somatosensory processing. This leads to increased sensory activation at the level of the spinal cord and decreased cortical inhibition of unwanted actions. Histological and functional imaging data together suggest that RLS exhibits a "hyperdopaminergic" presynaptic state characterized by increased synthesis and release of dopamine that is balanced by a "hypodopaminergic" postsynaptic state with decreased D2 receptor expression, though it remains unclear to what extent the pre and postsynaptic changes in RLS are primary, secondary, or compensatory [10].

3.2. Presentation. Patients present with nonpainful, irresistible urges to move their legs. Patients report their symptoms as a pulling, crawling, itching, or stretching sensation in the calves that happen at rest and is improved with leg movement. Studies show that the incidence of RLS is twice as high in women compared to men, which might suggest that hormones play a role in RLS [11].

3.3. Treatment. Drugs from various classes have been used off-label to treat the symptoms of RLS over the years. Multiple drugs that target the dopaminergic system have been used to treat RLS, which supports the hypothesis that central dopamine abnormalities play a significant role in the pathophysiology of RLS [12]. Double blind, placebo controlled studies demonstrated effectiveness of carbidopa/levodopa, propoxyphene, dopamine agonists, and pramipexole in reducing RLS symptoms [13–15]. Evidence from an evidence-based review by the International Parkinson and Movement Disorder Society found levodopa, ropinirole, pramipexole, cabergoline, pergolide, and gabapentin all are efficacious in treating RLS. However, augmentation, an iatrogenic worsening of RLS symptoms following treatment with dopaminergic agents, has been recognized as an important issue in the management of RLS [16]. Other studies have shown that benzodiazepines and baclofen are clinically effective in treating RLS [17, 18].

Gabapentin was shown to be efficacious in treating the symptoms of RLS. One study found that 600 mg of gabapentin enacarbil was efficacious for Japanese patients up to 12 weeks [16]. There are no major safety concerns with gabapentin. Side effects are common, and older patients may experience dizziness, somnolence, and peripheral edema [12]. These sedative side effects of gabapentin might suggest using the drug before or during sleep.

Clonidine has been reported in multiple studies as showing effective results in treating RLS. One study reported that the use of clonidine (mean = 0.05 mg/day) is useful in patients who experience delayed sleep onset due to leg sensations [19]. The study showed that clonidine decreased rapid movement sleep pattern (REM) sleep and increased REM latency, but did not change total sleep duration, stage 1 and 2 sleep, sleep efficiency, awakenings, arousals, or periodic limb movements in sleep. Another double-blind study conducted in 20 patients with chronic renal failure showed complete relief of RLS symptoms in 8 out of 10 patients upon treatment with clonidine for 3 days. Whereas only 1 out of 10 patients has mild alleviation in RLS symptoms in the placebo group [20].

Dexmedetomidine is a full α2-adrenoceptor (α2-AR) agonist that is similar to the partial α2-adrenoceptor agonist, clonidine. It is used in several clinical settings in view of its diverse actions which include sedation, analgesia, anxiolysis, perioperative sympatholysis, cardiovascular stabilizing effects, reduced anesthetic requirements, and preservation of respiratory function [21]. Dexmedetomidine is 8 to 10 times more selective towards α2-AR than clonidine [22]. Binding to the different subtypes of α2-AR allows dexmedetomidine to exert its diverse effects. Dexmedetomidine may cause decreasing the heart rate and vasoconstriction of the peripheral vasculature [23]. Dexmedetomidine also exerts a biphasic effect on the blood pressure by binding to two different subtypes of adrenergic receptors (AR). Dexmedetomidine evokes a short hypertensive phase mediated by its binding to α-2B adrenergic receptors followed by a hypotensive phase by binding to α-2B adrenergic receptors. Dexmedetomidine binds to α2A-AR subtype of α2-AR causing transient hypertension and to α2B-AR subtype leads to hypotension [24]. Dexmedetomidine causes its sedative effects by acting on the α2A-AR in the Locus ceruleus in the brain stem [23].

In addition, the adrenergic effects of dexmedetomidine produces antinociceptive effects and reduces release of the spinal neurotransmitter glutamate at the postsynaptic membrane [25, 26]. Of note, dexmedetomidine was recently shown to be effective in treating RLS exacerbation. In a case study report, a 22-year woman with suspected RLS was scheduled for bilateral sagittal split ramus osteotomy under general anesthesia [22]. During the surgery, general anesthesia included dexmedetomidine (0.2 μg/kg/h), which was also administered at the same rate for postoperative sedation and analgesia. After the surgery, the patient began experiencing urges to move her legs described as "ants creeping on both ankles," which resembled her previous RLS-like symptoms. The symptoms gradually became more severe (10/10) and spread to the upper extremities despite massaging the ankles. Dexmedetomidine infusion was increased from 0.2 to 0.4 μg/kg/h for optimal bed rest and allowed her to sleep for 3 hours. Upon waking, the patient was able to walk and stretch and reported resolution of RLS symptoms, which suggested a role for dexmedetomidine in alleviating RLS exacerbations [22].

3.4. Proposed Mechanism of RLS after Dexmedetomidine Administration. The alpha 2 effect of dexmedetomidine in the dorsal horn would be expected to reduce the nociceptive sensory input related to RLS, which should reduce the motor response to the noxious sensations that normally trigger them.

In fact, we may have been observing not RLS but periodic limb movement disorder (PLMD), which is closely associated with RLS and produces spontaneous periodic leg movements during sleep. Even if the patient had RLS with PMLD, there is no immediately obvious explanation for symptom worsening with dexmedetomidine from a pharmacologic perspective as PLMD seems to be treated similarly to RLS, with dopaminergic agents, gabaergic agents, or gabapentinoids.

Our best explanation for how dexmedetomidine could worsen uncontrolled periodic movements centers on dopaminergic circuits; because these movements occurred regardless of sedation depth, it is unlikely that the movements were related to sensory phenomena as seen in RLS but were more analogous to the dyskinesias and athetosis in Parkinson's disease patients treated with dopaminergic agents. Interestingly, there is evidence that adrenergic agents can influence dyskinesias. Idazonax, an alpha-2 antagonist, has been shown to decrease dyskinesias in both PD humans and MPTP monkeys treated with L-dopa without worsening parkinsonian symptoms [27].

There are multiple typologies of movement disorders associated with L-dopa administration in PD patients [28]. Marconi et al. offered a proposal that, after a dose of L-dopa, the increasing secretion of dopamine in the striatum first begins to stimulate the dorsal putamen neurons before it is able to relieve parkinsonian symptoms, because this area usually has the greatest nigrostriatal hence may have the most hypersensitivity to dopamine (DA). This putamen area corresponds to cortico-striatal output to the lower extremity and also is rich in the D2 neurons that form the origin of the "indirect pathway" [29], resulting in the onset of dyskinesias and ballistic movements in the lower extremities. At least one study has demonstrated RLS patients have decreased 18F-dopamine uptake in the putamen with reduced D2 binding [30], and D2 receptor loss in the putamen was also demonstrated in RLS patients in an autopsy study [31].

In summary, while no literature exists that the authors are able to find, it may be that dexmedetomidine may worsen RLS. Mechanisms for this are unclear, but the authors present the following hypothesis that must be validated. Dexmedetomidine provides sedation without respiratory depression and analgesia. However, in order to produce these pharmacologic actions, it might deactivate the neural pathways that provide descending input to the peripheral nerves as well as centrally. This may in turn block the normal mechanism that RLS patients use to prevent leg movement consciously, although not completely prevent unintended leg movements. Blocking this descending neural pathway may explain why dexmedetomidine may worsen RLS in some patients, yet improve it in others, where the neural block for ascending pathways is sufficient to prevent leg movements.

4. Conclusion

We report a case of a 71-year-old patient with significant comorbidities and no history of RLS, who developed severe RLS symptoms after receiving sedation for a podiatric surgical procedure [32]. The symptoms were not improved by any therapy, and the surgical team was able to compensate for the movement, but the foot not undergoing surgery that did not have regional anesthesia was problematic in management. It may be that the dexmedetomidine exacerbated the symptoms of previously undiagnosed RLS or PLMD. Had this diagnosis been present preoperatively, given the intraoperative course, dexmedetomidine might have been avoided with possibly improved surgical conditions.

Consent

Consent is not applicable as no identifiable attributes are given for patient.

Disclosure

This work was presented in part by Sandra Iskandar at the 2022 Western Anesthesia Resident's Conference hosted by Harbor/UCLA Department of Anesthesiology with the same title and authors as current manuscript.

Authors' Contributions

All authors contributed to this submission, and all agree with contents.

References

[1] A. Mansur, P. R. Castillo, F. Rocha Cabrero, and S. R. A. Bokhari, "Restless legs syndrome," in *StatPearls*, StatPearls Publishing, Treasure Island (FL), 2021, https://www.ncbi.nlm.nih.gov/books/NBK430878/.

[2] S. T. O'keeffe, J. Noel, and J. N. Lavan, "Restless legs syndrome in the elderly," *Postgraduate Medical Journal*, vol. 69, no. 815, pp. 701–703, 1993.

[3] N. Ohshita, A. Yamagata, K. Kaneda et al., "Anesthetic management of a patient with restless legs syndrome: a case report," *Anesthesia Progress*, vol. 67, no. 4, pp. 226–229, 2020.

[4] M. Miyamoto, T. Miyamoto, M. Iwanami, K. Suzuki, and K. Hirata, "Pathophysiology of restless legs syndrome," *Brain Nerve*, vol. 61, no. 5, pp. 523–532, 2009.

[5] V. Dhawan, M. Ali, and K. R. Chaudhuri, "Genetic aspects of restless legs syndrome," *Postgraduate Medical Journal*, vol. 82, no. 972, pp. 626–629, 2006.

[6] J. Winkelmann, B. Schormair, P. Lichtner et al., "Genome-wide association study of restless legs syndrome identifies common variants in three genomic regions," *Nature Genetics*, vol. 39, no. 8, pp. 1000–1006, 2007.

[7] N. K. Banerji and L. J. Hurwitz, "Restless legs syndrome, with particular reference to its occurrence after gastric surgery," *British Medical Journal*, vol. 4, no. 5738, pp. 774-775, 1970.

[8] M. M. Ohayon and T. Roth, "Prevalence of restless legs syndrome and periodic limb movement disorder in the general population," *Journal of Psychosomatic Research*, vol. 53, no. 1, pp. 547–554, 2002.

[9] S. Y. Koh, M. S. Kim, S. M. Lee, J. M. Hong, and J. H. Yoon, "Impaired vascular endothelial function in patients with restless legs syndrome: a new aspect of the vascular pathophysiology," *Journal of Neurology*, vol. 359, no. 1-2, pp. 207–210, 2015.

[10] C. J. Earley, G. R. Uhl, S. Clemens, and S. Ferré, "Connectome and molecular pharmacological differences in the dopaminergic system in restless legs syndrome (RLS): plastic changes and neuroadaptations that may contribute to augmentation," *Sleep Medicine*, vol. 31, pp. 71–77, 2017.

[11] K. Berger, J. Luedemann, C. Trenkwalder, U. John, and C. Kessler, "Sex and the risk of restless legs syndrome in the general population," *Archives of Internal Medicine*, vol. 164, no. 2, pp. 196–202, 2004.

[12] J. Winkelmann, R. P. Allen, B. Högl et al., "Treatment of restless legs syndrome: evidence-based review and implications for clinical practice (revised 2017)," *Movement Disorders*, vol. 33, no. 7, pp. 1077–1091, 2018.

[13] C. Brodeur, J. Montplaisir, R. Godbout, and R. Marinier, "Treatment of restless legs syndrome and periodic movements during sleep with L-dopa: a double-blind, controlled study," *Neurology*, vol. 38, no. 12, pp. 1845–1848, 1988.

[14] A. S. Walters, W. A. Hening, N. Kavey, S. Chokroverty, and S. Gidro-Frank, "A double-blind randomized crossover trial of bromocriptine and placebo in restless legs syndrome," *Annals of Neurology*, vol. 24, no. 3, pp. 455–458, 1988.

[15] L. Jama, K. Hirvonen, M. Partinen et al., "A dose-ranging study of pramipexole for the symptomatic treatment of restless legs syndrome: polysomnographic evaluation of periodic leg movements and sleep disturbance," *Sleep Medicine*, vol. 10, no. 6, pp. 630–636, 2009.

[16] Y. Inoue, K. Hirata, N. Uchimura, K. Kuroda, N. Hattori, and M. Takeuchi, "Gabapentin enacarbil in Japanese patient with restless legs syndrome: a 12-week, randomized, double-blind, placebo controlled, parallel-group study," *Current Medical Research and Opinion*, vol. 29, no. 1, pp. 12–21, 2014.

[17] R. Peled and P. Lavie, "Double-blind evaluation of clonazepam on periodic leg movements in sleep," *Journal of Neurology, Neurosurgery, and Psychiatry*, vol. 50, no. 12, pp. 1679–1681, 1987.

[18] C. Guilleminault and W. Flagg, "Effect of baclofen on sleep-related periodic leg movements," *Annals of Neurology*, vol. 15, no. 3, pp. 234–239, 1984.

[19] M. L. Wagner, A. S. Walters, R. G. Coleman, W. A. Hening, K. Grasing, and S. Chokroverty, "Randomized, double-blind, placebo-controlled study of clonidine in restless legs syndrome," *Sleep*, vol. 19, no. 1, pp. 52–58, 1996.

[20] M. Ausserwinkler and P. Schmidt, "Successful clonidine treatment of restless leg syndrome in chronic kidney insufficiency," *Schweiz Med Wochenschr*, vol. 119, no. 6, pp. 184–186, 1989.

[21] K. M. Kemp, L. Henderlight, and M. Neville, "Precedex: is it the future of cooperative sedation?," *Nursing*, vol. 38, Suppl Critical, pp. 7-8, 2008.

[22] D. S. Wagner and C. M. Brummett, "Dexmedetomidine: as safe as safe can be," *Seminars in Anesthesia, Perioperative Medicine and Pain*, vol. 25, no. 2, pp. 77–83, 2006.

[23] M. Kaur and P. M. Singh, "Current role of dexmedetomidine in clinical anesthesia and intensive care," *Anesthesia: Essays and Researches*, vol. 5, no. 2, pp. 128–133, 2011.

[24] M. Philipp, M. Brede, and J. Hein Lam, "Physiological significance of alpha (2)-adrenergic receptor subtype diversity: one receptor is not enough," *American Journal of Physiology-Regulatory, Integrative and Comparative Physiology*, vol. 283, no. 2, pp. R287–R295, 2002.

[25] X. Li and J. C. Eisenach, "alpha2A-adrenoceptor stimulation reduces capsaicin-induced glutamate release from spinal cord synaptosomes," *The Journal of Pharmacology and Experimental Therapeutics*, vol. 299, no. 3, pp. 939–944, 2001.

[26] A. Bekker and M. K. Sturaitis, "Dexmedetomidine for neurological surgery," *Neurosurgery*, vol. 57, 1 Supplement, pp. 1–10, 2005, discussion 1-10.

[27] O. Rascol, I. Arnulf, H. P.-S. Paul et al., *Idazoxan, an Alpha-2 Antagonist, and L-Dopa-Induced Dyskinesias in Patients with parkinson's Disease*, International Parkinson and Movement Disorder Society, 2001.

[28] R. Marconi, D. Lefebvre-Caparros, A.-M. Bonnet, M. Vidailhet, B. Dubois, and Y. Agid, *Levodopa-Induced Dyskinesias in parkinson's Disease Phenomenology and Pathophysiology*, International Parkinson and Movement Disorder Society, 2004.

[29] P. Calabresi, B. Picconi, A. Tozzi, V. Ghiglieri, and M. di Filippo, "Direct and indirect pathways of basal ganglia: a critical reappraisal," *Nature Neuroscience*, vol. 17, no. 8, pp. 1022–1030, 2014.

[30] N. Turjanski, A. J. Lees, and D. J. Brooks, "In vivo studies on striatal dopamine D_1 and D_2 site binding in L-dopa-treated Parkinson's disease patients with and without dyskinesias," *Neurology*, vol. 49, no. 3, pp. 717–723, 1997.

[31] C. James, X. Wang, R. Allen et al., "Altered dopaminergic profile in the putamen and substantia nigra in restless leg syndrome," *Brain*, vol. 132, Part 9, pp. 2403–2412, 2009.

[32] S. Iskandar, M. S. Martins, A. Hudson, J. Hirsch, and J. S. Jahr, "Does dexmedetomidine improve or worsen restless leg syndrome under sedation: a case report and extensive review," in *Abstract presented at the 2022 Western Anesthesia Resident's Conference*, Harbor/UCLA Department of Anesthesiology, 2022https://secured.societyhq.com/warc/2022/abstracts/instructions.iphtml.

38

Dantrolene Administration in the Management of the Prehospital Patient with Methylenedioxymethamphetamine Overdose

Kia Nikoomanesh,[1,2] **Alexander T. Phan**,[2,3] **Julian Choi**,[1,2] **Sarkis Arabian**,[1,2] **and Michael M. Neeki**[2,4]

[1]*Department of Critical Care Medicine, Arrowhead Regional Medical Center, Colton, CA 92324, USA*
[2]*California University of Science and Medicine, Colton, CA 92324, USA*
[3]*Department of Internal Medicine, Arrowhead Regional Medical Center, Colton, CA 92324, USA*
[4]*Department of Emergency Medicine, Arrowhead Regional Medical Center, Colton, CA 92324, USA*

Correspondence should be addressed to Alexander T. Phan; phana1@armc.sbcounty.gov

Academic Editor: Seda B. Akinci

Methylenedioxymethamphetamine (MDMA) is a psychoactive substance that is used commonly as a recreational drug at rave music festivals. MDMA intoxication can cause a myriad of symptoms and side effects including the manifestation of hyperpyrexia in patients. Hyperpyrexia can mimic a heat stroke and ultimately lead to various forms of end-organ damage. The most common methods used in treating MDMA-induced hyperpyrexia focus on the rapid reduction of core body temperature. Various off-label medications have also been used in combating MDMA-induced hyperpyrexia. Dantrolene is one such medication, although its role in the treatment of MDMA intoxication remains uncertain. This case series preliminarily examines the efficacy of dantrolene in mitigating MDMA-induced hyperpyrexia and potentially reducing the risk of end-organ damage in patients suffering from MDMA overdose. This study focuses on nine patients who presented after ingesting various forms of MDMA at "rave" music events. All patients were found to be hyperthermic in the field with a maximum core body temperature of 109 degrees Fahrenheit. All patients were immediately managed by cooling measures, and seven patients additionally received dantrolene in the field before being transferred to Arrowhead Regional Medical Center. Upon arrival to the hospital, nearly every patient was found to have significantly decreased body temperatures when compared to previously measured body temperatures out in the field. However, nearly all patients in the study were also noted to have laboratory abnormalities consistent with various forms of end-organ damage. The degree and severity of end-organ damage observed in MDMA-induced hyperpyrexia seem to be a function of initial core body temperature. Higher core body temperature tends to correlate with more forms of end-organ damage and a higher severity of end-organ damage. Intervention with dantrolene and cooling measures appeared to have no effect on reducing the risk of developing end-organ damage in this patient population.

1. Introduction

Methylenedioxymethamphetamine (MDMA), also known as "ecstasy" or "molly," is a psychoactive substance commonly abused at electronic dance music festivals, "raves," dance clubs, and other social venues. MDMA is an amphetamine derivative that also has some pharmacological properties of mescaline. The amphetamine properties of MDMA amplify the user's sympathetic nervous system, while its mescaline properties provide both hallucinogenic and psychogenic effects. MDMA ingestion can lead to several side effects ranging from minor clinical symptoms to potentially fatal complications. These complications are grouped into four categories of toxicity: hepatic, cardiovascular, cerebral, and hyperpyrexic [1]. The hyperpyrexic pattern of toxicity has been hypothesized to be the most dangerous. It is believed to be the product of increased adrenergic, serotonergic, and dopaminergic responses in the body. The adrenergic response leads to peripheral vasoconstriction which in turn decreases heat dissipation. Meanwhile, increased serotonergic and dopaminergic effects disrupt the body's central hypothalamic thermoregulation and induce serotonin syndrome, which can thereby increase thermogenesis [2, 3]. These mechanisms induce hyperthermia, which is often exacerbated by overcrowded club and party settings where MDMA is taken [4, 5]. Patients thereby suffer from hyperpyrexia which can mimic a heat stroke, leading to rhabdomyolysis, disseminated intravascular coagulation (DIC), liver damage, and acute renal failure [2, 6].

Current standard methods of treating MDMA-induced hyperpyrexia include the use of supportive measures and active cooling techniques, such as chilled intravenous fluids, ice baths, and cooling blankets. In addition, multiple off-label medications have been trialed in the context of treating MDMA-induced hyperpyrexia. Dantrolene is one such medication. Over the years, many case reports and studies have investigated the efficacy of dantrolene in reducing mortality in patients with MDMA-induced hyperpyrexia. One systematic review of 71 cases of MDMA-induced hyperpyrexia cited a reduction in mortality from 44% to 19% when patients were given dantrolene [7]. Although this systematic review alluded to the possibility that dantrolene could also reduce the risk of severe sequelae, there have not been many other studies showing causality between the medication and reduced risks of end-organ damage in the context of MDMA overdose.

The following case series serves to further examine the role of dantrolene in the management of MDMA toxicity. Specifically, this case series focuses on the role of dantrolene in reducing the risk of end-organ damage as related to MDMA ingestion. To investigate this, we highlight the cases of 9 patients who presented to Arrowhead Regional Medical Center (ARMC) with hyperpyrexia after ingestion of MDMA at a local "rave" festival.

2. Methods

2.1. Study Population, Setting, and Data. We included patients who were admitted to Arrowhead Regional Medical Center (ARMC) between January 1, 2016, and December 31, 2018. Nine patients between the ages of 19 and 28 years of age were identified from our institution. Confirmatory testing for MDMA intoxication use was performed via urinalysis. Prisoners and individuals under the age of 18 were excluded from the study. This study was approved by the Institutional Review Board at ARMC, and researchers analyzed only deidentified data.

2.2. Study Definitions. Coexisting conditions were ascertained from physician documentation. Measures of end-organ damage in this study were defined by elevated creatinine (creatinine of greater than or equal to 1.5 milligrams/deciliter (mg/dL)), elevated transaminases (AST or ALT values greater than three times 40 units/liter (U/L)), elevated troponin I (troponin I > 0.3 U/L), evidence of seizures, and elevated creatine phosphokinase (CPK) levels (CPK > 1500 U/L).

3. Results

3.1. Patient Characteristics. During the period from January 1, 2016, to December 31, 2018, we identified nine patients who presented to ARMC following ingestion of MDMA in various forms including "Blue Pikachu," "Red Winnie the Pooh," and "Red Supreme." The mean age was 24 (range, 19 to 28). All patients exhibited evidence of hyperpyrexia in the field following MDMA overdose. Appropriate medical evaluation and various forms of cooling measures were subsequently initiated at the event site for every patient. Seven patients received intravenous (IV) infusion of dantrolene, doses unknown, in the field in addition to external cooling measures, which included the use of ice packs and cooling blankets. All patients were orotracheally intubated due to a low Glasgow Coma Scale (GCS) score of less than 8. After initial stabilization in the field, patients were transported to ARMC's emergency department (ED). Upon arrival to the ED, patients were reevaluated and the resuscitation continued per existing protocols. Relevant labs were drawn, and patients underwent imaging studies such as chest X-ray and computerized tomography (CT) scans. All nine patients did not have any existing past medical history and were all young, healthy adults. All patients were then admitted to AMRC's medical intensive care unit for further management. Eventually, all nine patients were successfully extubated, survived, and were either discharged from the hospital or left against medical advice several days after admission. We were unable to follow these patients past their admissions in the hospital. We therefore could not monitor any trend in their lab values to determine if end-organ damage was acute or if it eventually became chronic.

3.2. Laboratory and Radiologic Findings. All pertinent vitals and lab values from our patients have been included in Table 1. Radiologic findings did not show evidence of acute abnormalities. All of the patients in our case series exhibited evidence of hyperpyrexia and 8 out of 9 experienced some degree of end-organ damage on arrival to the hospital. Recorded body temperatures in the field prior to cooling measures and/or dantrolene administration ranged between 102.6 F (degrees Fahrenheit) and 109.0 F. The most common forms of end-organ damage experienced by patients included acute kidney injury (66.67%), rhabdomyolysis (66.67%), and elevated troponin I (55.56%). Additionally, two patients experienced seizures, and three patients suffered from transaminitis. Six out of seven patients in the dantrolene plus cooling measure group experienced a decrease in their temperature to less than 100.0 F by the time they arrived to the hospital's ED. One of the two patients who did not receive dantrolene also had a decrease in body temperature to less than 100 F by the time they arrived to the ED. All seven of the patients who received dantrolene experienced at least one type of end-organ damage.

Furthermore, subgroup analysis (Table 2) was performed based on initial core body temperature prior to intervention. In the subgroup of five patients with an initial core body temperature of at least 108.0 F, all patients suffered from at least two forms of end-organ damage (mean

TABLE 1: All patient data for dantrolene administration, body temperatures, serum creatinine, serum sodium, serum AST, serum ALT, serum troponin, serum CPK, evidence of seizures, evidence of end-organ damage, number of organs affected, and mortality.

Patient	Dantrolene (yes/no)	Temp (F) in field	Temp (F) ED arrival	Cr (mg/dL)	Sodium (mEq/L)	AST (U/L)	ALT (U/L)	Troponin (U/L)	CPK (U/L)	Seizure (yes/no)	End-organ damage (yes/no)	Number of organs affected	Mortality
Patient 1	Yes	106	99.5	1.7	138	44	48	<0.3	664	No	Yes	1	None
Patient 2	No	108	102.9	2.7	144	79	19	0.63	65730	No	Yes	3	None
Patient 3	Yes	106	95.7	2.4	137	195	293	2.27	1311	Yes	Yes	4	None
Patient 4	Yes	108	104	2.2	130	413	512	0.95	41262	No	Yes	4	None
Patient 5	Yes	109	88.1	1.6	138	29	20	2.56	60669	Yes	Yes	4	None
Patient 6	No	102.6	97	1.1	138	78	52	<0.3	473	No	No	0	None
Patient 7	Yes	108.3	89.9	1.5	137	40	49	0.45	2553	No	Yes	3	None
Patient 8	Yes	107.5	93.3	1.1	137	64	40	<0.3	6408	No	Yes	1	None
Patient 9	Yes	108.3	96.1	1	133	306	296	<0.3	11332	No	Yes	2	None

Legend: F: Fahrenheit; mEq/L: milliequivalents per liter; mg/dL" milligrams per deciliter; U/L: units per liter; Cr: creatinine; AST: aspartate transaminase; ALT: alanine transaminase; CPK: creatine phosphokinase.

Table 2: Comparison of variables between the initial core body temperature groups (<108 F vs. ≥108 F).

	Initial core body temperatures < 108 F ($n = 4$)	Initial core body temperatures ≥ 108 F ($n = 5$)
Creatinine (mg/dL)	1.4 (1.1, 2.05)	1.6 (1.5, 2.2)
Sodium (mEq/L)	137.5 (137, 138)	137 (133, 138)
AST (U/L)	71 (54, 136.5)	79 (40, 306)
ALT (U/L)	50 (44, 172.5)	49 (20, 296)
Troponin levels (U/L)	2.27 (0, 1.135)	0.63 (0.45, 0.95)
CPK (U/L)	987.5 (568.5, 3859.5)	41262 (11332, 60669)
Mean number of organs affected	1.5 (0.5, 2.5)	3.2 (2.5, 4)
Number of patients with end-organ damage	3	5
Mortality	0	0

Legend: F: Fahrenheit; mEq/L: milliequivalents per liter; mg/dL: milligrams per deciliter; U/L: units per liter; Cr: creatinine; AST: aspartate transaminase; ALT: alanine transaminase; CPK: creatine phosphokinase.

number of organs damaged was 3.25). We compared this to a subgroup of patients who had initial core body temperatures of less than 108.0 F and found that only one of these four patients suffered from more than one form of end-organ damage (mean number of organs damaged was 1.5). *P* values for all data in Table 2 were >0.1. Additionally, the highest creatinine, CPK, troponin, and transaminase levels all decreased to normal limits over the hospital course in the subgroup of patients with initial core body temperatures of at least 108.0 F.

4. Discussion

Unlike many other toxicological emergencies, MDMA overdose lacks a concrete algorithm for management. Treatment of hyperpyrexia related to MDMA ingestion starts with supportive measures including chilled IV fluids, ice baths, and cooling blankets. Cooling measures are the gold standard for reduction of core body temperature, as prolonged hyperpyrexia is associated with end-organ damage. In the case of MDMA toxicity, standard cooling measures may not adequately reduce core body temperature at an appropriate rate, which warrants the investigation of pharmacological intervention. However, the role of pharmacologic agents in this setting has yet to be formally established. Physicians have trialed various medications in attempts to reduce morbidity and mortality as related to MDMA overdose. Case reports have documented the use of cyproheptadine [8], chlorpromazine, and more extensively, dantrolene [9–12] to help mitigate MDMA-induced hyperpyrexia. These medications have all shown varying degrees of success in reducing mortality and sequelae related to MDMA overdose. However, given the lack of clinical trials and observational studies, no single medication has been favored over the rest.

To further explore the role of pharmacological intervention in the setting of MDMA overdose, our case series focused on the use of the medication dantrolene in the prehospital resuscitation arena. Founded in the 1960s, dantrolene is a skeletal muscle relaxant which works by blocking calcium release from the sarcoplasmic reticulum of a myocyte [13]. This leads to a decrease in intracellular calcium concentrations that ultimately results in excitation-contraction decoupling and reduced muscle tone. A reduction in muscle tone translates into a lack of heat production, which can then lead to a decrease in core body temperature in a variety of clinical contexts. Common adverse effects of dantrolene include drowsiness, dizziness, weakness, fatigue, and diarrhea. While the mechanism of action makes theoretical sense, the clinical application of dantrolene has been slightly more controversial. In a review by Hadad et al., animal and human subjects with elevated body temperatures or clinically defined heat stroke were given dantrolene; the results demonstrated a mixed picture with either an increase or no change in cooling rate [14]. The largest human study from the review ($n = 52$) showed dantrolene did not increase the rate of cooling when added to evaporative cooling techniques in heat stroke patients [15]. Therefore, the role of dantrolene in clinical practice has historically been called into question.

Our investigation centered on the previous hypothesis that early administration of dantrolene would rapidly reduce core body temperature and thereby reduce the risk of severe sequelae in MDMA overdose [7]. We identified seven cases of MDMA-related hyperpyrexia that were treated with both dantrolene and cooling measures in the field and two cases that were only treated with cooling measures. Since hyperpyrexia is associated with end-organ damage, the most optimal time to administer dantrolene would be upon presentation to medical care. Our patients all received variable doses of intravenous dantrolene by emergency medical services and were immediately transferred to our hospital for higher level of care. While almost all patients in the dantrolene plus cooling measure group experienced a rapid drop in their temperatures, it is difficult to attribute this temperature correction specifically to the use of dantrolene alone due to the small sample size of patients who did not receive dantrolene and the observation that patient 6 had a reduction in body temperature to less than 100.0 F without dantrolene administration. Furthermore, despite the early administration of dantrolene in the field, all patients who received the medication suffered from some form of end-organ damage. Although these patients went on to survive, it appears that dantrolene had no overall effect on the rate of end-organ damage. Dantrolene may have contributed to the rapid correction of body temperature in patients who received the medication, but this did not appear to correlate with any reduction in the overall degree of end-organ damage.

Of the group of patients transported to ARMC, the one patient who did not experience end-organ damage (patient 6 in table 1) did not receive dantrolene in the field. This was also the patient with the lowest initial core body temperature (102.6 F). It is therefore possible that initial core body temperature is a better predictor of end-organ damage than the degree of temperature reduction precipitated by medications like dantrolene. This theory is supported by one systematic review on MDMA overdose which delineated patients into categories based on their initial core temperature [7]. In this systematic review, it was noted that patients with initial core temperatures of 40.0 to 41.9 C (104.0 F to 107.4 F) had a higher number of both severe and mild-to-moderate complications in comparison to the group of patients with initial temperatures of 38.0 to 39.9 C (100.4 F to 103.8 F), irrespective of dantrolene administration. Our subgroup analysis supplements these findings by reflecting more forms of end-organ damage in patients with core body temperatures of ≥108.0 F (mean number of organs damaged = 3.2) when compared to patients with core body temperatures of <108.0 F (mean number of organs damaged = 1.5), again, irrespective of dantrolene administration.

The highest degree of end-organ damage was observed in the group of five patients who presented with temperatures of at least 108 F, irrespective of dantrolene administration. In the subgroup of patients with body temperatures of at least 108 F, the one patient who did not receive dantrolene experienced damage to 3 organs, while the three patients who received dantrolene experienced damage to a mean of 3.25 organs. From this limited data, it appears that dantrolene did not have a significant role in the reduction of end-organ damage. Rather, our observations, although statistically insignificant, support the theory that sequelae from MDMA overdose are more likely a function of the degree of initial hyperpyrexia.

The primary limitation to our study is that our sample size was small, and this is due to the dearth of patient cases of MDMA-induced hyperpyrexia noted at our institution, as it is a relatively rare disease process. Although we cannot draw definitive conclusions based on a sample size of nine patients, our results support the findings of Grunau et al. and provide preliminary evidence that may aid in future studies that assess the efficacy of dantrolene administration on end-organ damage in the setting of MDMA overdose. In the future, a multi-institutional study may produce a larger sample size to better quantify and statistically analyze the efficacy of this pharmacologic agent. A second limitation includes a lack of data regarding the dosing of dantrolene provided to our patients in the field. Future studies may attempt to correlate morbidity and mortality with the dosing and route of dantrolene administration provided to patients suffering from MDMA overdose.

5. Conclusions

The purpose of this case series was to provide more preliminary data regarding the use of dantrolene in the setting of MDMA overdose and MDMA-induced hyperpyrexia. Many case reports and a number of systematic reviews have previously linked possible improved mortality with the administration of dantrolene in this setting. However, few case reports and systematic reviews have specifically touched upon the subject of morbidity. Our case series showed no significant improvement or prevention of end-organ damage when dantrolene is provided to patients with MDMA-induced hyperpyrexia. We believe that the degree of end-organ damage suffered by patients with MDMA intoxication is more likely a function of initial core body temperature, irrespective of dantrolene administration. Future studies would benefit from having a larger sample size and including a larger number of patients who did not receive dantrolene prior to admission into the hospital, as this would be ideal for comparative purposes. Additionally, further analyses of a larger sample size can be performed to determine the optimal dosing of dantrolene in the setting of MDMA toxicity.

Consent

Consent was obtained or waived by all participants in this study. This is a case series based on retrospective chart review, and the informed consent was waived by the Arrowhead Regional Medical Center Institutional Review Board.

Acknowledgments

The authors would like to thank and express their gratitude to Arrowhead Regional Medical Center's exceptional medical staff for their clinical support.

References

[1] H. Kalant, “The pharmacology and toxicology of "ecstasy" (MDMA) and related drugs,” *CMAJ*, vol. 165, no. 7, pp. 917–928, 2001.

[2] A. P. Hall and J. A. Henry, “Acute toxic effects of “Ecstasy” (MDMA) and related compounds: overview of pathophysiology and clinical management,” *British Journal of Anaesthesia*, vol. 96, no. 6, pp. 678–685, 2006.

[3] M. E. Liechti, “Effects of MDMA on body temperature in humans,” *Temperature*, vol. 1, no. 3, pp. 192–200, 2014.

[4] R. I. Dafters, “Hyperthermia following MDMA administration in rats: effects of ambient temperature, water consumption, and chronic dosing,” *Physiology and Behavior*, vol. 58, no. 5, pp. 877–882, 1995.

[5] E. A. Kiyatkin, A. H. Kim, K. T. Wakabayashi, M. H. Baumann, and Y. Shaham, “Critical role of peripheral vasoconstriction in fatal brain hyperthermia induced by MDMA (Ecstasy) under conditions that mimic human drug use,” *Journal of Neuroscience.*, vol. 34, no. 23, pp. 7754–7762, 2014.

[6] P. Halpern, J. Moskovich, B. Avrahami, Y. Bentur, D. Soffer, and K. Peleg, "Morbidity associated with MDMA (ecstasy) abuse: a survey of emergency department admissions," *Human and Experimental Toxicology*, vol. 30, no. 4, pp. 259–266, 2011.

[7] B. E. Grunau, M. O. Wiens, and J. R. Brubacher, "Dantrolene in the treatment of MDMA-related hyperpyrexia: a systematic review," *CJEM*, vol. 12, no. 5, pp. 435–442, 2010.

[8] F. Chu, A. K. M. Yim, and S. W. Ng, "A case series of life-threatening MDMA poisoning in an electronic dance music party in Hong Kong," *Asia Pacific Journal of Medical Toxicology*, vol. 7, no. 3, pp. 79–83, 2018.

[9] C. Singarajah and N. G. Lavies, "An overdose of ecstasy. A role for dantrolene," *Anaesthesia*, vol. 47, no. 8, pp. 686-687, 1992.

[10] K. J. Dar and M. E. McBrien, "MDMA induced hyperthermia: report of a fatality and review of current therapy," *Intensive Care Medicine*, vol. 22, no. 9, pp. 995-996, 1996.

[11] A. S. Logan, B. Stickle, N. O'Keefe, and H. Hewitson, "Survival following 'Ecstasy' ingestion with a peak temperature of 42°C," *Anaesthesia*, vol. 48, no. 11, pp. 1017-1018, 1993.

[12] J. Moon and J. Cros, "Role of dantrolene in the management of the acute toxic effects of Ecstasy (MDMA)," *British Journal of Anaesthesia*, vol. 99, no. 1, p. 146, 2007.

[13] T. Krause, M. U. Gerbershagen, M. Fiege, R. Weisshorn, and F. Wappler, "Dantrolene - a review of its pharmacology, therapeutic use and new developments," *Anaesthesia*, vol. 59, no. 4, pp. 364–373, 2004.

[14] E. Hadad, Y. Cohen-Sivan, Y. Heled, and Y. Epstein, "Clinical review: treatment of heat stroke: should dantrolene be considered?," *Critical Care*, vol. 9, no. 1, pp. 86–91, 2005.

[15] A. Bouchama, A. Cafege, E. B. Devol, O. Labdi, K. El-Assil, and M. Seraj, "Ineffectiveness of dantrolene sodium in the treatment of heatstroke," *Critical Care Medicine*, vol. 19, no. 2, pp. 176–180, 1991.

Postoperative 'STEMI' in Intracerebral Hemorrhage due to Arteriovenous Malformation: A Case Report and Review of Literature

Ravinder Datt Bhanot,[1,2] Jasleen Kaur,[1] Shitiz Sriwastawa,[3] Kendall Bell,[1] and Kushak Suchdev[3]

[1]*Department of Internal Medicine, Wayne State University, Detroit, MI, USA*
[2]*Division of Pulmonary and Critical Care, St Mary's Of Michigan Medical Center Saginaw, MI, USA*
[3]*Department of Neurology, Wayne State University, Detroit, MI, USA*

Correspondence should be addressed to Ravinder Datt Bhanot; ravinder.bhanot@ascension.org

Academic Editor: Kurt Lenz

Electrocardiogram (ECG) changes suggestive of cardiac ischemia are frequently demonstrated in patients with ischemic stroke and subarachnoid hemorrhage. However, little is known of such changes particularly acute ST segment myocardial infarction (STEMI) in patients with intracerebral hemorrhage (ICH), especially after neurosurgery. We present a patient with intraparenchymal hemorrhage due to cerebral arteriovenous malformation (AVM) who exhibited acute STEMI after neurosurgery. Serial cardiac biomarkers and echocardiograms were performed which did not reveal any evidence of acute myocardial infarction. The patient was managed conservatively from cardiac stand point with no employment of anticoagulants, antiplatelet therapy, fibrinolytic agents, or angioplasty and recovered well with minimal neurological deficit. This case highlights that diffuse cardiac ischemic signs on the ECG can occur in the setting of an ICH after neurosurgery, potentially posing a difficult diagnostic and management conundrum.

1. Background

A number of patients with stroke and aneurysmal subarachnoid hemorrhage (aSAH) have changes on electrocardiogram (ECG) [1]. They can be in the form of T wave inversions, QT interval prolongation, and others. Most of the patients who demonstrate ECG changes also have concomitant heart disease and hypertension which makes it difficult to attribute the ECG changes to the cerebral event alone. Rarely, intracranial hemorrhage (ICH) can also be associated with ECG changes similar to patients with stroke [2]. We present a patient with intraparenchymal hemorrhage due to cerebral arteriovenous malformation (AVM) who exhibited acute ST segment elevation suggestive of myocardial infarction in ECG after neurosurgery. Serial cardiac biomarkers and echocardiograms were performed which did not reveal any evidence of acute coronary event and the ECG changes resolved spontaneously. Acute cerebrovascular events can be associated with fleeting ECG changes or lead to fatal arrhythmias. The mechanism for these changes is poorly understood. Our case represents an uncommon clinical scenario with ICH patients and the challenges in treatment. This case is discussed here for its rarity with a brief review of the literature.

2. Case Report

A 42-year-old male, nonsmoker, with medical condition significant for hypertension presented to the emergency department after a fall followed by two episodes of seizures. On presentation physical examination was notable for altered level of consciousness and mild symmetrical decrease in power of 4/5 in all four limbs. Laboratory workup including complete blood count, electrolytes, coagulation panel, lipid profile, urine, and serum drug screen was unremarkable. CT scan head revealed a 1.5 cm left temporoparietal lobe intraparenchymal hemorrhage with surrounding edema as shown in (Figure 1(a)). As part of the diagnostic workup, an ECG was also performed on admission which was normal. The patient was admitted to the neurointensive

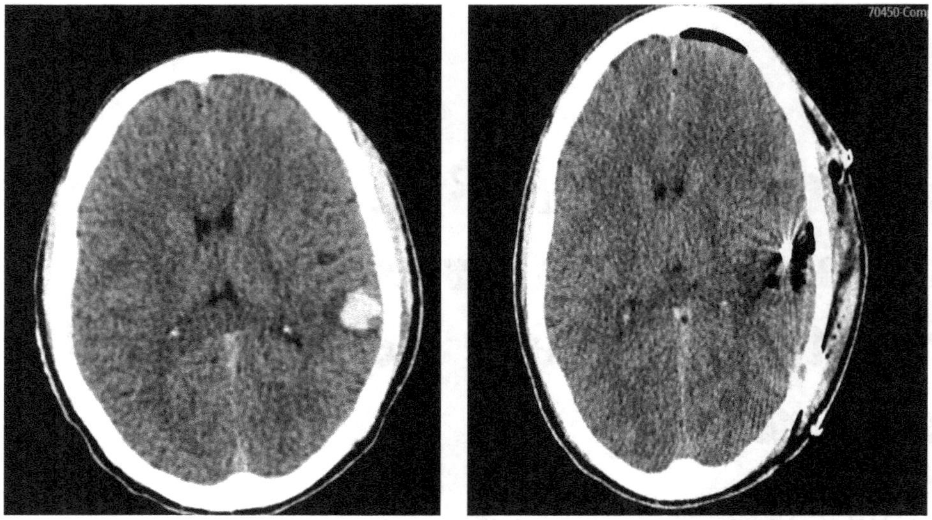

(a) CT scan head showing a 1.5 cm left temporoparietal lobe intraparenchymal hemorrhage with surrounding edema

(b) CT scan head after craniotomy and surgical resection of the AVM

FIGURE 1

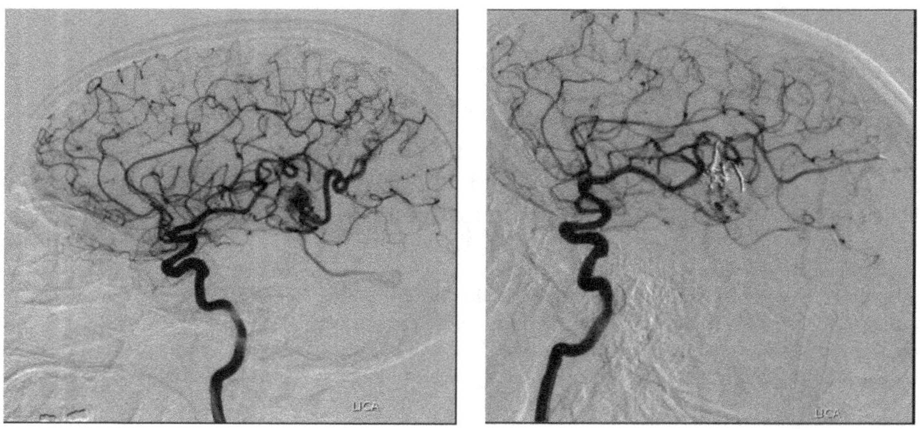

(a) Cerebral angiogram showing an arteriovenous malformation with blood supply arising from 2 branches of MCA (Middle Cerebral Artery)

(b) Cerebral angiogram showing partial embolization of the arteriovenous malformation

FIGURE 2

care unit (NICU) for further management. A computerized tomography angiogram was performed, which showed early draining veins at the site of the lesion, suspicious for an underlying vascular malformation. Subsequently a cerebral angiogram was performed which confirmed the presence of an AVM underlying the hemorrhage (Figure 2(a)). A partial embolization of the AVM was performed, and the patient was boarded for surgical resection (Figure 2(b)).

On day 3 of admission, the patient complained of sudden-onset chest pain. He described it as left sided, retrosternal, sharp, nonradiating pain, worsened when lying down on left side, lasted 2-3 minutes and then resolved spontaneously. It did not recur however prompted an ECG which showed sinus rhythm with nonspecific ST segment elevation in leads V3-V6 (Figure 3). Cardiology was consulted who deemed the ECG changes as J point elevation suggestive of benign early repolarization and not a true acute coronary event. A high sensitivity cardiac troponin assay done immediately and repeated two times at 6 hours and 12 hours from the onset of symptoms remained negative (<0.017 ng/ml; normal value <0.057 ng/ml). A transthoracic echocardiogram (TTE) performed later that day revealed no regional wall motion abnormalities or left ventricular dysfunction. The next day, patient was taken for craniotomy and surgical resection of the AVM (Figure 1(b)). The surgery was uneventful. A follow-up ECG on the postoperative day 1 revealed pronounced ST elevation with new T wave inversions (in leads V2-V6) highly suggestive of acute STEMI (Figure 4). The patient

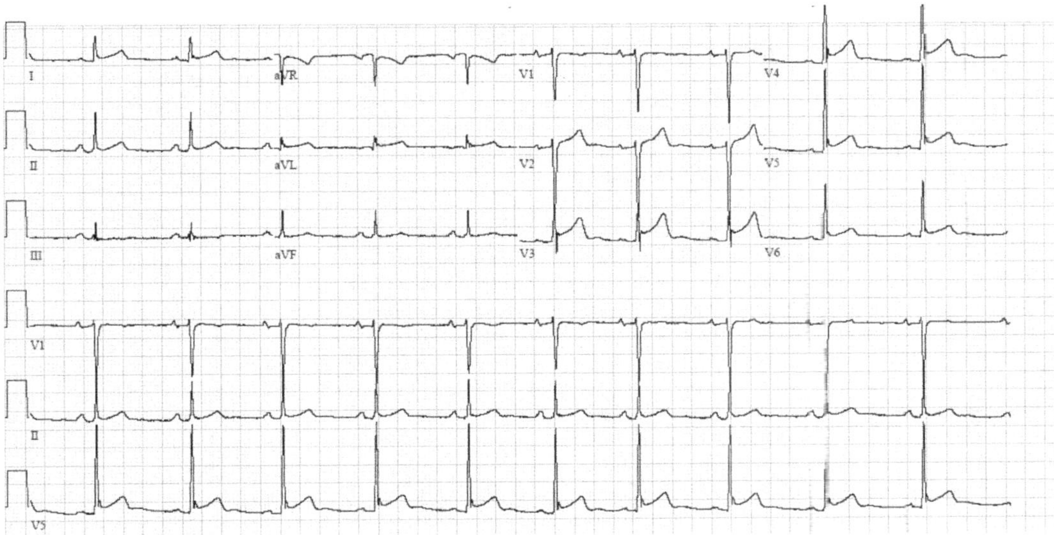

FIGURE 3: ECG prior to the surgery showing ST segment elevation in leads V3-V6.

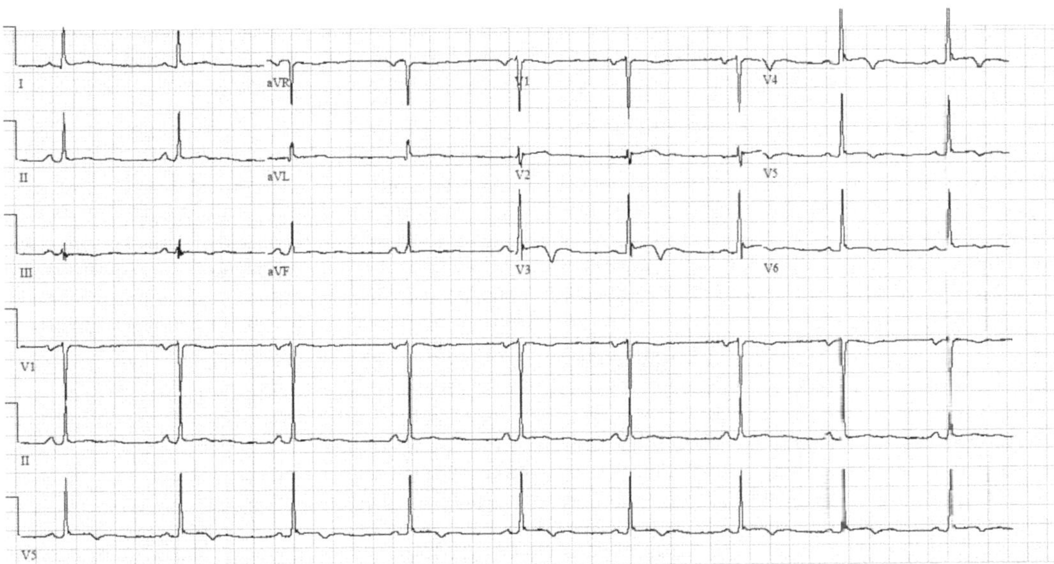

FIGURE 4: ECG postoperative day 1 showing ST elevation with new T wave inversions in leads V2-V6.

was completely asymptomatic with no chest pain or other cardiac symptoms. Serial estimation of high sensitivity cardiac troponin was again negative (<0.017 ng/ml) and a repeat TTE was unremarkable. Given these findings and the absence of the symptoms, no intervention was done and he was monitored in the NICU.

The patient did not have any further untoward event(s) and continued to do well postoperatively with normalization of his ECG changes over the next 48 hours (Figure 5). He improved neurologically and was transferred out of the ICU on day 7. He was subsequently discharged on day 12 with home health physical therapy, neurosurgery, and cardiology follow-up appointments. An exercise stress test was eventually performed 3 months' after discharge which did not reveal any evidence of coronary artery disease.

3. Discussion

The electrocardiogram (ECG) is one of the most frequently performed investigations in clinical practice for chest pain. While it is true that an acute myocardial infarction resulting from an occlusive thrombus is recognized on an ECG by ST segment elevation, there are several other conditions and diseases that can simulate or mimic these changes. It can present as a normal finding in some young healthy young men or in a certain pattern commonly referred to as early repolarization. Left bundle branch block, left ventricular hypertrophy, acute pericarditis and myocarditis, stress cardiomyopathy (Takotsubo cardiomyopathy), and certain electrolyte disturbances like hyperkalemia are some of the other nonischemic etiologies of ST elevation. Coronary artery

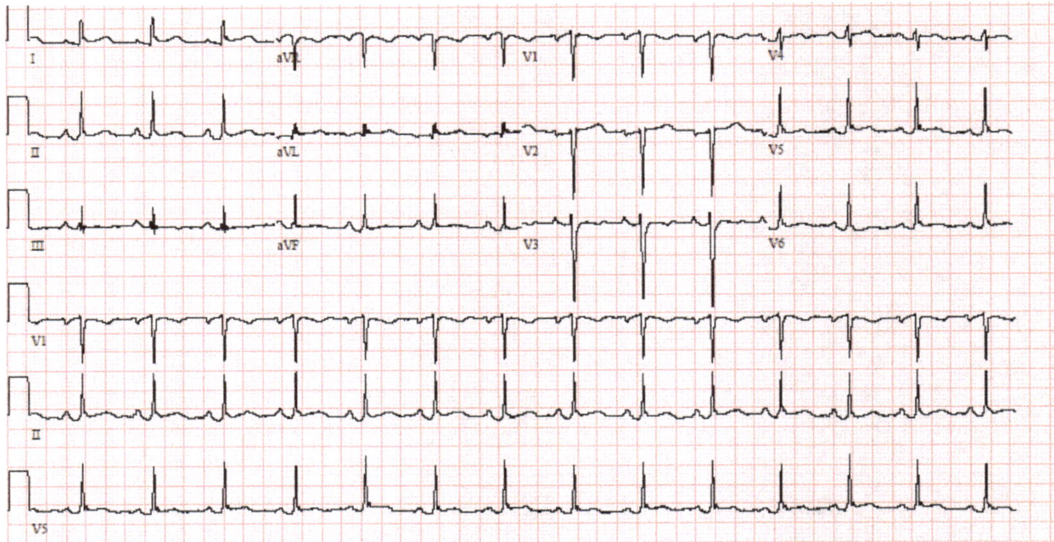

FIGURE 5: ECG postoperative day 3 showing resolution of ST elevation and T wave inversions in leads V2-V6.

vasospasm can also manifest with indistinguishable ECG changes often warranting a coronary angiogram. Our patient had negative serial cardiac biomarkers and echocardiograms and no significant risk factors other than hypertension (nonsmoker, nondiabetic, normal lipid profile, no cardiac family history, etc.). Hence, a coronary intervention was not deemed necessary and underlying ICH, although not common, was considered responsible for the ECG changes.

ECG abnormalities are commonly seen in association with aSAH and ischemic stroke [3, 4]. Rarely ECG changes and elevated troponins can be seen with ICH. One case series found increased troponins levels in 20% of supratentorial hemorrhages but without confirmatory ECG changes [5]. A recent study by Takeuchi et al. [2] did show that ECG abnormalities can be common in patients with ICH with most frequently observed abnormalities as ST depression (24%) along with T wave inversion and QTc prolongation (both 19%) but not ST elevation (6%) as seen in our patient. Some previous studies also found that these abnormalities particularly QTc prolongation were frequently observed in the acute phase of ICH [6]. However, we did not find any of these or other studies reporting ST elevation in an ICH patient after neurosurgery.

There is some evidence that ECG changes in stroke, including ICH, are caused by over activity of the sympathetic limb of the autonomic nervous system, with insular cortex playing a major in its regulation [7, 8]. These data also indicate some lateralization of cardiovascular representation with sympathetic predominance of cardiovascular regulation being a right insular function, and parasympathetic cardiac neural regulation relating to the left insula [8]. In our patient, the hemorrhage was in the left temporoparietal region involving the left insular cortex. We believe that suppression of left insular outflow likely shifted the autonomic balance towards the right insula and sympathetic predominance. This uninterrupted sympathetic activity may have led to initial ECG changes. These changes became more pronounced with ST elevation and T wave inversion postoperatively due to stress of anesthesia and neurosurgery causing increased levels of circulating catecholamines.

Nonetheless, these ECG findings cause considerable diagnostic problems and management dilemmas in the acute setting. Quite often these ECG changes are benign and self-limiting but lack of information leads to misdiagnosis and unwarranted treatment. This is especially worrisome in patients with ICH because treatment of ischemic heart disease consists of anticoagulants, antiplatelet therapy, or fibrinolytic agents with or without angioplasty which can profoundly worsen the prognosis in these patients [9]. Therefore, sequential evaluation by not only ECG but also serial cardiac biomarkers estimation and echocardiographic assessment is considered necessary for determination of the appropriate therapeutic approach. The same approach was employed in our patient with no untoward effect.

In summary, this case highlights the unique association of an acute cerebrovascular injury and surgical intervention with diffuse 'ischemic' changes on the ECG. Although the exact reason behind this association is not known, dysregulation of the brain cardiac axis is the probable explanation. Future studies are needed which will help us understand the various unknowns about the brain heart relationship and provide insights into the management of such cases.

References

[1] A. P. Patel, B. I. Ibrahim, and F. Dockery, "The ischaemic ECG: is it all in the head?" *BMJ Case Reports*, vol. 2013, Article ID bcr2013009854, 2013.

[2] S. Takeuchi, K. Nagatani, N. Otani, K. Wada, and K. Mori, "Electrocardiograph abnormalities in intracerebral hemorrhage," *Journal of Clinical Neuroscience*, vol. 22, no. 12, pp. 1959–1962, 2015.

[3] K. A. Bybee and A. Prasad, "Stress-related cardiomyopathy syndromes," *Circulation*, vol. 118, no. 4, pp. 397–409, 2008.

[4] K. C. Johnston, J. Y. Li, P. D. Lyden et al., "Medical and neurological complications of ischemic stroke: experience from the RANTTAS trial," *Stroke*, vol. 29, no. 2, pp. 447–453, 1998.

[5] B. V. Maramattom, E. M. Manno, J. R. Fulgham, A. S. Jaffe, and E. F. M. Wijdicks, "Clinical importance of cardiac troponin release and cardiac abnormalities in patients with supratentorial cerebral hemorrhages," *Mayo Clinic Proceedings*, vol. 81, no. 2, pp. 192–196, 2006.

[6] C. Tatschl, C. Stöllberger, K. Matz et al., "Insular involvement is associated with QT prolongation: ECG abnormalities in patients with acute stroke," *Cerebrovascular Disease*, vol. 21, no. 1-2, pp. 47–53, 2006.

[7] H. Christensen, G. Boysen, A. F. Christensen, and H. H. Johannesen, "Insular lesions, ECG abnormalities, and in outcome in acute stroke," *Journal of Neurology, Neurosurgery & Psychiatry*, vol. 76, no. 2, pp. 269–271, 2005.

[8] O. Stephen, "Cerebrogenic cardiac arrhythmias: cortical lateralization and clinical significance," *Clinical Autonomic Research*, vol. 16, no. 1, pp. 6–11, 2006.

[9] M. D. R. Van Bree, Y. B. W. E. M. Roos, I. A. C. Van Der Bilt et al., "Prevalence and characterization of ECG abnormalities after intracerebral hemorrhage," *Neurocritical Care*, vol. 12, no. 1, pp. 50–55, 2010.

A Case of Linezolid Toxicity Presenting as a Sepsis Mimic

Rashmi Mishra [1] Harish Patel [2,3] Bindu Goel,[4] and Trupti Vakde [3,5]

[1]*Department of Medicine, Penn Highlands Healthcare, PA, USA*
[2]*Division of the Gastroenterology, BronxCare Health System, NY, USA*
[3]*Department of Medicine, BronxCare Health System, NY, USA*
[4]*Mercy Medical Center, IA, USA*
[5]*Division of the Pulmonary and Critical care Medicine, BronxCare Health System, NY, USA*

Correspondence should be addressed to Harish Patel; hpatel@bronxleb.org

Academic Editor: Kenneth S. Waxman

Linezolid is an efficacious and well tolerated antimicrobial but can have serious adverse effects including myelo-suppression, serotonin syndrome, neuropathy, hypoglycemia, liver dysfunction, and lactic acidosis. The side effects are generally duration dependent; linezolid use is not recommended for more than 28 days. *Case.* A 59-year-old female presented with malaise, loss of appetite, and altered mentation. She had multiple medical comorbidities and required long-term anticoagulation with warfarin for venous thromboembolism. She had multiple medication allergies. Prior to admission, she was on linezolid for cellulitis of foot due to Methicillin-resistant *Staphylococcus aureus* (MRSA). On physical exam, she was drowsy and required endotracheal intubation for airway protection. Initial laboratory parameters showed lactic acidosis, thrombocytopenia, supra-therapeutic coagulation profile, low blood glucose, and transaminitis. Her altered mentation was due to hypoglycemia. The interaction with warfarin led to altered coagulation profile. She developed shock and vasopressors were initiated. Given her presentation, she was managed as severe sepsis. There were no active infectious foci attributing to decline of her clinical status. Linezolid was discontinued and she was managed with intravenous polymyxin B, aztreonam, and vancomycin. Her hemodynamic status improved within one day. She was extubated on Day 5 of her presentation. Her laboratory parameters showed gradual improvement over 12 days after discontinuation of linezolid. Retrospective evaluation revealed linezolid toxicity as possible cause of presentation. Linezolid toxicity can present as sepsis mimic and should be considered as a differential diagnosis while managing sepsis with other antimicrobial agents.

1. Introduction

Linezolid is an oxazolidinedione antibiotic approved for use against serious Gram-positive infections, including methicillin-resistant *Staphylococcus aureus* (MRSA) and vancomycin-resistant enterococcus faecium [1]. It is generally well tolerated, but can have serious adverse effects including myelosuppression [2], thrombocytopenia [3], serotonin syndrome [4], neuropathy [5], liver dysfunction [6], hypoglycemia, and lactic acidosis. However, rare but potential warfarin interaction leading to hypercoaguable state has been reported [7].

Antibiotics are used for the management of the bacterial infection. The antimicrobial induced adverse events, like lactic acidosis, can be confused with presentation of severe sepsis. It is imperative to recognize the cluster of adverse events to guide optimal treatment. A rare triad of toxicity of the hypoglycemia, lactic acidosis, and acute pancreatitis from linezolid has been reported [8]. We present a novel case of the linezolid toxicity presenting with a rare constellation of adverse events in the form of thrombocytopenia, lactic acidosis, hypoglycemia, and warfarin toxicity. It is imperative to include linezolid toxicity in differential diagnosis of sepsis and use alternative antibiotics for the management of possible bacterial infection.

2. Case

A 59-year-old female presented with malaise and low appetite for one day. Her family brought her to emergency room (ER) in view of altered mentation. Her medical comorbid conditions included coronary artery disease, hypertension, diabetes mellitus, and multiple venous thromboembolism requiring long-term anticoagulation with warfarin, chronic renal insufficiency, and steroid dependent asthma.

TABLE 1: Demonstrates laboratory parameters at the time of admission and the improvement after discontinuation of linezolid.

Parameters	Day 1	Day 3	Day 5	Day 12	Day 114
Hemoglobin (g/dL)	8.4	6.6	7.9	7.9	
WBC (k/μL)	16	2.9	6.7	21.1	
Platelets (k/μL)	26	17	11	190	
INR	8.4	1.9	1.6	1.4	
Creatinine (mg/dL)	3.3	3.1	2.3	1.0	
AST (U/l)	1289	559	101	346	19
ALT (U/l)	897	688	418	669	33
LDH (units/ml)	479				
Bilirubin (gm/ml)	2.1	1.3	1.4	0.9	
Lactic acid (mMol/L)	12.4	6.5	4.4		
Blood gas (pH)	7.06	7.4	7.38		
Blood glucose (mg/dL)	54	139	207	260	
Fibrinogen (mg/dL)	225				

Few weeks prior to her index presentation, she was hospitalized for foot infection. Her evaluation did not reveal osteomyelitis. She developed cellulitis near the ulcer and wound culture revealed growth of Methicillin resistant *Staphylococcus aureus* (MRSA). The antibiotics susceptibility revealed sensitivities to vancomycin and moxifloxacin. Infectious disease consultation was obtained and in view of the allergy to moxifloxacin and renal insufficiency, 3 weeks of the linezolid was recommended. She was initiated on intravenous linezolid 600 mg twice daily. She was followed up in the infectious disease ambulatory clinic. She was followed up in the anticoagulation monitoring clinic, and she did not require any alteration in warfarin dose. Glucose monitoring diary maintained by visiting nurse service revealed a controlled diabetes state. There was interval improvement in cellulitis and foot ulcer. She presented to our ER few days after the clinic assessment.

She had multiple medication allergies. She was allergic to azithromycin, penicillin, moxifloxacin, aspirin, ibuprofen, and ketorolac. She had unclear history of allergy to vancomycin. However, further evaluation during index hospitalization revealed the reaction to be rate dependent infusion reaction.

Her initial vitals were blood pressure of 90/46 mm Hg, oxygen saturation of 97% on room air, heartrate of 110 beats per minute, and she was afebrile. Her physical examination was significant for respiratory distress and drowsiness. The foot exam revealed interval healing of the foot ulcer. There were no meningeal signs. Neurological exam did not reveal any focal deficits. Her abdomen was soft and nontender. Cardiac auscultation did not reveal any new murmur.

Initial laboratory parameters showed lactic acidosis, thrombocytopenia, supra-therapeutic international normalized ratio (INR), low blood glucose, transaminitis, and normal fibrinogen levels (Table 1).

Imaging studies did not reveal any infective foci. There was no intracranial bleeding on Computerized tomography (CT) of the head. X-ray chest at the time of admission revealed clear lung fields with no pulmonary infiltrates. Ultrasound of abdomen revealed acalculus gallbladder and normal dimension of the common bile duct.

Given her altered mentation she required intubation and mechanical ventilation. In view of prior MRSA infection she was managed initially for sepsis. The initial impression of her presentation was sepsis, and required further evaluation for source of infection. Infection disease consultation recommended trough monitored intravenous vancomycin along with polymyxin B and aztreonam. Interdisciplinary discussion between clinical pharmacy, infectious disease consultant, and intensivist recommended further evaluation of records for vancomycin allergy versus allergic reaction. Patient received polymyxin B and aztreonam. She further developed shock. Her periphery was cold; despite fluid resuscitation she required the vasopressor for a brief period. The clinical pharmacist recommended vancomycin use, and her hemodynamic status improved with one day. Lactic acidosis can be from hypotension at presentation, but the improvement was not in conjunction to recovery of shock. This late recovery of serum chemistry led to investigate alternate etiology for lactic acidosis. Infectious disease follow-up recommended vancomycin levels to guide subsequent dose and bacterial cultures for titration of antibiotics. However, her blood culture and wound culture from infection site were negative for any bacterial growth. Both cultures were obtained at time of presentation prior to antibiotics administration. Hematology consultation opined that the hypercoaguable state was warfarin induced rather than sepsis induced. A normal fibrinogen level supported this conclusion. She completed the course of linezolid and hence it was not given at time of admission. She was extubated on Day 5 of admission. Her laboratory parameters showed gradual improvement over 12 days after discontinuation of linezolid (Table 1). Given the absence of septic foci, the clinical scenario supported the presentation to be a constellation of adverse events from linezolid and she did not require the additional antibiotics therapy.

3. Discussion

Linezolid binds to bacterial RNA and prevents formation of a functional 70S initiation complex which is important for the bacterial translocation process. It has been hypothesized that due to the similarities between human and bacterial ribosomes [9], linezolid inhibits the human mitochondrial ribosome by a similar mechanism. Henceforth, the deficiency of mitochondria encoded proteins can lead to lactic acidosis [10–12]. A longer duration of therapy of more than 6 weeks, has been associated with higher rates of lactic acidosis [1]. A systemic review of 47 cases of linezolid identified male gender as a risk factor for development of lactic acidosis, rather than duration of antimicrobial use and patient age [13]. Sepsis, thiamine deficiency, and liver cirrhosis have been associated with the higher incidence of the linezolid associated lactic acidosis [14]. Tissue hypoxia leads to increase in lactate production. Hypotension affects the lactate clearance and hence leads to hyperlactate state [15]. Although, hypo perfusion can be a cause for lactic acidosis in our patient. Lactic acid levels improve with sepsis management, correction of hypotension, and it is correlated with better prognosis [16, 17]. In our case, the lactate recovery did not correlate to shock management and achievement of re-perfusion status. Lactic acid recovery with linezolid toxicity is prolonged and its can take more than 10 days for the lactate levels to normalize [18]. Metformin is also known to cause lactic acidosis, specifically in patients with the renal and hepatic insufficiency [19]. Metformin can limit mitochondrial cellular respiration leading to lactic acidosis [20]. However, our patient was not on metformin. Hence, possible explanation of a prolonged plateau to normalization of lactate level can be explained by linezolid toxicity.

The literature has depicted an association of linezolid with myelosuppression [3, 14, 21, 22]. No increased risk of agranulocytosis or other irreversible blood dyscrasias was found [21]. More than 2 weeks of therapy has been found to be a risk factor for linezolid induced thrombocytopenia [21, 22]. Thrombocytopenia secondary to linezolid is reversible upon discontinuation of drug [22]. Patients with renal impairment may develop higher plasma linezolid concentration, and hence more likely to develop thrombocytopenia as result of the linezolid toxicity [3, 14]. Vitamin B6 supplementation has been reported to reverse linezolid associated cytopenia [21]. Frequent blood cell count monitoring is suggested for individuals on more than two weeks of the linezolid therapy.

Linezolid related nonselective monoamine oxidase (MAO) inhibition could induce hypoglycemia [23]. This phenomenon is further supported by the higher incidence of hypoglycemia in the individuals on MAO and insulin or sulfonylurea concurrently [24, 25].Our patient was on insulin for the management of her diabetes, but there was no evidence for the use of MAO inhibitors. The bacterial infection can lead to brittle diabetes status, but we did not identify any active bacterial infection while managing her acute presentation. Her diabetes was well controlled at the time of ambulatory visit assessment prior to ER presentation. Medications with dopamine (D2) receptor agonist activity, like bromocriptine, are utilized for antihyperglycemic effect and can cause side effects of hypoglycemia. Linezolid may increase the levels of dopamine via its MAO inhibition activity, hence leading to hypoglycemia [23]. Another mechanism of the hypoglycemia is from linezolid induced mitochondrial dysfunction leading to pancreatic beta-cell related insulin secretion dysregulation [8].

Initial reports of the potential interaction between warfarin and linezolid surfaced in 2015 [7]. Linezolid can have the antimicrobial activity against Bifidobacterium, hence compromising the vitamin K production in the gut [7]. It is hypothesized that linezolid can decrease vitamin K production and potentiate the warfarin toxicity. Our patient had a stable coagulation profile on a stable dose of warfarin until linezolid initiation and there were no other interaction attractable to the hypercoagulable state.

Transaminitis related to linezolid (drug) induced liver injury has been well reported [6, 10]. The liver histopathology in these cases reveals diffuse microvesicular hepatosteatosis [6]. Ischemic hepatitis can be alternative explanation, but would require the clinical acumen to differentiate between the two etiologies. In ischemic hepatitis there is delayed peaking of bilirubin with ALT/LDH ration of lower than 1.5 [26]. In index case, the bilirubin levels peaked at presentation and ALT/LDH ratio was 1.8. Sepsis can be an alternate explanation, but a clear infectious etiology could not be demonstrated.

The hemodynamic status in our patient improved rapidly. However, the resolution of other parameters like transaminitis, thrombocytopenia, and hyperlactatemia required multiple days leading to prolonged hospitalization.

In view of pancytopenia and neuro-toxicity the European Medicines Agency (EMEA) and U.S. Food and Drug Administration have suggested to limit linezolid use to 28 days [27, 28]. Linezolid remains an effective antimicrobial for MRSA related infections. A prolonged duration (>4 weeks) of linezolid use, though not well tolerated, has been reported for management of bone infection [29]. In our patient, in view of her multiple drug allergies and renal insufficiency linezolid remains the preferred antibiotic. We faced challenges in management of possible MRSA infection in view of unclear history of vancomycin allergy. Mitochondrial genetics has been studied in linezolid toxicity, specifically for those related to shorter duration of therapy [30]. In presented cases, mitochondrial genetic can explain presentation of lactic acidosis. However, etiology of other side effect was unrelated.

4. Conclusion

Prolonged use of the linezolid has been associated with lactic acidosis, hypoglycemia, thrombocytopenia, and interaction with warfarin. This case brings to light the need for physicians to be aware of linezolid toxicity being a sepsis mimic during course of management. Alternative antimicrobial agents should be considered for management of suspected bacterial infection.

Abbreviations

MRSA: Methicillin-resistant *Staphylococcus aureus*

INR: International normalized ratio.

Disclosure

No specific grant from funding agencies in the public, commercial, or not-for-profit sectors was received for writing this case report.

References

[1] J. H. Im, J. H. Baek, H. Y. Kwon, and J. S. Lee, "Incidence and risk factors of linezolid-induced lactic acidosis," *International Journal of Infectious Diseases*, vol. 31, pp. 47–52, 2015.

[2] J. Deng, L. X. Su, Z. X. Liang et al., "Effects of vitamin B6 therapy for sepsis patients with linezolid-associated cytopenias: a retrospective study," *Current Therapeutic Research, Clinical and Experimental*, vol. 74, pp. 26–32, 2013.

[3] D. Echeverria-Esnal, A. Retamero, S. L. Pardos, and S. Grau, "Severe thrombocytopenia caused by linezolid poisoning in an underweight critically ill patient with renal impairment treated with the recommended doses," *Enfermedades Infecciosas y Microbiologia Clinica*, vol. 34, no. 3, pp. 213–214, 2016.

[4] D. K. Quinn and T. A. Stern, "Linezolid and serotonin syndrome," *Primary Care Companion to The Journal of Clinical Psychiatry*, vol. 11, no. 6, pp. 353–356, 2009.

[5] J. P. Rho, I. G. Sia, B. A. Crum, M. B. Dekutoski, and R. T. Trousdale, "Linezolid-associated peripheral neuropathy," *Mayo Clinic Proceedings*, vol. 79, no. 7, pp. 927–930, 2004.

[6] L. De Bus, P. Depuydt, L. Libbrecht et al., "Severe drug-induced liver injury associated with prolonged use of linezolid," *Journal of Medical Toxicology*, vol. 6, no. 3, pp. 322–326, 2010.

[7] Y. Sakai, T. Naito, C. Arima et al., "Potential drug interaction between warfarin and linezolid," *Internal Medicine*, vol. 54, no. 5, pp. 459–464, 2015.

[8] P. C. Johnson, M. Vaduganathan, K. M. Phillips, and W. J. O'Donnell, "A triad of linezolid toxicity: hypoglycemia, lactic acidosis, and acute pancreatitis," *Baylor University Medical Center Proceedings*, vol. 28, no. 4, pp. 466–468, 2015.

[9] A. Santini, D. Ronchi, M. Garbellini, D. Piga, and A. Protti, "Linezolid-induced lactic acidosis: the thin line between bacterial and mitochondrial ribosomes," *Expert Opinion on Drug Safety*, vol. 16, no. 7, pp. 833–843, 2017.

[10] E. Potolidis, E. Gousi, D. Delios, E. Bei, and C. Mandros, "Linezolid induced lactic acidosis and hepatic failure," *International Journal of Case Reports and Images*, vol. 3, no. 12, pp. 79–81, 2012.

[11] A. S. De Vriese, R. Van Coster, J. Smet et al., "Linezolid-induced inhibition of mitochondrial protein synthesis," *Clinical Infectious Diseases*, vol. 42, no. 8, pp. 1111–1117, 2006.

[12] J. Carson, J. Cerda, J. H. Chae, M. Hirano, and P. Maggiore, "Severe lactic acidosis associated with linezolid use in a patient with the mitochondrial DNA A2706G polymorphism," *Pharmacotherapy*, vol. 27, no. 5, pp. 771–774, 2007.

[13] Y. Mao, D. Dai, H. Jin, and Y. Wang, "The risk factors of linezolid-induced lactic acidosis: a case report and review," *Medicine*, vol. 97, no. 36, p. e12114, 2018.

[14] F. K. Gould, "Linezolid: safety and efficacy in special populations," *The Journal of Antimicrobial Chemotherapy*, vol. 4, pp. iv3–iv6, 2011.

[15] S. M. Lee and W. S. An, "New clinical criteria for septic shock: serum lactate level as new emerging vital sign," *Journal of Thoracic Disease*, vol. 8, no. 7, pp. 1388–1390, 2016.

[16] T. C. Jansen, J. van Bommel, F. J. Schoonderbeek et al., "Early lactate-guided therapy in intensive care unit patients," *American Journal of Respiratory and Critical Care Medicine*, vol. 182, no. 6, pp. 752–761, 2010.

[17] B. Suetrong and K. R. Walley, "Lactic acidosis in sepsis: it's not all anaerobic: implications for diagnosis and management," *Chest*, vol. 149, no. 1, pp. 252–261, 2016.

[18] A. A. Apodaca and R. M. Rakita, "Linezolid-induced lactic acidosis," *New England Journal of Medicine*, vol. 348, no. 1, pp. 86–87, 2003.

[19] S. R. Salpeter, E. Greyber, and G. A. Pasternak, E. E. Salpeter, "Risk of fatal and nonfatal lactic acidosis with metformin use in type 2 diabetes mellitus," *The Cochrane Database of Systematic Reviews*, vol. 1, p. Cd002967, 2010.

[20] K. T. Kopec and M. J. Kowalski, "Metformin-associated lactic acidosis: case files of the Einstein Medical Center medical toxicology fellowship," *Journal of Medical Toxicology*, vol. 9, no. 1, pp. 61–66, 2013.

[21] G. French, "Safety and tolerability of linezolid," *Journal of Antimicrobial Chemotherapy*, vol. 51, no. 90002, pp. 45–53, 2003.

[22] S. L. Gerson, S. L. Kaplan, J. B. Bruss et al., "Hematologic effects of linezolid: summary of clinical experience," *Antimicrobial Agents and Chemotherapy*, vol. 46, no. 8, pp. 2723–2726, 2002.

[23] T. Bodnar, K. Starr, and J. E. Halter, "Linezolid-associated hypoglycemia in a 64-year-old man with type 2 diabetes," *The American Journal of Geriatric Pharmacotherapy*, vol. 9, no. 1, pp. 88–92, 2011.

[24] A. J. Cooper and G. Ashcroft, "Potentiation of insulin hypoglycaemia by M.A.O.I. antidepressant drugs," *The Lancet*, vol. 1, no. 7434, pp. 407–409, 1966.

[25] P. I. Adnitt, "Hypoglycemic action of monoamineoxidase inhibitors," *Diabetes*, vol. 17, no. 10, pp. 628–633, 1968.

[26] J. F. L. Cobbold, J. A. Summerfield, L. S. Friedman, and E. B. Keeffe, "Chapter 22—The liver in systemic disease," in *Handbook of Liver Disease*, pp. 297–307, W. B. Saunders, Philadelpia, 3rd edition, 2012.

[27] Information. Z-P., "Access data food and drug administration," 2000.

[28] A. M. Bressler, S. M. Zimmer, J. L. Gilmore, and J. Somani, "Peripheral neuropathy associated with prolonged use of linezolid," *The Lancet Infectious Diseases*, vol. 4, no. 8, pp. 528–531, 2004.

[29] E. Senneville, L. Legout, M. Valette et al., "Effectiveness and tolerability of prolonged linezolid treatment for chronic osteomyelitis: a retrospective study," *Clinical Therapeutics*, vol. 28, no. 8, pp. 1155–1163, 2006.

[30] G. Garrabou, À. Soriano, T Pinós et al., "Influence of mitochondrial genetics on the mitochondrial toxicity of linezolid in blood cells and skin nerve fibers," *Antimicrobial Agents and Chemotherapy*, vol. 61, no. 9, pp. e00542–e00517, 2017.

41

The Considerations and Controversies in using High-Flow Nasal Oxygen with Self-Prone Positioning in SARS-CoV-2 COVID-19 Disease

Kieran P. Nunn,[1,2] Murray J. Blackstock,[1,2] Ryan Ellis,[1] Gauhar Sheikh,[1] Alastair Morgan,[1,2] and Jonathan K. J. Rhodes[1,2,3]

[1]*Intensive Care Unit, Western General Hospital, Crewe Road South, Edinburgh EH4 2XU, UK*
[2]*Intensive Care Unit, Royal Infirmary of Edinburgh, 51 Little France Crescent, Edinburgh EH16 4SA, UK*
[3]*Edinburgh Critical Care Research Group (ECCRG), The University of Edinburgh, The Royal Infirmary of Edinburgh, 51 Little France Cres., Edinburgh EH16 4SA, UK*

Correspondence should be addressed to Kieran P. Nunn; kieran.nunn@doctors.org.uk

Academic Editor: Zsolt Molnár

Evidence exists for the use of high-flow nasal oxygen (HFNO) in the general critical care population for acute hypoxemic respiratory failure. There is discord between guidelines for hypoxemia management in COVID-19. Both noninvasive management and intubation present risk to patients and staff and potentially overwhelm hospital mechanical ventilator capacity. The use of HFNO has been particularly controversial in the UK, with oxygen infrastructure failure. We discuss our experience of managing COVID-19 with HFNO and awake self-prone positioning. We focus upon the less-usual case of an eighteen-year-old female to illustrate the type of patient where HFNO may be used when perhaps earlier intubation once was. It is important to consider the wider implications of intubation. We have used HFNO as a bridge to intubation or as definitive management. As we await clinical trial evidence, HFNO with self-prone positioning has a role in COVID-19 for certain patients. Response parameters must be set and reviewed, oxygen infrastructure considered, and potential staff droplet exposure minimised.

1. Introduction

Pandemic SARS-CoV-2 infection's most immediately life-threatening feature is the novel interstitial lung disease (COVID-19) causing hypoxemic respiratory failure due to viral pneumonitis and ARDS (Acute Respiratory Distress Syndrome). Health systems are pressurised in preparing for anticipated surges in patient numbers requiring respiratory support. There were early concerns about ventilator availability. We may face this again. Patients present with variable, fluctuating hypoxemic respiratory failure, often in the absence of dyspnoea. The pathophysiology of dyspnoea is complex, involving multiple chemo- and mechanoreception afferents. So, the absence of dyspnoea does not necessarily mean that hypoxemia is benign. Significant uncertainty exists over the optimal therapeutic target when correcting hypoxemia in COVID-19 respiratory failure. Tolerable levels of hypoxemia versus concern over pulmonary oxygen toxicity in acute lung injury must also be balanced against local logistical factors concerning the means to deliver different types of supplemental oxygen therapy safely and the infrastructure these require. In a trial stopped for safety after 205 patients were enrolled, it emerged that conservative oxygen targets in the early management phase of ARDS, PaO_2 55 mmHg–70 mmHg (oxygen saturation (SpO_2) 88-92%), compared to liberal PaO_2 90 mmHg–105 mmHg ($SpO_2 > 95\%$), could be harmful [1]. The Surviving Sepsis group recommend targeting SpO_2 92%-96% in adults with COVID-19 [2, 3].

The decision-making when treating hypoxemia is complex and controversial in COVID-19 for many reasons. Recently in the UK, we have seen hospital oxygen supply infrastructure failures with consequent Incident Reporting & Investigation Centre reports (IM/2020/005) [4] and National Patient Safety Alerts (NatPSA/2020/002/NHSPS)

Table 1: A comparison of major organisation recommendations for CPAP/NIV and HFNO.

Body	Noninvasive ventilation	High-flow nasal oxygen
SCCM (USA) [6]	Consider if HFNO failed	Yes
NIH (USA) [6]	Consider if HFNO unavailable	Yes
ANZICS (Australia & New Zealand) [8–10]	No	Yes
WHO (Switzerland) [7]	Yes	Yes
FICM, RCoA, ICS, & AAGBI (UK) [11]	Bridge to intubation	No
ESICM (Europe/UK) [2]	Consider if HFNO failed	Yes
Surviving Sepsis Campaign [2]	Consider if HFNO failed	Yes
NHS England [40]	Yes	No

SCCM: Society of Critical Care Medicine; NIH: National Institutes of Health; ANZICS: Australian and New Zealand Intensive Care Society; WHO: World Health Organisation; FICM: Faculty of Intensive Care Medicine; RCoA: Royal College of Anaesthetists; ICS: Intensive Care Society; AAGBI: Association of Anaesthetists of Great Britain and Ireland; ESICM: European Society of Intensive Care Medicine.

[5]. Noninvasive options for advanced supplemental oxygen delivery, including continuous positive airway pressure (CPAP) and high-flow nasal oxygen (HFNO), are inconsistently recommended. And there are concerns about both variable consumption and excessive use of oxygen in addition to the potential risk of cross-infection to other patients and staff. In the USA, the Society of Critical Care Medicine along with the National Institutes of Health (NIH) [6], the European Society of Intensive Care Medicine, the Australian and New Zealand Intensive Care Society, and the World Health Organisation recommends HFNO with effective infection control measures including personal protective equipment (PPE) when supplemental oxygen via nasal canulae or simple facemask systems are ineffective and immediate intubation is not required [2, 7–10]. In the UK, the Faculty of Intensive Care Medicine, the Intensive Care Society, the Association of Anaesthetists of Great Britain and Ireland, and the Royal College of Anaesthetists do not support the use of HFNO or similar devices [11]. A lot of this COVID-19-specific guidance is understandably based on early information and experience (Table 1). Because of this, these organisations have established web resources which are frequently updated.

We present an illustrative case of COVID-19 pneumonitis that was managed with HFNO and self-prone positioning. We summarise HFNO in the management of 16 COVID-19 patients admitted to our Intensive Care Unit (ICU) (Table 2). This was in line with our pre-COVID-19 treatment of some mild ARDS patients. A recent network meta-analysis of noninvasive oxygenation strategies and all-cause mortality in non-COVID-19 acute hypoxemic respiratory failure is reassuring of the use of these strategies pre-COVID-19. Yet even before COVID-19, the relative benefits of each strategy were not clear [12]. In considering our management, a systematic literature search was conducted through June 2020 to identify any publication of patients with COVID-19 treated with HFNO. The following electronic bibliographic databases were searched from 1974 until June 16, 2020, using a comprehensive search strategy developed by an information specialist: Embase, Medline, DynaMed, and The Right Decision. We separately searched society, professional body, and government guidelines as well as identified references. The full texts of all articles identified as relevant during title and abstract screening were obtained and reviewed. The comprehensive search strategy is described in the online supplement (available here). As anticipated, it is too early to have trial evidence. But it remains important to discuss experience whilst decisions on oxygen treatment are being made every day.

2. Case Presentation

An 18-year-old female presented in the early hours of the morning on day 1. Having previously consulted primary care services, she was confirmed SARS-CoV-2 COVID-19 positive 3 days prior to hospitalisation through community testing. She had followed Scottish COVID-19 lockdown guidance, but she did work directly with the public in a UK supermarket chain that was also taking distancing and protection precautions. She had become short of breath at rest: respiratory rate (RR) 43 breaths per minute and SpO_2 85% on air. She described a productive cough and pleuritic chest pain. She also gave a history of intermittent fever, blocked nose and sore throat, bad taste, and reduced appetite. Seventeen hours later, she was admitted to ICU. Her weight had been stable (104 kg BMI 36). She had a history of chronic widespread pain, migraines, fibromyalgia, anxiety, and irritable bowel syndrome. Her medication history was medroxyprogesterone 10 mg, fluoxetine 20 mg, propranolol modified release 80 mg, almotriptan 12.5 mg, and nortriptyline 30 mg. She had never smoked and did not consume alcohol at all. She studied full time at university up until COVID-19 closure and lockdown.

Initial ward management included supplemental oxygen fraction (FiO_2) 35% by a fixed performance mask. Her observations at this stage were SpO_2 96%, blood pressure (BP) 138/73 mmHg, heart rate (HR) 118/min, and temperature 38.4°C. She reported feeling better, but she looked unwell from the end of the bed, appearing pale, clammy, and tachypnoeic. Her peripheries were warm with normal heart sounds and no oedema; calves were soft and nontender. She remained unable to complete most sentences. Chest X-ray showed bilateral peripheral nodular opacification, most marked in the left mid zone, in keeping with consolidation (Figure 1). The arterial blood gas (ABG) confirmed hypoxaemia PaO_2 75 mmHg (P:F 215 mmHg), $PaCO_2$ 29 mmHg, H^+ 34 nmol/L, and base excess -2.8 mmol/L. A prompt referral to critical care was made, and when that consult occurred, SpO_2

Table 2: A case series of our patients treated with high-flow nasal oxygen during the first wave of the COVID-19 pandemic.

Age (years)	Gender	Comorbidities	ICU admission P:F (mmHg)	Initial HFNO P:F (mmHg)	Intubated	Preintubation P:F on HFNO (mmHg)	Proned (i = intubated)	Preprone P:F (mmHg)	Postprone P:F (mmHg)	Preextubation P:F (mmHg)	Outcome
63	M	HTN, BMI, DM	96	113 (FiO_2 0.6, flow 40 L/min)	Y	57 (FiO_2 1.0, flow 50 L/min)	Y (i)	98 (FiO_2 0.7)	222 (FiO_2 0.45)	Tracheostomy	I
44	M	BMI, DM	66	93 (FiO_2 1.0, flow 60 L/min)	Y	50 (FiO_2 1.0, flow 60 L/min)	Y (i)	101 (FiO_2 0.55)	140 (FiO_2 0.45)	187 (FiO_2 0.4)	D/C
60	M		61	71 (FiO_2 0.9, flow 65 L/min)	Y	60 (FiO_2 1.0, flow 60 L/min)	Y (i)	128 (FiO_2 0.5)	88 (FiO_2 0.75)	N/A	Died
68	M	HTN, BMI, PAF, CMT	183	165 (FiO_2 0.6, flow 60 L/min)	Y	135 (FiO_2 0.55, flow 50 L/min)	Y (i)	113 (FiO_2 0.9)	285 (FiO_2 0.55)	N/A	Died
66	M	TIA, HT	68	59 (FiO_2 1.0, flow 60 L/min)	Y	N/A (immediate progression)	Y (i)	N/A (immediate progression)	135 (FiO_2 0.55)	N/A	Died
66	M	DM, A	116	116 (FiO_2 0.5, flow 60 L/min)	N	N/A	Y	90 (FiO_2 0.5)	103 (FiO_2 0.6)	N/A	D/C
65	M	HTN, BMI, DM	105	144 (FiO_2 0.9, flow 50 L/min)	N	N/A	Y	105 (FiO_2 0.6)	104 (FiO_2 0.8)	N/A	D/C
67	M	NHL-R	112	116 (FiO_2 0.65, flow 40 L/min)	Y	143 (FiO_2 60%, flow 40 L/min)	N	N/A	N/A	N/A	Died
53	F	HTN, BMI, DM, S, RA-R	81	126 (FiO_2 0.60, flow 50 L/min)	N	N/A (immediate progression)	Y	Not available	Not available	187 (FiO_2 0.35)	D/C
47	M	DM, GPA-R	77	65 (FiO_2 0.8, flow 60 L/min)	Y	67 (FiO_2 0.8, flow 50 L/min)	Y (i)	11	83 (FiO_2 0.9)	Tracheostomy	D/C
53	M		99	117 (FiO_2 0.6, flow 50 L/min)	N	N/A	Y	Not available	Not available	N/A	D/C
45	M	BMI, G	90	104 (FiO_2 0.7, flow 50 L/min)	Y	62 (FiO_2 0.9, flow 60 L/min)	N	N/A	N/A	210 (FiO_2 0.35)	D/C
54	M	AML	54	HFNC applied for palliation	N	N/A	N	N/A	N/A	N/A	Died
30	M	BMI, A	150	101 (FiO_2 0.55, flow 50 L/min)	Y	49 (FiO_2 0.75, flow 45 L/min)	Y (i)	105 (FiO_2 0.5)	128 (FiO_2 0.55)	Tracheostomy	D/C
18	F	BMI, F, D	107	108 (FiO_2 0.6, flow 60 L/min)	N	N/A	Y	161 (FiO_2 0.7)	329 (FiO_2 0.4)	N/A	D/C
51	M	A	141	95 (FiO_2 0.8, flow 60 L/min)	N	N/A	Y	Not available	Not available	N/A	D/C

Legend: HTN: hypertension; BMI: BMI > 25; DM: type 2 diabetes; A: asthma; S: smoker; PAF: paroxysmal atrial fibrillation; CMT: Charcot-Marie-Tooth; TIA: transient ischaemic attack; HT: hypothyroid; NHL-R: non-Hodgkin lymphoma-taking rituximab; RA-R: rheumatoid arthritis-taking rituximab; GPA-R: granulomatosis with polyangiitis-taking rituximab; G: gout; AML: acute myeloid leukaemia; F: fibromyalgia; D: depression. Our preference and new admissions were treated with HFNO using the Optiflow+ setup detailed in the case report. If there was a demand on equipment or the patient was later in the phase of weaning or being extubated to HFNO, then we did also deliver HFNO by the Dräger Evita® Infinity® V500 ventilator. I = inpatient; D/C = discharged home; died = death in intensive care.

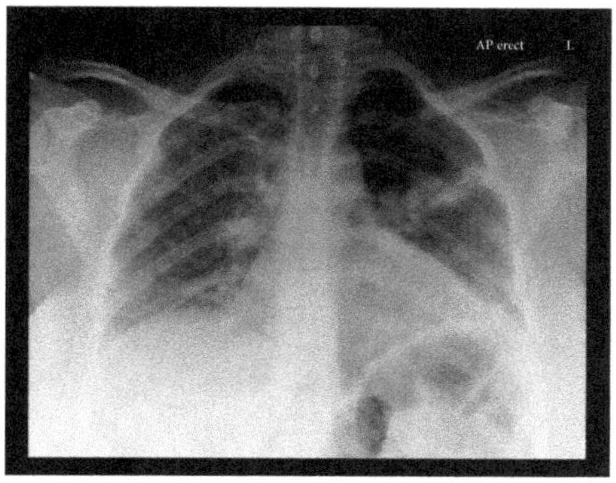

Figure 1: Chest X-ray on admission to the hospital prior to intubation.

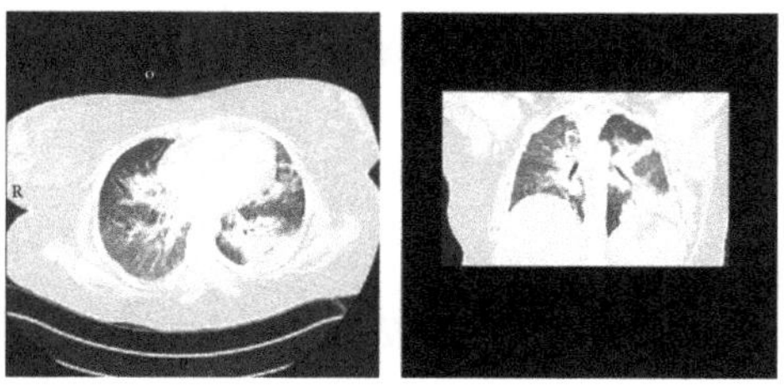

Figure 2: CTPA demonstrated COVID-19 pneumonitis throughout and left consolidation. Appearances in the left lung may suggest superadded bacterial consolidation on a background of bilateral COVID-19 pneumonitis. Appearances in the right lung are more suggestive of COVID-19 pneumonitis.

was maintained at 94-96% with FiO_2 40% and the temperature was 38.4°C. C-reactive protein (CRP) was 163 mg/L, and full blood count, liver function and urea, and electrolytes were normal. She had received intravenous amoxicillin. After initial improvement however, she was admitted to our mixed level 2/3 critical care having deteriorated to SpO_2 96% on FiO_2 60% by a fixed performance mask and RR 35/min unstressed but 38°C with mean arterial pressure (MAP) 60 mmHg. On route to the ICU, a CT pulmonary angiogram (CTPA) was performed (Figure 2). This excluded a pulmonary embolism and confirmed COVID-19 changes with left upper lobe consolidation. On admission into a single occupancy room, an arterial line was sited, intravenous crystalloid in targeted boluses used, HFNO started (Optiflow+ (Fisher & Paykel Healthcare), Courtaboeuf, France; heat and moisture exchanger (HME) filter; MR850 heater humidification device and MR290 autofill chamber (Fisher & Paykel Healthcare); and an air/oxygen blender capable of 100% O_2 and up to 70 L/min flow (Bio-Med Devices, Guilford, CT, USA)), and 0.1 mg/kg oral morphine given with encouragement to self-prone. PaO_2 was 45 mmHg on 15 L/min O_2 (mask) and improved over the first period in intensive care on 60% FiO_2 at 60 L/min HFNO with PaO_2 65 mmHg, $PaCO_2$ 31 mmHg, SpO_2 94%, MAP 77 mmHg, and HR 120/min.

We aimed for $SpO_2 > 92\%$, PaO_2 equal or over 60 mmHg, and mean arterial pressure 65 mmHg. Self-prone positioning was encouraged when the P:F ratio was under 150 mmHg (20 kPa). Clarithromycin was added to amoxicillin. Prophylactic low-molecular weight heparin (LMWH) was prescribed with LMWH (anti-Xa) assay monitoring, aiming for 0.1–0.4 μ/mL. We asked her to lie on her front for as long as possible. She was able to tolerate this most of the time, only turning supine for care, meals, and interventions. We did not stipulate a maximum prone time as the advantage of being awake is that patients can self-adjust pressure areas as well as engage more fully with physiotherapy and nursing intervention.

On day 2, the HFNO was titrated between 40 and 70 L/min. The trend in FiO_2, SpO_2, PaO_2, and P:F ratio throughout her time in critical care shows improvement and fluctuation with time self-prone (Figure 3). Typically, her observations were stable at RR 34/min, SpO_2 95%, PaO_2 157 mmHg, and $PaCO_2$ 35 mmHg with self-prone positioning and her PaO_2 was under 60 mmHg when supine. She would desaturate to a low SpO_2 80%-88% range on movement for nursing care. The use of the broad-spectrum antimicrobial cover was continued in line with daily microbiologist input. On day 3, the HFNO support was reduced to 40–50 L/min, FiO_2 40%, RR 22/min, and SpO_2 91%. Remaining prone (P:F ratio 140 mmHg, PaO_2 56 mmHg), she was comfortable, afebrile, RR 18-24/min, alert, and orientated. Her heart rate had settled to 67 bpm and BP 114/65. She continued to self-prone through day 4. Part of the success of this strategy was to ensure her comfort with measures such as extra pillows under pressure points of her pelvis. She remained in positive spirits, and overall, she found the patient interface of HFNO acceptable and did not like the idea of CPAP or invasive ventilation. On day 5, she completed co-amoxiclav, HFNO flow was reduced to a minimum, and FiO_2 was 40%; eventually, she was liberated from HFNO onto a 24-28% fixed performance oxygen mask. On day 6, she was discharged back to infectious diseases having not been intubated. She reported feeling physically much better but remained anxious and found it difficult to process the events of the last few days. She remained tired and lethargic but subjectively less short of breath, and all chest pain had resolved. By day 7, tiredness and the cough were the main complaints but the cough was now nonproductive. Assistance was required when walking to the toilet. Mobility gradually improved. Psychiatry was consulted and felt that she seemed to have coped well with being in the hospital, including ICU, but had raised concern about remembering any new detail that may become hard to process pertaining to this spell of hospitalisation and ill health. Strategies for managing this were provided. On day 9, with RR 19/min, SpO_2 98% on room air, BP 101/67 mmHg, HR 104/min, temperature 36.5°C, and feeling well, she was discharged home.

3. Discussion

We were initially deterred from our usual practice with HFNO in hypoxemic type 1 respiratory failure by the early rhetoric in COVID-19. Prior to COVID-19, in hypoxemic type 1 respiratory failure, we used HFNO for some patients as a bridge to intubation or as definitive treatment where response and sustained improvement was demonstrated. It remains important not to delay inevitable intubation. We intubated 75% of COVID-19 patients admitted to ITU which

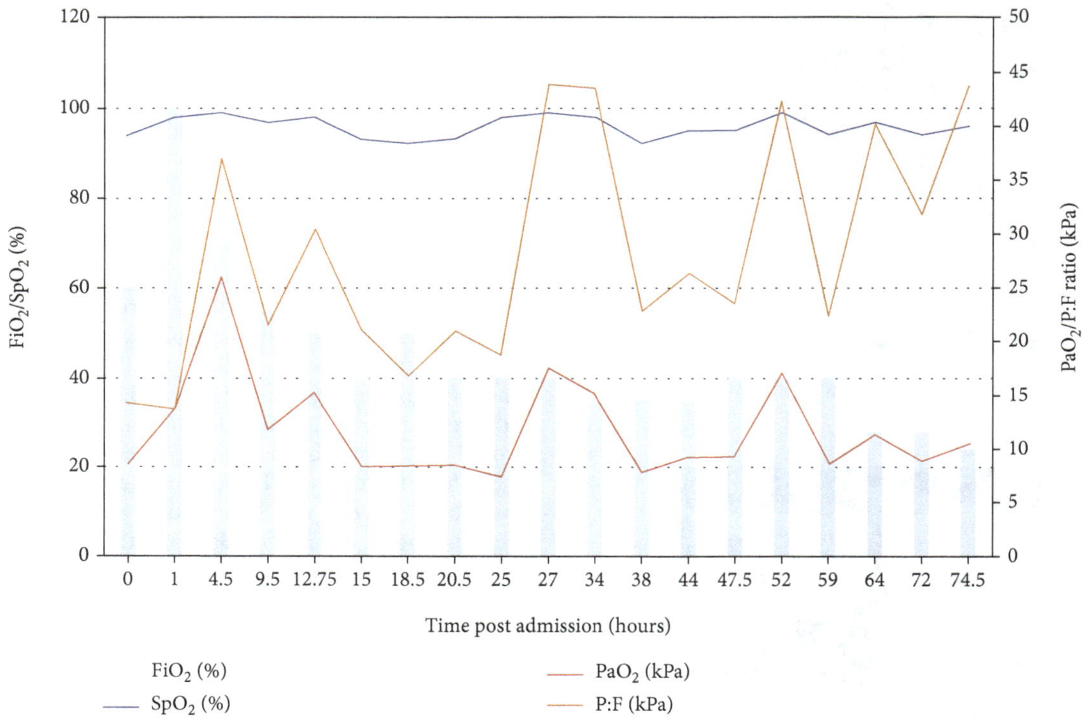

FIGURE 3: The patient trend in FiO_2, SpO_2, PaO_2, and P:F ratio throughout her time in critical care (P:F 40 kPa = 300 mmHg, P:F 26.7 kPa = 200 mmHg, and P:F 13.3 kPa = 100 mmHg). Self-prone positioning was encouraged when the P:F ratio was under 150 mmHg (20 kPa). We did not stipulate a maximum prone time; this was determined by patient comfort, tolerance, and between-care episodes requiring the patient to be supine.

dropped to 57% when we started using HFNO. The relatively high COVID-19 mortality in our HFNO group (31%) compared to our overall COVID-19 mortality (20%) comes from a relatively small sample from which general inferences cannot be made. Yet, it is important to acknowledge that this mortality was made up from patients who went on to be intubated and then died or where an active decision not to intubate had been made.

The case discussed highlights the importance of accounting for patient, hospital, and staff safety factors and of considering patient demographics and history, including psychiatric history in the decision between NIV, including HFNO, and intubation. We know that the ITU psychological burden is especially high with intubation and sedation [13, 14]. We fortuitously have not had any staff testing COVID-19 positive, and we are deeply saddened by the morbidity and mortality amongst healthcare workers worldwide. Notwithstanding, this is in accord with the prior opinion that aerosolization from HFNO may be insignificant when infection control practice and PPE are optimal [15–18].

All currently available guidelines were considered for an individualised patient approach. In some cases, HFNO allowed time for the appropriateness of escalation to invasive ventilation to be determined as being in the patients' best interest. This is a crucial bridging role of HFNO. We have found that HFNO is a comfortable, tolerable patient interface in both the supine and prone positions and has not had compliance issues allowing constant usage. COVID-19 pneumonitis causes a heterogenous lung due to ventilation-perfusion ratio ($\dot{V}/\dot{Q}$) mismatching, a significant shunt fraction, and contributing lung microthrombi causing impaired hypoxic pulmonary vasoconstriction [19]. Prone positioning is beneficial in invasively ventilated ARDS patients, and there is emerging evidence for awake self-prone positioning [19, 20]. When we have used CPAP by the mask interface, compliance has been an issue in some cases. This has previously been reported [21–23]. A mask limits head position in a self-prone strategy. HFNO device tolerance and thus, by implication, better compliance and reduced frustration-led patient interface disconnections are also likely to confer relative healthcare worker protection. Prior to COVID-19, it was not our usual practice to use CPAP in this setting and this may have influenced our perception. Similar cases have started to be reported [24–31]. HFNO cannot change the natural course of viral pneumonia, but neither can intubation, and CPAP/NIV has not previously been recommended [32]. In patients not responding to supplemental oxygen with improved PaO_2, there is more likely to be a significant intrapulmonary shunt and invasive ventilation is probably required imminently, but in supplemental oxygen responders, the pathophysiology is predominantly ventilation-perfusion mismatching. Arterial oxygenation can be safely sustained with oxygen therapy in this latter group [33].

The early National Institute for Health and Care Excellence (NICE) COVID-19 rapid guideline advised that when an adult is admitted to hospital, an early assessment of frailty is made which can be either individualised or by the Clinical Frailty Scale score [34] as part of determining disposition.

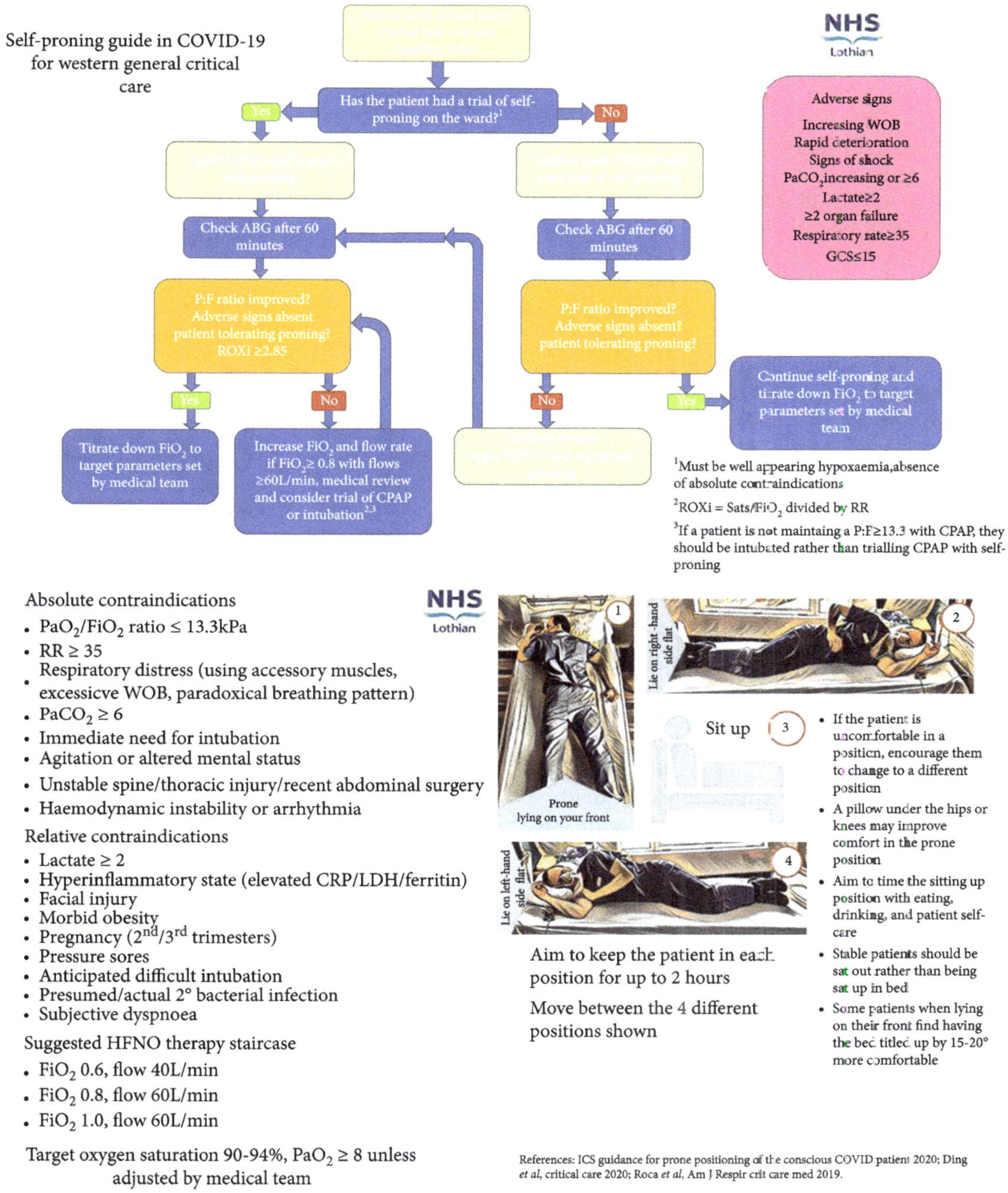

FIGURE 4: Western General Hospital, Edinburgh, NHS Lothian, NHS Scotland. Awake self-prone guideline.

HFNO is established in critical care [12, 35, 36]. Combination therapy in ARDS with prone positioning is described [37]. FLORALI publication in 2015 made it clear that intubation should not be delayed [12, 38]. Persistence with noninvasive methods can result in patient self-inflicted lung injury [7, 19, 39]. A key question from the FLORALI papers was whether HFNO could prevent intubation. However, it is important to consider that most patients in this trial had pneumonia and did not all meet the current criteria for ARDS. Therefore, the results may not be generalisable to all patients with hypoxemic respiratory failure. Yet this study did suggest that HFNO is noninferior to other oxygen delivery methods including noninvasive ventilation (NIV/CPAP) in reducing the subsequent need for intubation. HFNO reduced ICU and 90-day mortality compared with other strategies. It also subjectively improved dyspnoea and respiratory discomfort, important for patient experience, at 1 hour compared with the other oxygen delivery devices [38].

The UK National Health Service (NHS) has published COVID-19 guidance [40, 41]. It is recommended that NIV (including HFNO) is delivered in a negative pressure room with air exchanges greater than 10 cycles per hour or in an air-cycled neutral pressure room or side room. In anticipation of the first COVID-19 patients being admitted, our unit was sealed and modified for full droplet precaution. We use filtering facepiece 3 (FFP3) plus visor and fluid-resistant gown PPE and have greater than 50% of beds in single occupancy rooms.

Where there is no adequate response, where clinical decline continues, or where patient tolerance limits use, early intubation and mechanical ventilation should be pursued where appropriate. In COVID-19 with full FFP3 PPE, human factor challenges are compounded by staff training challenges (redeployment in the pandemic), fatigue, and the visual and hearing cue limitations associated with masks and visors. This amalgamates to make ICU intubation more difficult and possibly more hazardous than usual. Where intubation is not needed, it can be argued that consequently the clinician is protected from intubation risks and we can consider the resource-saving benefit to the broader population. The ROX index may play a predictive role in identifying failing HFNO and need for intubation. Whilst it lacks external validity, it utilises three bedside observations (SpO_2, FiO_2, and RR) to standardise the degree of hypoxic respiratory failure [42–44]. We consider this to be additionally helpful in our local guidance for trialling self-prone positioning in critical care (Figure 4), based on Intensive Care Society guidance [45].

We have not used HFNO outside of critical care. This helped both in the monitoring of total hospital oxygen usage and in the advocated approach of using it as a targeted, duration-limited therapy with a clear escalation or deescalation exit strategy based on both clinical judgement and understanding of oxygen infrastructure. HFNO should be confined to use where regular review and goal setting are possible. Consideration needs to be given to current patient numbers on oxygen in the hospital and the hospital infrastructure including the capacity of the Vacuum Insulated Evaporator (VIE) and cylinder manifolds as well as the hospital pipework flow capacity. In an audit of our own unit's oxygen consumption, we found marked differences between invasively ventilated patients and those on HFNO, FiO_2 0.43 (IQR 0.41-0.45) vs. 0.55 (IQR 0.48-0.60) ($p = 0.029$) for invasive ventilation vs. HFNO, respectively, and fresh oxygen flow rates of 3.0 (IQR 2.6-3.2) vs. 18.4 (IQR 14.4-25.9) L/min ($p = 0.029$) for invasive ventilation vs. HFNO, respectively. Clearly, the use of HFNO has significant resource implications and may not be deliverable in all infrastructures. Indeed, the latent heat of vaporisation of oxygen to convert from liquid to gas through the superheater takes atmospheric energy to change the oxygen phase, with the air-water vapour losing so much energy that it condenses and in excess freezes. Under normal operating conditions, the VIE utilises this latent heat to keep cool, but if usage is high, the temperature in the evaporator will fall too much so that the regulators governing the pipeline pressure will no longer function correctly. The excess demand due to overwhelming case numbers in the COVID-19 pandemic has led to reports of hospital oxygen systems freezing and failing [4, 46, 47].

Organised trials are now needed. RECOVERY-RS (ISRCTN16912075) will look at three different approaches to providing ventilatory support, including HFNO, to patients suspected or confirmed COVID-19. Hopefully, many of the uncertainties of how best to provide noninvasive respiratory support will be answered in a relatively homogeneous population, at least compared with previous studies in ARDS.

4. Conclusions

A one-size-fits-all approach to hypoxemic respiratory failure is not possible. We provide data to show that HFNO has a role in selected units and patients alongside real-time oxygen infrastructure consideration. HFNO is possibly suited to and more efficacious with self-prone positioning. A clear plan must be in place to determine the threshold for the failure of HFNO and escalation to intubation and invasive mechanical ventilation, if appropriate. In deciding not to use HFNO due to potential aerosolization concerns, the clinician is committing to alternative therapies that have their own associated risks including aerosolization [48–50].

Consent

Written consent for publication was obtained from the patient for the publication of the case report.

Authors' Contributions

The contributions of the authors involved in this study are as follows: Kieran P Nunn: conceptualization, writing–original draft preparation, and verified data; Murray J Blackstock: writing–reviewing and editing; Ryan Ellis: visualization, investigation, writing, and verified data; Gauhar Sheikh: visualization, investigation, and verified data; Alastair Morgan: reviewing and wrote our self-prone critical care guideline; and Jonathan KJ Rhodes: writing–reviewing and editing, supervision, and verified data.

Acknowledgments

The authors acknowledge the following: evidence search: High Flow Nasal Oxygen in treating SARS-CoV-2 COVID-19 Disease (coronavirus); Amanda Wright (COVID19 Knowledge Service) (date search completed: 17.06.20), NHS Greater Glasgow & Clyde Library Network; and Dr. Alan Simms, Consultant Radiologist, Department of Radiology, Western General Hospital Edinburgh, advising and preparing anonymised images for publication.

References

[1] L. Barrot, P. Asfar, F. Mauny et al., "Liberal or conservative oxygen therapy for acute respiratory distress syndrome," *The New England Journal of Medicine*, vol. 382, no. 11, pp. 999–1008, 2020.

[2] W. Alhazzani, M. H. Møller, Y. M. Arabi et al., "Surviving Sepsis Campaign: guidelines on the management of critically ill adults with coronavirus disease 2019 (COVID-19)," *Intensive Care Medicine*, vol. 46, no. 5, pp. 854–887, 2020.

[3] S. R. Wilcox, "Management of respiratory failure due to COVID-19," *BMJ*, vol. 369, article m1786, 2020.

[4] Incident Reporting & Investigation Centre (IRIC) NHS National Services Scotland, "Safety Action Notice. Protection of hospital oxygen pipeline systems through managed distribution of oxygen-dependent patients (COVID-19). SAN(SC)20/05," 2020. http://www.nhsnss.org.

[5] 2020, https://www.google.com/url?sa=t&rct=j&q=&esrc=s&source=web&cd=4&cad=rja&uact=8&ved=2ahUKEwjBoaXzmrbpAhUNRhUIHV33BykQFjADegQIBBAB&url=https%3A%2F%2Fwww.england.nhs.uk%2Fwp-content%2Fuploads%2F2020%2F04%2FFINAL-NatPSA-Interuption-of-HFNO-during-transfer-April-2020-v3.pdf&usg=AOvVaw0U8M3Ncs18FR7aqtsHtvHk.

[6] COVID-19 Treatment Guidelines Panel, "Coronavirus disease 2019 (COVID-19) treatment guidelines. National Institutes of Health," 2020, https://www.covid19treatmentguidelines.nih.gov/.

[7] World Health Organization, "Clinical management of severe acute respiratory infection (SARI) when COVID-19 disease is suspected," 2020, http://www.who.int/publications-detail/clinical-management-of-severe-acute-respiratory-infection-when-novel-coronavirus-(ncov)-infection-is-suspected.

[8] ANZICS COVID-19 Working Group, "The Australian and New Zealand Intensive Care Society COVID-19 guidelines (version 1)," 2020, http://www.anzics.com.au/wp-content/uploads/2020/03/ANZICS-COVID-19-Guidelines-Version-1.pdf.

[9] ANZICS COVID-19 Working Group, "The Australian and New Zealand Intensive Care Society COVID-19 guidelines (version 2)," 2020, http://www.anzics.com.au/wp-content/uploads/2020/03/ANZICS-COVID-19-Guidelines-Version-1.pdf.

[10] "2020 National COVID-19 Clinical Evidence Taskforce," 2020, https://covid19evidence.net.au/.

[11] Faculty of Intensive Care Medicine, Intensive Care Society, Association of Anaesthetists and Royal College of Anaesthetists, "Critical care preparation and management in the COVID-19 pandemic," 2020, http://www.icmanaesthesiacovid-19.org/critical-care-preparation-and-management-in-the-covid-19-pandemic.

[12] B. L. Ferreyro, F. Angriman, L. Munshi et al., "Association of noninvasive oxygenation strategies with all-cause mortality in adults with acute hypoxemic respiratory failure: a systematic review and meta-analysis," *JAMA*, vol. 324, no. 1, pp. 57–67, 2020.

[13] K. A. Samuelson, D. Lundberg, and B. Fridlund, "Stressful memories and psychological distress in adult mechanically ventilated intensive care patients - a 2-month follow-up study," *Acta Anaesthesiologica Scandinavica*, vol. 51, no. 6, pp. 671–678, 2007.

[14] H. Myhren, O. Ekeberg, K. Tøien, S. Karlsson, and O. Stokland, "Posttraumatic stress, anxiety and depression symptoms in patients during the first year post intensive care unit discharge," *Critical Care*, vol. 14, no. 1, article R14, 2010.

[15] A. Agarwal, J. Basmaji, F. Muttalib et al., "High-flow nasal cannula for acute hypoxemic respiratory failure in patients with COVID-19: systematic reviews of effectiveness and its risks of aerosolization, dispersion, and infection transmission," *Canadian Journal of Anesthesia/Journal canadien d'anesthésie*, vol. 67, no. 9, pp. 1217–1248, 2020.

[16] D. S. Hui, B. K. Chow, T. Lo et al., "Exhaled air dispersion during high-flow nasal cannula therapy *versus* CPAP *via* different masks," *European Respiratory Journal*, vol. 53, no. 4, article 1802339, 2019.

[17] J. Li, J. B. Fink, and S. Ehrmann, "High-flow nasal cannula for COVID-19 patients: low risk of bio-aerosol dispersion," *European Respiratory Journal*, vol. 55, no. 5, article 2000892, 2020.

[18] C. Lyons and M. Callaghan, "The use of high-flow nasal oxygen in COVID-19," *Anaesthesia*, vol. 75, no. 7, pp. 843–847, 2020.

[19] I. Telias, B. H. Katira, and L. Brochard, "Is the prone position helpful during spontaneous breathing in patients with COVID-19?," *JAMA*, vol. 323, no. 22, pp. 2265–2267, 2020.

[20] X. Elharrar, Y. Trigui, A. M. Dols et al., "Use of prone positioning in nonintubated patients with COVID-19 and hypoxemic acute respiratory failure," *JAMA*, vol. 323, no. 22, pp. 2336–2338, 2020.

[21] P. G. Catcheside, "Predictors of continuous positive airway pressure adherence," *F1000 Medicine Reports*, vol. 2, 2010.

[22] J. S. Virk and B. Kotecha, "When continuous positive airway pressure (CPAP) fails," *Journal of Thoracic Disease*, vol. 8, no. 10, pp. E1112–E1121, 2016.

[23] British Thoracic Society Standards of Care Committee, "Non-invasive ventilation in acute respiratory failure," *Thorax*, vol. 57, no. 3, pp. 192–211, 2002.

[24] A. J. Ciment and L. M. Ciment, "A 55-year-old COVID-19-positive man managed with self-regulation of high-flow oxygen by high-velocity nasal insufflation therapy," *Respirol Case Rep.*, vol. 8, no. 5, article e00591, 2020.

[25] C. Despres, Y. Brunin, F. Berthier, S. Pili-Floury, and G. Besch, "Prone positioning combined with high-flow nasal or conventional oxygen therapy in severe Covid-19 patients," *Critical Care*, vol. 24, no. 1, p. 256, 2020.

[26] S. Geng, Q. Mei, C. Zhu et al., "High flow nasal cannula is a good treatment option for COVID-19," *Heart & Lung*, vol. 49, no. 5, pp. 444-445, 2020.

[27] G. He, Y. Han, Q. Fang et al., "Clinical experience of high-flow nasal cannula oxygen therapy in severe COVID-19 patients," *Journal of Zhejiang University (Medical Science)*, vol. 49, no. 2, pp. 232–239, 2020.

[28] V. Karamouzos, F. Fligou, C. Gogos, and D. Velissaris, "High flow nasal cannula oxygen therapy in adults with COVID-19 respiratory failure. A case report," *Monaldi Archives for Chest Disease*, vol. 90, no. 2, 2020.

[29] A. S. Rali, K. R. Nunna, C. Howard, J. P. Herlihy, and K. K. Guntupalli, "High-flow nasal cannula oxygenation revisited in COVID-19," *Cardiac Failure Review*, vol. 6, 2020.

[30] the Critical Care Western Research Group, M. Slessarev, J. Cheng, M. Ondrejicka, and R. Arntfield, "Patient self-proning with high-flow nasal cannula improves oxygenation in COVID-19 pneumonia," *Canadian Journal of Anesthesia/Journal canadien d'anesthésie*, vol. 67, no. 9, pp. 1288–1290, 2020.

[31] Q. Xu, T. Wang, X. Qin, Y. Jie, L. Zha, and W. Lu, "Early awake prone position combined with high-flow nasal oxygen therapy in severe COVID-19: a case series," *Critical Care*, vol. 24, no. 1, p. 250, 2020.

[32] S. A. Namendys-Silva, "Respiratory support for patients with COVID-19 infection," *The Lancet Respiratory Medicine*, vol. 8, no. 4, 2020.

[33] M. J. Tobin, "Basing respiratory management of COVID-19 on physiological principles," *American Journal of Respiratory and Critical Care Medicine*, vol. 201, no. 11, pp. 1319-1320, 2020.

[34] "National Institute for Health and Care Excellence (NICE) COVID-19 rapid guideline: critical care in adults," 2020, https://www.nice.org.uk/guidance/ng159.

[35] B. K. Patel, J. P. Kress, and J. B. Hall, "Alternatives to invasive ventilation in the COVID-19 pandemic," *JAMA*, vol. 324, no. 1, pp. 43-44, 2020.

[36] B. Rochwerg, D. Granton, D. X. Wang et al., "High flow nasal cannula compared with conventional oxygen therapy for acute hypoxemic respiratory failure: a systematic review and meta-analysis," *Intensive Care Medicine*, vol. 45, pp. 563–572, 2019.

[37] L. Ding, L. Wang, W. Ma, and H. He, "Efficacy and safety of early prone positioning combined with HFNC or NIV in moderate to severe ARDS: a multi-center prospective cohort study," *Critical Care*, vol. 24, no. 1, p. 28, 2020.

[38] J. P. Frat, A. W. Thille, A. Mercat et al., "High-flow oxygen through nasal cannula in acute hypoxemic respiratory failure," *The New England Journal of Medicine*, vol. 372, no. 23, pp. 2185–2196, 2015.

[39] L. Brochard, A. Slutsky, and A. Pesenti, "Mechanical ventilation to minimize progression of lung injury in acute respiratory failure," *American Journal of Respiratory and Critical Care Medicine*, vol. 195, no. 4, pp. 438–442, 2017.

[40] NHS England and NHS Improvement, "Guidance for the role and use of non-invasive respiratory support in adult patients with coronavirus (confirmed or suspected) 26 March 2020 Version 2," 2020, https://www.england.nhs.uk/coronavirus/wp-content/uploads/sites/52/2020/03/CLEARED_Specialty-guide_-NIV-respiratory-support-and-coronavirus-v2-26-March-003.pdf.

[41] NHS England, *Specialty guides for patient management during the coronavirus pandemic. Guidance for the role and use of non-invasive respiratory support in adult patients with COVID-19 (confirmed or suspected) 6 April 2020, Version 3*, https://www.england.nhs.uk/coronavirus/secondary-care/other-resources/specialty-guides/.

[42] O. Roca, B. Caralt, J. Messika et al., "An index combining respiratory rate and oxygenation to predict outcome of nasal high-flow therapy," *American Journal of Respiratory and Critical Care Medicine*, vol. 199, no. 11, pp. 1368–1376, 2019.

[43] O. Roca, J. Messika, B. Caralt et al., "Predicting success of high-flow nasal cannula in pneumonia patients with hypoxemic respiratory failure: the utility of the ROX index," *Journal of Critical Care*, vol. 35, pp. 200–205, 2016.

[44] E. Spinelli, O. Roca, and T. Mauri, "Dynamic assessment of the ROX index during nasal high flow for early identification of non-responders," *Journal of Critical Care*, vol. 58, no. 19, pp. 130-131, 2020.

[45] P. Bamford, A. Bentley, J. Dean, D. Whitmore, and N. Wilson-Baig, *ICS guidance for prone positioning of the conscious COVID patient 2020*, Intensive Care Society, London, 2020.

[46] NHS England and NHS Improvement Estates & Facilities Patient Safety Alert 2020/001, "Use of hospital CPAP during coronavirus epidemic," 2020, https://www.cas.mhra.gov.uk/ViewandAcknowledgment/ViewAlert.aspx?AlertID=103013.

[47] R. Moonesinghe, A. Menzies-Gow, and A. Eggleton, "Estates and Facilities Alert. NHSE/I – 2020/001," 2020, https://www.cas.mhra.gov.uk/ViewandAcknowledgment/ViewAttachment.aspx?Attachment_id=103492.

[48] J. C. Winck and N. Ambrosino, "COVID-19 pandemic and non invasive respiratory management: every Goliath needs a David. An evidence based evaluation of problems," *Pulmonology*, vol. 26, no. 4, pp. 213–220, 2020.

[49] R. Canelli, C. W. Connor, M. Gonzalez, A. Nozari, and R. Ortega, "Barrier enclosure during endotracheal intubation," *The New England Journal of Medicine*, vol. 382, no. 20, pp. 1957-1958, 2020.

[50] K. El-Boghdadly, D. J. N. Wong, R. Owen et al., "Risks to healthcare workers following tracheal intubation of patients with COVID-19: a prospective international multicentre cohort study," *Anaesthesia*, vol. 75, no. 11, pp. 1437–1447, 2020.

42

Use of Continuous Intravenous Anakinra Infusion in Multisystem Inflammatory Syndrome in Children

Abdulaziz Alolayan,[1] Abdullah S. Aldamegh,[2] and Azzah Alkhayrat[1]

[1]*Pharmacy Department, Prince Sultan Military Medical City, Saudi Arabia*
[2]*Pediatrics Department, Unaizah College of Medicine and Medical Sciences, Al-Qassim University, Saudi Arabia*

Correspondence should be addressed to Abdulaziz Alolayan; azoz.alolayan@hotmail.com

Academic Editor: Luca Gallelli

Coronavirus disease (COVID-19) is an emergency pandemic with a high mortality rate worldwide. One of its complications in children is developing multisystemic inflammatory syndrome related to cytokine storm. Anakinra is a recombinant human interleukin-1 (IL-1) receptor antagonist used to suppress the exaggerated inflammatory response in such conditions, and it is potentially lifesaving in a cytokine storm. We present the case of a patient with critical COVID-19 associated with multisystem inflammatory syndrome in children (MIS-C) successfully treated with anakinra intravenous (IV) infusion.

1. Introduction

During the COVID-19 pandemic, there has been an increase in reports of the pediatric severe acute respiratory syndrome (SARS) related to multi-inflammatory disorders. Moreover, it is known as MIS-C associated with COVID-19, which shares some clinical characteristics with Kawasaki disease (KD) [1–3]. Kawasaki disease's clinical characteristics are persistent fever, bulbar conjunctivitis, skin rash, or mucosal involvement [4]. They present with respiratory and gastrointestinal symptoms in the form of severe disease action. At the same time, some cases are ending in macrophage activation syndrome (MAS) [5–10]. It has implied that the syndrome results from hyperinflammation caused by a cytokine storm [11]. Anakinra is an IL-1 receptor antagonist used for some rheumatoid diseases and other inflammatory conditions [12, 13]. Updated published data announced the effectiveness and safety of anakinra in reducing mortality and acute care admission in patients with COVID-19 associated with MIS-C. Anakinra dose studied for MIS-C is from 5-10 mg/kg/day subcutaneously (SC) daily or in divided doses, and higher doses might be considered [14–17]. Some studies showed that the feasibility of using IV administration of anakinra instead of SC supported its efficacy and safety [18, 19]. Monteagudo et al. demonstrated that the utilization of continuous IV anakinra infusion dose reached up to 2400 mg/day resulting in rapid serologic and subsequent clinical improvement in adult patients with MAS. Their study notified that anakinra has short and unclear stability in solution based on the manufacture leaflet. Therefore, the prepared solution was infused over a maximum of 8 hours [20]. Due to the lack of evidence, we report our experience using continuous IV infusion of anakinra for refractory MIS-C in a tertiary care hospital center.

2. Case Report

On January 16, 2022, a fourteen-month girl was brought to the emergency room of Prince Sultan Military Medical City (PSMMC) with a history of fever and cough for four days that worsened in the last two days and was associated with a decrease in the level of activity. She had a positive history of contact with sick family members with respiratory symptoms; however, it was not investigated for COVID-19. The fever initially subsided by paracetamol IV (15 mg/kg/dose) every 6 hours and then became persistent, ranging from 39–40°C. She has a known case of craniosynostosis, gastroesophageal reflux disease, and global developmental delay

TABLE 1: Laboratory characteristics of patient.

	Day 1 Hospital admission	Day 3 Pediatric ICU admission	Day 14 2nd steroid pulse therapy	Day 26 Discharge from pediatric ICU
WBC count (×109/L)	3.20	6.0	16.9	13.34
Lymphocyte count (×109/L)	1.16	1.43	7.1	2.77
Hemoglobin (g/L)	11.5	9.1	9.2	10.2
PLT count (×109/L)	60	95	178	224
Ferritin (mg/L)	2028	901	6933	413
CRP (mg/dL)	141	34	8.52	7.72
AST (U/L)	526	195	112	44
ALT (U/L)	206	80	114	36
GGT (U/L)	242	227	207	430
LDH (U/L)	>1800	1295	602	281
Fibrinogen (g/L)	5.3	2.5	4	3.9
D-dimer ng/mL)	4630	2080	2960	520

that are under investigation. Infection with COVID-19 was confirmed by reverse transcription polymerase chain reaction (RT-PCR) on the nasopharyngeal swab, and chest X-ray (CXR) showed infiltration mainly on the left side. The lab results are shown in Table 1.

The patient initially had been inserted on noninvasive ventilation, "high flow nasal cannula," supportive care and started on antimicrobials amoxicillin-clavulanic acid IV (90 mg/kg/day) as empirical therapy until full investigation become resulted and remdesivir IV (5 mg/kg as loading dose and then 2.5 mg/kg/daily) for viral infection. On day two, the patient had been successfully weaned from the nasal cannula (NC). However, later, the patient's condition had been worsened as oxygen saturation reached 78%, and CXR showed a collapse in her left lower lob and consolidation of the right mid and lower zones. Therefore, she had been admitted to the pediatric intensive care unit (PICU) and started on continuous positive airway pressure (CPAP) at 8 and fractional inspired oxygen (FiO2) at 100%; antibiotic was upgraded from amoxicillin-clavulanic acid to piperacillin-tazobactam IV (300 mg/kg/day) to treat hospital-acquired infection because the patient's condition was seemed to be a picture of sepsis. CXR was repeated and showed bilateral collapse. CPAP increased to nine, and FiO_2 was 100%. Later, the patient's oxygen was desaturated (75%-80%), with significant suprasternal and subcostal retractions. As a result, she had been intubated through high-frequency oscillatory ventilation (HFOV) because the patient's condition deteriorated with a picture of acute respiratory distress syndrome (ARDS). The patient had been paralyzed and sedated. Antibiotics were upgraded to meropenem IV (60 mg/kg/day) and vancomycin IV (60 mg/kg/day), and the rheumatology team had been consulted for possible complications of COVID-19 with MIS-C. Methylprednisolone pulse therapy had been suggested to start and was already given (30 mg/kg) by IV due to the deterioration of the patient's condition.

On day three, systolic blood pressure dropped to 50, diastolic to 28, and mean arterial pressure became 37. Vasopressors had been given for one day only. An echocardiogram was done and showed moderate pericardial effusion, and pro-BNP reached 2093 pg/mL. MIS-C was confirmed based on the lab results and clinical condition. IV immunoglobulin (IVIG) had been given on day three for a total of two doses. Methylprednisolone pulse therapy had been completed for five days and then shifted to maintenance dose. On day four, the patient's condition still had not improved. So the rheumatology team recommended to start anakinra SC (8 mg/kg/day), and by the next day, the dose had been titrated up, and the route of administration shifted to IV push. On day 10, the patient still had not improved. Based on Monteagudo et al.'s study, the dose and the route of anakinra had been shifted from IV push to IV infusion to (12 mg/kg/day) over 24 hours. Furthermore, due to the instability of IV preparation, the medication had been prepared in separate bags to be run for 8 hours and diluted in sodium chloride 0.9%. On day 14, another corticosteroid pulse therapy had been given for three days. On day 22, the patient's condition had been improved, and the respiratory therapy had been shifted from HFOV to synchronized intermittent mandatory ventilation(SIMV). On day 25, the patient was extubated to NC. A sharp reduction of inflammatory markers and ferritin is observed in Table 1.

Respiratory parameters had been improved, followed by a favorable radiographic evolution. On day 26, the patient discharged from the ICU. Tapering of methylprednisolone dose was planned, and anakinra shifted to the SC (4 mg/kg/daily). Recently, the patient was discharged on room air and has been followed up with the rheumatology team as outpatient clinic. During the ICU admission, full panel of septic work up had been requested including virus PCRs, and patient infected only with *Stenotrophomonas maltophilia* through tube as secondary to COVID-19 infections, and treated with co-trimoxazole IV (20 mg/kg/day). Meropenem and vancomycin were discontinued after finding the final results. Antifungal also had been started from day seven for eight days to rule out fungal infection due to worsening condition.

3. Discussion

To our knowledge, this is the first report of a severe case of COVID-19 related to MIS-C effectively treated with anakinra IV infusion. Lately, a cytokine storm has been associated with the critical stage of COVID-19, resulting in hyperinflammatory effects, with suspicion of poor prognosis [21]. Hyperinflammatory syndrome is described by life-threatening hypercytokinemia leading to multiorgan failure. A retrospective multicenter study found that the mortality rate of 190 confirmed COVID-19 cases in Wuhan was associated with COVID-19-driven hyperinflammation [22]. In cytokine storms, IL-1β appears to be one of the significant proinflammatory markers. Anakinra is an antagonist of the IL-1β receptor, which inhibits the release of IL-1β from macrophages. Schmitz et al.'s study shows that the blockage of IL-1 has been associated with the reversal of acute lung injury in avian influenza [23]. Fingerhutová et al.'s study demonstrated that aggressive therapy of MAS using continuous IV anakinra infusions in higher doses successfully reverses the cytokine storm, especially in the pediatric population [24]. In the case of our patient, treatment with different modalities like upgrading antibiotics, two courses of corticosteroid, IVIG, and SQ with IV push of anakinra did not provide clinical improvement immediately. In contrast, using anakinra IV infusion with a higher dose showed a synergic effect in improvement. However, a possible benefit due to the late effect of these modalities, late effect cannot be ruled out. Although the solid evidence-based studies of anakinra did not test the feasibility of using IV infusion, our case report showed promising efficacy of anakinra IV infusion, and no severe side effects appeared during ICU admission.

4. Conclusion

During COVID-19, whether moderate or severe, there are many challenges in the way of therapeutic plans, and using anakinra is one of them. Our case suggests that administering IV infusion of anakinra in cytokine storm related to MIS-C contributed to a significant clinical improvement, is workable, and has a safe profile.

Consent

Written informed consent was obtained from legal guardian.

Acknowledgments

This research was supported by the Prince Sultan Military Medical City, Research Center.

References

[1] K. Chiotos, H. Bassiri, E. M. Behrens et al., "Multisystem inflammatory syndrome in children during the coronavirus 2019 Pandemic: a case series," *Journal of the Pediatric Infectious Diseases Society*, vol. 9, no. 3, pp. 393–398, 2020.

[2] Centre for Disease Control and Prevention, *Emergency preparedness and response multisystem in ammatory syndrome in children (MIS-C) associated with coronavirus disease 2019*, 2020.

[3] Royal College of Pediatrics and Child Health, "Guidance: paediatric multisystem inflammatory syndrome temporally associated with COVID-19," in Paediatric multisystem inflammatory syndrome temporally associated with covid-19 (PIMS) - guidance for clinicians, 2020, https://www.rcpch.ac.uk/sites/default/files/2020-05/COVID-19-Paediatric-multisystem-inflammatorysyndrome-20200501.pdf.

[4] L. R. Feldstein, E. B. Rose, S. M. Horwitz et al., "Multisystem inflammatory syndrome in U.S. children and adolescents," *The New England Journal of Medicine*, vol. 383, no. 4, pp. 334–346, 2020.

[5] L. Verdoni, A. Mazza, A. Gervasoni et al., "An outbreak of severe Kawasaki-like disease at the Italian epicentre of the SARS-CoV-2 epidemic: an observational cohort study," *The Lancet*, vol. 395, no. 10239, pp. 1771–1778, 2020.

[6] Z. Belhadjer, M. Méot, F. Bajolle et al., "Acute heart failure in multisystem inflammatory syndrome in children in the context of global SARS-CoV-2 pandemic," *Circulation*, vol. 142, no. 5, pp. 429–436, 2020.

[7] M. Grimaud, J. Starck, M. Levy et al., "Acute myocarditis and multisystem inflammatory emerging disease following SARS-CoV-2 infection in critically ill children," *Annals of Intensive Care*, vol. 10, no. 1, p. 69, 2020.

[8] A. Wolfler, S. Mannarino, V. Giacomet, A. Camporesi, and G. Zuccotti, "Acute myocardial injury: a novel clinical pattern in children with COVID-19," *The Lancet Child & Adolescent Health*, vol. 4, no. 8, pp. e26–e27, 2020.

[9] E. Whittaker, A. Bamford, J. Kenny et al., "Clinical characteristics of 58 children with a pediatric inflammatory multisystem syndrome temporally associated with SARS-CoV-2," *Journal of the American Medical Association*, vol. 324, no. 3, pp. 259–269, 2020.

[10] J. Toubiana, C. Poirault, A. Corsia et al., "Kawasaki-like multisystem inflammatory syndrome in children during the COVID-19 pandemic in Paris, France: prospective observational study," *BMJ*, vol. 369, article m2094, 2020.

[11] T. Tanner and D. M. Wahezi, "Hyperinflammation and the utility of immunomodulatory medications in children with COVID-19," *Paediatric Respiratory Reviews*, vol. 35, pp. 81–87, 2020.

[12] J. Ramírez and J. D. Cañete, "Anakinra for the treatment of rheumatoid arthritis: a safety evaluation," *Expert Opinion on Drug Safety*, vol. 17, no. 7, pp. 727–732, 2018.

[13] C. J. Fisher Jr., J.-F. A. Dhainaut, S. M. Opal et al., "Recombinant human interleukin 1 receptor antagonist in the treatment of patients with sepsis syndrome. Results from a randomized, double-blind, placebo-controlled trial. Phase III rhIL-1ra Sepsis Syndrome Study Group," *JAMA: The Journal of the American Medical Association*, vol. 271, no. 23, pp. 1836–1843, 1994.

[14] T. Huet, H. Beaussier, O. Voisin et al., "Anakinra for severe forms of COVID-19: a cohort study," *The Lancet Rheumatology*, vol. 2, no. 7, pp. e393–e400, 2020.

[15] G. Cavalli, G. De Luca, C. Campochiaro et al., "Interleukin-1 blockade with high-dose anakinra in patients with COVID-19, acute respiratory distress syndrome, and hyperinflammation: a retrospective cohort study," *The Lancet Rheumatology*, vol. 2, no. 6, pp. e325–e331, 2020.

[16] G. Dimopoulos, Q. de Mast, N. Markou et al., "Favorable anakinra responses in severe COVID-19 patients with secondary hemophagocytic lymphohistiocytosis," *Cell Host & Microbe*, vol. 28, no. 1, pp. 117–23.e1, 2020.

[17] E. Khani, M. Shahrabi, H. Rezaei, F. Pourkarim, H. Afsharirad, and M. Solduzian, "Current evidence on the use of anakinra in COVID-19," *International Immunopharmacology*, vol. 111, article 109075, 2022.

[18] J. Galea, K. Ogungbenro, S. Hulme et al., "Intravenous anakinra can achieve experimentally effective concentrations in the central nervous system within a therapeutic time window: results of a dose-ranging study," *Journal of Cerebral Blood Flow and Metabolism*, vol. 31, no. 2, pp. 439–447, 2011.

[19] E. V. Granowitz, R. Porat, J. W. Mier et al., "Pharmacokinetics, safety and immunomodulatory effects of human recombinant interleukin-1 receptor antagonist in healthy humans," *Cytokine*, vol. 4, no. 5, pp. 353–360, 1992.

[20] L. A. Monteagudo, A. Boothby, and E. Gertner, "Continuous intravenous anakinra infusion to calm the cytokine storm in macrophage activation syndrome," *ACR Open Rheumatology*, vol. 2, no. 5, pp. 276–282, 2020.

[21] C. Huang, Y. Wang, X. Li et al., "Clinical features of patients infected with 2019 novel coronavirus in Wuhan, China," *The Lancet*, vol. 395, no. 10223, pp. 497–506, 2020.

[22] G. Grasselli, A. Pesenti, and M. Cecconi, "Critical care utilization for the COVID-19 outbreak in Lombardy, Italy," *JAMA*, vol. 323, no. 16, p. 1545, 2020.

[23] N. Schmitz, M. Kurrer, M. F. Bachmann, and M. Kopf, "Interleukin-1 is responsible for acute lung immunopathology but increases survival of respiratory influenza virus infection," *Journal of Virology*, vol. 79, no. 10, pp. 6441–6448, 2005.

[24] Š. Fingerhutová, E. Jančová, and P. Doležalová, "Anakinra in paediatric rheumatology and periodic fever clinics: is the higher dose safe?," *Frontiers in Pediatrics*, vol. 10, 2022.

A Rare Cause of a Rare Disorder: *E. coli*-Induced Purpura Fulminans Secondary to Urinary Tract Infection

Jacob Lowry[1] and Edva Noel[2]

[1]*Department of General Surgery, Atrium Health Navicent, 777 Hemlock St, Macon, GA 31201, USA*
[2]*Department of Nephrology, Temple University Hospital, 3440 N. Broad Street, Kresge West, Suite 100, PA 19004, USA*

Correspondence should be addressed to Edva Noel; edvanoel@gmail.com

Academic Editor: Silvia Natoli

Purpura fulminans is a devastating thrombotic disorder infrequently encountered in medical practice and amongst the medical literature. It is a hematologic emergency in which prompt recognition and initiation of treatment are critical to mitigate its significant morbidity and mortality. Surgical evaluation is commonly required, since the debilitating skin and soft tissue necrosis often degenerate into necrotizing fasciitis, critical limb ischemia, warranting surgical interventions in either a staged or single-step approach. Purpura fulminans can be neonatal, infectious, or idiopathic. Infection-induced purpura fulminans is less common, and only a few microorganisms have been associated with this condition: *Meningococcus* spp., *Pneumococcus* spp., or *Staphylococcus* spp. This report presents a rare case of *Escherichia coli*-induced purpura fulminans. Apart from the unfortunate partial amputation of all left-hand five digits, our patient made a full recovery following effective infectious source control, supportive care with volume resuscitation, anticoagulation, and wound care.

1. Introduction

Purpura fulminans (PF) is a rapidly progressive thrombotic disorder that primarily affects the microvasculature of the integumentary system that quickly progresses to skin necrosis. It is associated with disseminated intravascular coagulation (DIC) with a thrombotic phenotype. Although DIC is commonly observed in the critical care setting (9-19% of patients), PF prevalence remains scarce overall [1, 2]. Neonatal, infectious, and idiopathic are the three known clinical presentations of PF. *Meningococcus* spp. and *Streptococcus* spp. account for most of the reported infectious cases [3]. PF represents a true hematologic emergency that, even if recognized and managed early, carries a mortality rate as high as 43% [4]. Current management focuses on supportive care and, in severe cases, surgical debridement or amputation secondary to serious cutaneous necrosis. We report a rare case of PF associated with *E. coli* septicemia along with a brief review of the pertinent literature regarding the pathophysiology, diagnosis, and management of PF.

2. Case Description

A 55-year-old African American female with medical history of hyperlipidemia, gastroesophageal reflux disease, and an anemia of unknown etiology who initially presented to an outlying hospital with complaints of left flank pain, dysuria, and malodorous urine for a few weeks. She is a nonsmoker, and her only home medications were dexlansoprazole and over-the-counter multiple vitamins. Her family history is remarkable for her father who died from heart disease and her mother and two siblings who are alive with no known health issues. Initial evaluation confirmed sepsis with a SOFA score of 1. Blood cultures and a urinalysis with reflex for culture were obtained, and empiric antibiotic with ceftriaxone was started. The remaining pertinent labs are summarized in Tables 1–3. A computed tomography scan of the abdomen and pelvis revealed a 5-mm obstructive left ureteral stone associated with hydronephrosis and perinephric stranding. A diagnosis of complicated pyelonephritis with sepsis was made. IV fluid resuscitation as per the sepsis

Table 1: Laboratory values upon initial presentation to our facility. Of note, patient remained on continuous heparin infusion during time of lab results.

Lab tests	Hospital day 1 (outlying hospital)	Hospital day 1 (this hospital)	Hospital day 5 (this hospital)	Units (normal range)
Hemoglobin	12.8	11.5	10.6	11.6-15 g/dL
Hematocrit	39.3	35.6	33.7	35.5-44.9%
White blood cell count	13.8 with 13% bands	55.96	19.9	3.4-10.8 K/mm^3
Platelets	203 (nadir 73)	92	288	150-379 K/mm^3
Sodium	140	143	137	135-145 mmol/L
Potassium	3.6	3.9	4.7	3.5-5 mmol/L
Chloride	110	111	104	95-105 mmol/L
Bicarbonate	24	24	24	23-29 mmol/L
Blood urea nitrogen	20	21	8	5-20 mg/dL
Creatinine	1.5	0.66	0.67	0.61.2 mg/dL
Albumin	4	2.7	2.9	3.5-4.8 g/dL
Aspartate aminotransferase	26	227	124	0-40 U/L
Alanine transferase	20	114	74	0-32 U/L
Lactate	6.8	1.5	2.2	Mmol/L
Creatinine phosphokinase	*	5976	1002	22-198 U/L
Activated partial thromboplastin time (PTT)	*	55.9 (on heparin drip)	65.5 (on heparin drip)	25-35 seconds
Prothrombin time (PT)	*	14.7	14.3	Seconds
International normalized ratio (INR)	*	1.2	1.15	N/a
D-dimer	*	13.95	3.66	<0.5 μg/mL
Total bilirubin	*	0.5	0.2	0.0-1.2 mg/dL
Fibrinogen	*	622	619	200-400 mg/dL
Haptoglobin	*	*	284	41-165 mg/dL
Antinuclear antibody (ANA) screen	*	*	Positive (RNP ab)	0.2 - 0.9 AU/mL
p/c-Antineutrophil cytoplasmic antibodies (ANCA)	*	*	0.2	<0.4 (negative)
Complement factors 3, 4	*	*	116, 21	82-193 mg/dL, 15-57 mg/dL
Protein S, functional:	*	*	79%	60-123%
Protein C, functional:	*	*	174%	70-130%

*Indicates lab value either not drawn or not available due to lab error.

Table 2: Urinalysis upon initial presentation to outside facility on April 19, 2021.

Urinalysis results	
Leukocyte esterase	Trace
WBC count	19/hpf
Nitrite	Negative
Bacteria	Trace

Table 3: Microscopic analysis of urine from initial sample at outside facility.

Microbiology and serology	
Urine culture	+*E. coli*
Blood culture	+*E. coli*
Hepatitis panel	Negative
HIV serology	Negative

guidelines was started. Urology service consulted and performed cystoscopy with ureteral stone removal and stent placement. Postoperatively, the patient became hypotensive requiring norepinephrine infusion; lactate increased to 6.8 mmol/L, with a SOFA score of 8. The antibiotics spectrum was broadened to piperacillin-tazobactam, and transfer to the critical care unit followed.

On admission day 2, the patient started developing purpuric skin lesions. On day 3, more acral ischemic discoloration was evident. The ischemia was worse on the left hand where a radial arterial line was inserted for accurate measurement of the blood pressure (Figure 1(a)). An arterial Doppler ultrasound confirmed a distal left radial thrombosis with preservation of the ulnar blood flow; the arterial line was discontinued, and intravenous infusion of heparin drip was started. The leukocytosis worsened to 43×10^3 /μL, platelets dropped to $73 \times 10^3/\mu$L, and D-dimer increased to 21.6 μg/mL, but fibrinogen remained elevated to 637 mg/dL. Due to her deteriorating condition, she was transferred to our hospital for vascular surgery evaluation and higher level of care.

Upon transferring to our hospital, she no longer required vasopressors. She was afebrile but in sinus tachycardia at 115 bpm. All repeat pertinent labs including urine and blood cultures are shown in Tables 1–3. The heparin infusion and the antibiotic regimen were continued. Microbiology data from the transferring hospital confirmed pan-sensitive *E. coli* in blood and urine cultures. The symmetric acral skin lesions rapidly spread proximally within hours and evolved into large hemorrhagic bullae. The clinical picture of anemia, thrombocytopenia, and abnormal coagulation panel was consistent with DIC. The typical purpuric skin lesions in the setting of *E. coli*-sepsis and DIC led to the diagnosis of PF. At this point, hematology, general surgery, and hand surgery consultations were obtained.

She was continued on antibiotic and completed 14 days of ceftriaxone from the first negative blood culture. After 14 days of presentation, the skin lesions began to regress and did not require extensive debridement. However, the left-hand ischemia progressed to dry gangrene of all five fingers. On hospital day 24, the patient underwent partial left-hand amputation of all five digits after full demarcation of the viable tissues (Figures 1(b)). The right-hand lesions were wholly resolved, and the bilateral lower extremities significantly improved but did require prolonged daily wound care. Figure 2 offers a timeline of the important events.

3. Discussion

Acute infectious PF most commonly occurs in the settings of an acute bacterial infection. *Meningococcus* spp., *Staphylococcus* spp., and *Pneumococcus* spp. in adults are the most common bacterial infections associated with PF [3]. Hyposplenia or asplenia may constitute an additional risk factor for *Pneumococcus* PF specifically. One study notes a 7-fold higher incidence of *S. pneumoniae*-induced PF than in eusplenia, despite vaccination in 35% of the patients with similar morbidity and mortality outcomes [5]. Rat models *in vivo* have also isolated one specific *Meningococcus* strain containing type IV pili that adheres to the endothelium with subsequent colony formation and microvascular thrombosis due to excessive protein C activation and a consumptive coagulopathy [6]. Type IV pili are found in 5 serotypes of *Neisseria meningitidis* A, B, C, W135, and Y, which may in part explain the petechial rash commonly observed [7]. Rare cases associated with measles virus, *Rickettsia* spp., and *Haemophilus influenzae* have also been reported in the medical literature [8]. *E. coli*-septicemia-associated PF is rare; only a handful of cases have been reported [9–11]. PF may occur because of an acute infection even in asymptomatic, afebrile, or otherwise well-appearing individuals from pediatrics to adults, but it may also transpire in the post-infectious setting. This would suggest that the severity of the disease, and therefore the quantitative load of microorganisms, is not as important as certain qualitative aspects of the microorganism that lead to the development of acute infectious FP.. In one isolated case report, pathogen-specific factors are hypothesized as a potential predisposition to PF with *E. coli* septicemia [10]. That report describes a case of *E. coli*-associated PF in a patient with a previous episode of *E. coli* bacteremia without DIC. While the source of the first bacteremia is not mentioned, the second episode is attributed to intestinal translocation favored by malnutrition following bariatric surgery. We did not run a genetic study on the pan-sensitive *E. coli* identified as the cause of the infection in our patient since this would not have affected our management. Our initial management focused on source controlled of the infection and anticoagulation.

Neonatal, idiopathic, and acute infectious purpura are the three clinical presentations described in this condition. Neonatal PF is associated with hereditary deficiency of innate anticoagulants, including protein S, Protein C, and antithrombin III. Idiopathic or chronic PF usually develops days to weeks following a bacterial or a viral infection. Although the exact pathophysiological mechanism responsible for triggering PF remains unclear, predisposing risk factors appear to be associated with either an inherited or acquired deficiency in the anticoagulation pathway. These deficiencies primarily affect protein S, protein C, and antithrombin III (AT-III).

The acquired deficiency in anticoagulant proteins in acute infectious PF appears to result from a combined effect of bacterial antigens and inflammatory cytokines [interleukin (IL)-1, IL-12, interferon gamma, and tumor necrosis factor (TNF)–α]. Similarly, autoimmune phenomena have been reported in the postinfectious pediatric population whereby IgG cross-reacts to protein S resulting in its severe deficiency [12]. Due to an unknown mechanism, autoimmune targeting of protein C appears to be quite rare [13]. Recombinant protein C has been successfully used in the treatment of acute infectious PF in case reports. It has also been the focus of a phase 2/3 prospective multicenter trial in patients with severe congenital protein C deficiency to treat hematological complications from the innate disease process, including PF, DIC, and other thromboembolic events [14–16]. The evidence suggests an efficacious advantage based on these results; however, significant concerns regarding hemorrhagic complications have been noted surrounding its use. Protein C recombinant therapy is an approved treatment only for congenital protein C deficiency and remains off-label in the management of PF currently.

Four key features of acute infectious PF are as follows: large purpuric skin lesions, fever, hypotension, and DIC. Any new skin lesion in the presence of DIC should raise high suspicion for PF and prompt immediate initiation of appropriate management (discussed below). The skin lesions in PF develop and evolve within hours. They are typically petechial initially then progress to large, non-blanching retiform purpura with skin necrosis and often large hemorrhagic bullae.

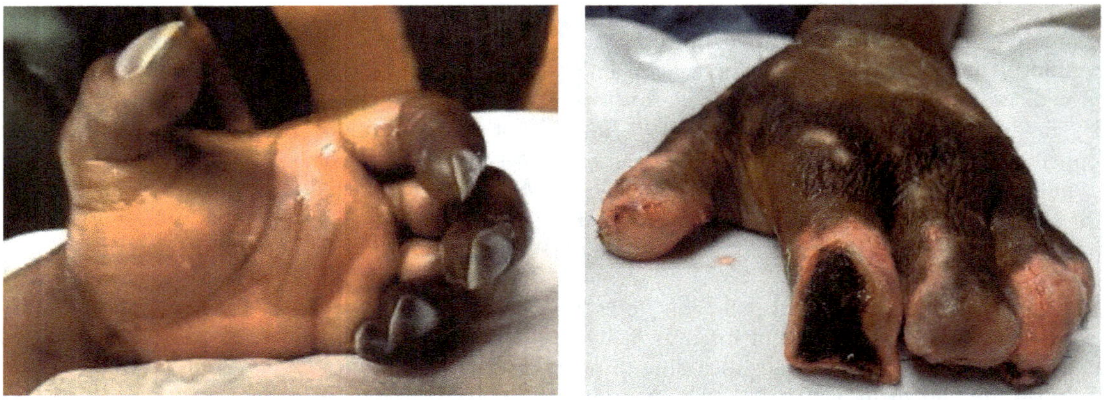

(a) (b)

FIGURE 1: (a) The left-hand ischemia with dry gangrene of all the five digits. Also noted is the bulla on the palmar aspect of the left hand. The dorsum aspect (not shown in this figure) also had a large bulla. (b) The left hand one week postamputation of all five digits.

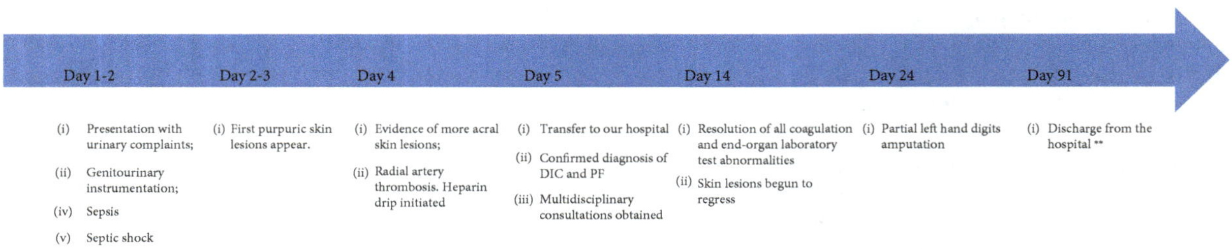

FIGURE 2: Timeline of the events summarizing the most important moments in the development and management of this patient. ** Prolonged discharge secondary to disposition issues.

The histopathology of these skin lesions often reveals thrombosis and extensive vascular damage: vascular congestion and dilation, endothelial necrosis, alteration of markers of endothelial integrity (CD31), and of the protein C pathway receptors (endothelial protein C receptor and thrombomodulin) [17]. It is worth underscoring that a skin biopsy is not necessary to make the diagnosis and may delay the prompt initiation of aggressive management of PF.

Our patient presented with flank pain due to ureterolithiasis and developed severe *E. coli* septicemia with shock requiring vasopressors following a urological instrumentation. Within 48 hours from the onset of sepsis, the first skin lesions appeared as a petechial rash. At that time, the patient was already exhibiting findings of DIC characterized by an elevated prothrombin time (PT) and aPTT, elevated D-dimer, and thrombocytopenia. In PF, the peripheral smear often shows a pattern of microangiopathic hemolytic anemia with schistocytes and helmet cells. Our patient's smear did not show schistocytes, but a DIC score per ISTH criteria was 5, which was high. The skin lesions rapidly evolved into large hemorrhagic bullae within 48 hours of appearance. TTP, HSP, and postinfectious thrombocytopenic purpura are all secondary skin lesions like PF but do not match the severity of the necrosis seen in our patient and therefore were ruled out. The case reported by Morales et al. is very similar to our case both in the presentation and the management [9]. Both cases highlight the importance of nurturing a high clinical suspicion for PF in the presence of purpuric skin lesions in septic patients even in the absence of a classic picture of DIC. In PF, the debilitating skin lesions often require extensive surgical debridement. In severe cases, limb amputation is necessary, resulting in significant disability, and in the worst cases, PF results in death [18].

For our patient, a multidisciplinary team composed of hematologists, surgeons, and wound care was assembled. Effective empiric antibiotic therapy was started along with aggressive volume resuscitation 30 mL/kg as per the sepsis guidelines. Initiation of systemic anticoagulation, preferably with heparin drip, has the potential to lessen the skin necrosis process, and the thrombotic burden in the medium-sized vessels is also pivotal in the management [19, 20]. Our patient was started on a continuous infusion of heparin that was monitored via aPTT with a target therapeutic range between 46 s and 70s. When a therapeutic aPPT level is difficult to attain despite a high dose of heparin, resistance to heparin should be considered. This situation, if it arises, should raise concerns for acquired protein C and ATIII deficiency. In such a case, co-administration of FFP or antithrombin III concentrate with protein C is reasonable [21]. We were able to easily achieve a therapeutic aPPT level in our patient. Hyperbaric oxygen (HBO) therapy has been used as an adjunctive treatment for chronic nonhealing wounds to promote healing [22]. Our patient's wounds progressed favorably with local care; they did not require extensive debridement; thus, we did not feel that HBO was necessary. In the medical literature, there is no mention of the type and duration of anticoagulation therapy for thrombosis in patients with PF without protein S or C or AT-III deficiency. Based on the current deep venous thrombosis management guidelines, our patient was continued on an oral direct thrombin inhibitor for an anticipated six months.

4. Conclusion

PF is an acute thrombotic hematologic emergency. Unfortunately, research has yet to establish the exact pathophysiological mechanism triggering its development. Current risk factors include infection by a select few microorganisms on the background of congenital or acquired anticoagulant deficiencies. In addition to its low overall incidence, diagnosis of PF, regardless of etiology, can prove difficult, especially in the critical care setting where skin lesions are frequent. The bacteria mentioned in this report demonstrate that the few encapsulated microorganisms with a well-documented link with PF may not be unique to this condition. Therefore, early recognition and treatment remain crucial to mitigate the devastating morbidity and mortality associated with this morbid complication. The mainstay of treatment currently is primarily supportive, including source control of infections, therapeutic anticoagulation, or any other justified therapies on an individualized basis.

Consent

A written consent was not obtained from the patient or a legal representative, but a waiver was provided by the Institutional Review Board of our hospital. Please view supplement files.

Authors' Contributions

All the authors substantially contributed to drafting and editing the manuscript and approved the final version for submission.

References

[1] T. Van der Linden, B. Souweine, L. Dupic, L. Soufir, and P. Meyer, "Management of thrombocytopenia in the ICU (pregnancy excluded)," *Annals of Intensive Care*, vol. 2, no. 1, p. 42, 2012.

[2] J. Nolan and R. Sinclair, "Review of management of purpura fulminans and two case reports," in *British Journal of Anesthesia*, Elsevier, 2017.

[3] T. Perera, "Purpura Fulminans," in *The American Surgeon*, U.S. National Library of Medicine, 2021.

[4] B. Childers and C. Cobanov, "Acute Infectious Purpura Fulminans: A 15-Year Retrospective Review of 28 Consecutive Cases," in *Stat Pearls*, U.S. National Library of Medicine, 2003.

[5] D. Contou, R. Coudroy, G. Colin et al., "Pneumococcal purpura fulminans in asplenic or hyposplenic patients: a French multicenter exposed-unexposed retrospective cohort study," *Critical Care*, vol. 24, no. 1, 2020.

[6] O. Join-Lambert, H. Lecuyer, F. Miller et al., "Meningococcal interaction to microvasculature triggers the tissular lesions of purpura fulminans," *The Journal of Infectious Diseases*, vol. 208, no. 10, pp. 1590–1597, 2013.

[7] A. I. Portilho, G. Trzewikoswki de Lima, and E. De Gaspari, "*Neisseria meningitidis*: analysis of pili and LPS in emerging Brazilian strains," *Therapeutic Advances in Vaccines and Immunotherapy*, vol. 8 article 2515135520919195, 2020.

[8] C. Dalugama and I. B. Gawarammana, "Rare presentation of rickettsial infection as purpura fulminans: a case report," *Journal of Medical Case Reports*, vol. 12, no. 1, 2018.

[9] M. D. M. Morales Hernandez, M. Carranza, B. Patel, J. Calvert, and G. Masri, "Purpura fulminans in a patient with septic shock due to Escherichia coli bacteremia with emphysematous pyelitis," *Cureus*, vol. 13, no. 2, article e13249, 2021.

[10] M. Ahmed, M. Samorowka, S. Habis, A. Mahmoud, and R. Saeed, "Escherichia coli bacteremia-induced purpura fulminans: a case report," *Cureus*, vol. 10, no. 11, article e3638, 2018.

[11] M. Amara, S. Bonacorsi, J. Bedel et al., "Group A Escherichia coli-related purpura fulminans: an unusual manifestation due to an unusual strain?," *Journal of Clinical Microbiology*, vol. 52, no. 12, pp. 4404–4406, 2014.

[12] C. Josephson, R. Nuss, L. Jacobson et al., "The varicella-autoantibody syndrome," *Pediatric Research*, vol. 50, no. 3, pp. 345–352, 2001.

[13] C. A. Mitchell, J. A. Rowell, L. Hau, J. P. Young, and H. H. Salem, "A fatal thrombotic disorder associated with an acquired inhibitor of protein C," *The New England Journal of Medicine*, vol. 317, no. 26, pp. 1638–1642, 1987.

[14] A. Kumar, N. Shah, V. Menon, and S. Nissen, "Purpura fulminans manifesting with Staphylococcus aureus endocarditis: a case report," *European Heart Journal-Case Reports*, vol. 3, no. 2, 2019.

[15] A. Veldman, D. Fischer, F. Y. Wong et al., "Human protein C concentrate in the treatment of purpura fulminans: a retrospective analysis of safety and outcome in 94 pediatric patients," *Critical Care*, vol. 14, no. 4, 2010.

[16] M. J. Manco-Johnson, L. Bomgaars, J. Palascak et al., "Efficacy and safety of protein C concentrate to treat purpura fulminans and thromboembolic events in severe congenital protein C deficiency," *Thrombosis and Haemostasis*, vol. 116, no. 1, pp. 58–68, 2016.

[17] B. J. Childers and B. Cobanov, "Acute infectious purpura fulminans: a 15-year retrospective review of 28 consecutive cases," *The American Surgeon*, vol. 69, no. 1, pp. 86–90, 2003.

[18] N. Lerolle, A. Carlotti, K. Melican et al., "Assessment of the interplay between blood and skin vascular abnormalities in adult purpura fulminans," *American Journal of Respiratory and Critical Care Medicine*, vol. 188, no. 6, pp. 684–692, 2013.

[19] N. Sakuragawa, H. Hasegawa, M. Maki, M. Nakagawa, and M. Nakashima, "Clinical evaluation of low-molecular-weight heparin (FR-860) on disseminated intravascular coagulation (DIC)–a multicenter co-operative double-blind trial in comparison with heparin," *Thrombosis Research*, vol. 72, no. 6, pp. 475–500, 1993.

[20] T. Pernerstorfer, U. Hollenstein, J. Hansen et al., "Heparin blunts endotoxin-induced coagulation activation," *Circulation*, vol. 100, no. 25, pp. 2485–2490, 1999.

[21] S. Gu, A. L. Miller, and E. P. Schmidt, "Acquired antithrombin deficiency and heparin resistance: the clot thickens," *American Journal of Respiratory and Critical Care Medicine*, vol. 197, p. 5313, 2018.

[22] S. Kaur, M. Pawar, N. Banerjee, and R. Garg, "Evaluation of the efficacy of hyperbaric oxygen therapy in the management of chronic nonhealing ulcer and role of periwound transcutaneous oximetry as a predictor of wound healing response: a randomized prospective controlled trial," *Journal of Anaesthesiology Clinical Pharmacology*, vol. 28, no. 1, pp. 70–75, 2012.

It is Always Early with Point-of-Care Ultrasound

Zouheir Ibrahim Bitar, Tamer Mohamed Zaalouk, Ossama Sajeh Maadarani, and Ragab Desouky Elshabasy

Critical Care Unit, Ahmadi Hospital, Kuwait Oil Company, P.O. Box 46468, 64015 Fahaheel, Kuwait

Correspondence should be addressed to Zouheir Ibrahim Bitar; zbitar2@hotmail.com

Academic Editor: Chiara Lazzeri

A 56-year-old male was admitted to the emergency department for acute pulmonary edema and septic shock, yet no clear source of infection was noted upon physical examination. Due to his unstable condition, bedside ultrasound was performed. A heterogeneous mass in the liver was noted; hence, a tentative diagnosis of liver abscess was made. The abscess was confirmed by abdominal magnetic resonance imaging. Drainage of the abscess was attempted and guided by early ultrasound. This case highlights that point-of-care ultrasound, when performed by an ultrasound-capable critical care physician, can significantly decrease the time to diagnosis for septic patients.

1. Case File

A 56-year-old male presented to our hospital's emergency department complaining of acute shortness of breath and 1 week of malaise. He complained of nausea and vomiting in that period, with mild abdominal pain, but no diarrhea, cough, chest pain, or dysuria. He was known to have diabetes mellitus requiring insulin, hypertension, an old myocardial infarction followed by left anterior descending artery and right coronary artery stenting with borderline impaired systolic function 6 months prior, and dyslipidemia.

Upon examination, he had a Glasgow Coma Scale of 15, was shivering, hypotensive (mean arterial blood pressure 40 mmHg), tachycardic (140 beats per minute), tachypneic (34 breaths/min), hypoxic (peripheral oxygen saturation 82% on room air), and febrile (temperature of 38.9°C). An arterial blood gas on 6 L/min of oxygen through a BiPAP machine revealed a compensated acute metabolic acidosis, with a pH of 7.404, pCO2 15 mmHg, pO2 101 mmHg, HCO3 15.4 mmol/L, and lactate 4 mmol/L. The patient was in a hyperosmolar state with high blood sugar 30 mml/L and normal blood ketones. He was admitted to the critical care unit upon diagnosis of acute pulmonary edema and suspicion of sepsis. The Rapid Assessment of Dyspnea with Ultrasound protocol [1] was immediately started and showed depressed systolic function of the left ventricle, with cardiac index 2 mL/min/m^2, and ultrasound of the chest showed severe bilateral ultrasonic B lines suggestive of acute pulmonary edema. Clinically, there was still no obvious source of infection: he had a bilateral pulmonary crepitation and there was no abdominal or costovertebral angle tenderness.

The patient's blood pressure was still low after dobutamine infusion followed by noradrenaline infusion and controlled intravenous fluid with insulin infusion; because the patient continued to be unstable, a bedside ultrasound examination for critically ill patients was performed to further look for a source of infection. Ultrasound revealed a heterogeneous mass seen in segments IV (at the level of the left portal vein of the left lobe), VIII and V (at the level of the right portal vein of the right liver lobe), and I (caudate lobe) of the liver with no obvious intrahepatic biliary dilatation. The largest mass measured 10 × 7 cm (Figure 1). A thickened wall of the gall bladder with gall stones and biliary mud was also seen suggestive of acute cholecystitis. A liver abscess was suspected. An abdominal magnetic resonance imaging scan was then performed, which confirmed the abscess with no obvious intrahepatic biliary dilatation; the mass measured 9.5 × 9.3 × 9.5 cm of volume 435 cc seen predominately involving segments IV and I (Figure 2). Piperacillin-tazobactam and metronidazole had already been administered. Urgent

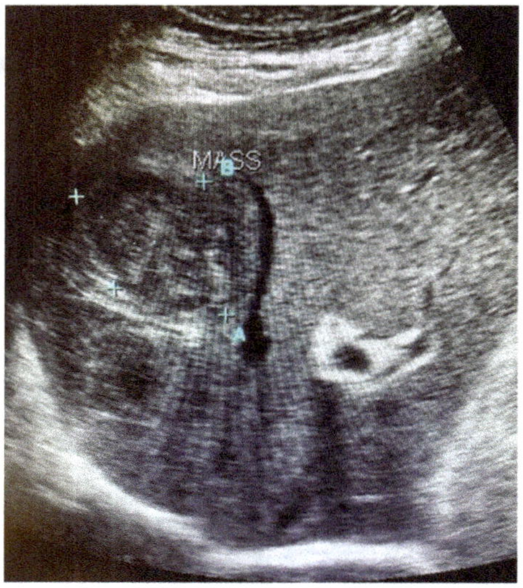

FIGURE 1: Ultrasound liver showing the heterogeneous mass suggestive of abscess.

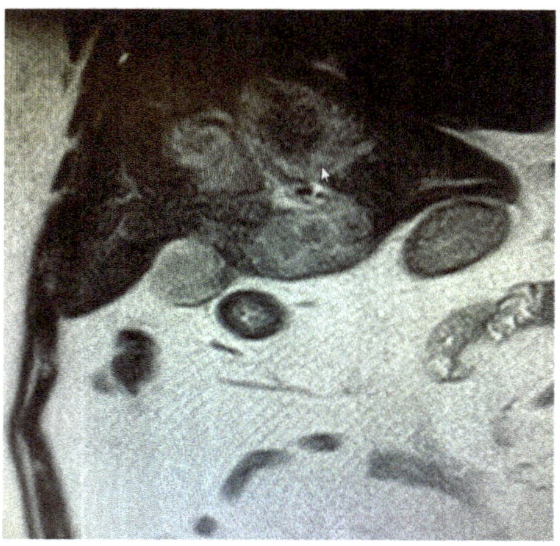

FIGURE 2: MRI abdomen showing T1 hypointense and T2 heterogeneous hyperintense thin-walled peripheral rim enhancing and intercommunicating cystic mass measuring predominately involving segments IV a, IV b, and I.

percutaneous ultrasound-guided drainage of the hepatic abscess revealed a thick purulent material, and then, with the help of the interventional radiologist, cholecystostomy was performed the next day; cultures later isolated *Enterococcus avium*. Cholecystostomy was performed because the patient was considered a high surgical risk for cholecystectomy. Abscess drainage and appropriate antibiotic therapy led to steady improvement, both clinically and on repeated imaging exams. The patient was discharged 2 weeks later with a stable condition, and laparoscopic cholecystectomy was performed 6 weeks later.

2. Discussion

Early recognition of septic shock and the initiation of appropriate antibiotics is the cornerstone treatment [2]. The optimal timing of source control is unknown but guidelines suggest no more than 6 to 12 hours after diagnosis since survival is negatively impacted by inadequate source control [3]. POCUS helps not only in the early identification of the source of infection but also in early interventions such as drainage or removal of the infectious source. However, because of the hemodynamic instability of septic shock patients [1], it is reasonable to carry out diagnostic and interventional ultrasound-guided procedures bedside.

Liver abscesses are the most common type of visceral abscess, and its risk factors include diabetes mellitus, underlying hepatobiliary or pancreatic disease and regular use of proton-pump inhibitors [4]. Ultrasound, computed tomography (CT), and magnetic resonance imaging are the diagnostic modalities typically used for identifying liver abscesses [5]. There is usually a delay of 1 week between the onset of symptoms and diagnosis, as most abscesses are nonspecific, and there are multiple occult sources of infection, such as silent gall bladder diseases and diverticulitis [6].

Streptococci, including *Enterococcus avium*, were the most common pathogen of pyogenic liver abscess in the United States [7]. Enteric gram-negative bacilli, particularly *K. pneumoniae*, are commonly identified pathogens in Asia and suggested an association with underlying colorectal cancer with a prevalence of colorectal cancer among pyogenic liver abscess patients 2.3 to 3.2 percent in long-term follow-up [8].

Percutaneous cholecystostomy in acute cholecystitis is indicated as the initial treatment, combined with antibiotics, for patients who are at high surgical risk such as being septic or critically ill [9]. Early cholecystostomy (<24 hours from symptom onset) was associated with a lower complication rate and a shorter hospital stay [10].

Identifying the source of infection can be challenging, yet important for managing the patient. A stepwise, structured POCUS approach helps to do so in a minimal amount of time.

Point-of-care ultrasound, in the hands of a critical care physician, significantly decreases the time to diagnosis for septic patients, potentially decreasing the time to source control.

Disclosure

The research was performed as part of the employment of the authors in Kuwait Oil Company.

Authors' Contributions

Zouheir I Bitar wrote the article, Tamer Mohamed Zaalouk and Ossama S. Maadarani shared in the discussion, and Ragab Desouky Elshabasy is in the collection of data and revision of the manuscript.

Acknowledgments

Our working website is http://www.kockw.com, Kuwait Oil Company, Ahmadi Hospital.

References

[1] W. Manson and N. M. Hafez, "The Rapid Assessment of Dyspnea with Ultrasound: RADiUS," *Ultrasound Clinics*, vol. 6, no. 2, pp. 261–276, 2011.

[2] D. C. Angus, A. E. Barnato, D. Bell et al., "A systematic review and meta-analysis of early goal-directed therapy for septic shock: the ARISE, ProCESS and ProMISe Investigators," *Intensive Care Medicine*, vol. 41, no. 9, pp. 1549–1560, 2015.

[3] A. Rhodes, L. E. Evans, W. Alhazzani et al., "Surviving sepsis campaign: international guidelines for management of sepsis and septic shock: 2016," *Intensive Care Medicine*, vol. 43, no. 3, pp. 304–377, 2017.

[4] C. J. Huang, H. A. Pitt, P. A. Lipsett et al., "Pyogenic hepatic abscess. Changing trends over 42 years," *Annals of Surgery*, vol. 223, no. 5, pp. 600–609, 1996.

[5] D. F. Zaleznik and D. L. Kasper, "Intra-abdominal abscesses," in *Gastrointestinal Infections: Diagnosis and Management*, J. T. Lamont, Ed., p. 397, Marcel Dekker, New York, 1997.

[6] M. Mavilia, M. Molina, and G. Y. Wu, "The evolving nature of hepatic abscess: a review," *Journal of Clinical and Translational Hepatology*, vol. 4, no. 2, pp. 158–168, 2016.

[7] L. Meddings, R. P. Myers, J. Hubbard et al., "A population-based study of pyogenic liver abscesses in the United States: incidence, mortality, and temporal trends," *The American Journal of Gastroenterology*, vol. 105, no. 1, pp. 117–124, 2010.

[8] W. Y. Kao, C. Y. Hwang, Y. T. Chang et al., "Cancer risk in patients with pyogenic liver abscess: a nationwide cohort study," *Alimentary Pharmacology & Therapeutics*, vol. 36, no. 5, pp. 467–476, 2012.

[9] M. M. Melin, M. G. Sarr, C. E. Bender, and J. A. van Heerden, "Percutaneous cholecystostomy: a valuable technique in high-risk patients with presumed acute cholecystitis," *The British Journal of Surgery*, vol. 82, no. 9, pp. 1274–1277, 1995.

[10] C. K. Chou, K. C. Lee, C. C. Chan et al., "Early percutaneous cholecystostomy in severe acute cholecystitis reduces the complication rate and duration of hospital stay," *Medicine (Baltimore)*, vol. 94, no. 27, article e1096, 2015.

Permissions

All chapters in this book were first published by Hindawi Publishing Corporation; hereby published with permission under the Creative Commons Attribution License or equivalent. Every chapter published in this book has been scrutinized by our experts. Their significance has been extensively debated. The topics covered herein carry significant findings which will fuel the growth of the discipline. They may even be implemented as practical applications or may be referred to as a beginning point for another development.

The contributors of this book come from diverse backgrounds, making this book a truly international effort. This book will bring forth new frontiers with its revolutionizing research information and detailed analysis of the nascent developments around the world.

We would like to thank all the contributing authors for lending their expertise to make the book truly unique. They have played a crucial role in the development of this book. Without their invaluable contributions this book wouldn't have been possible. They have made vital efforts to compile up to date information on the varied aspects of this subject to make this book a valuable addition to the collection of many professionals and students.

This book was conceptualized with the vision of imparting up-to-date information and advanced data in this field. To ensure the same, a matchless editorial board was set up. Every individual on the board went through rigorous rounds of assessment to prove their worth. After which they invested a large part of their time researching and compiling the most relevant data for our readers.

The editorial board has been involved in producing this book since its inception. They have spent rigorous hours researching and exploring the diverse topics which have resulted in the successful publishing of this book. They have passed on their knowledge of decades through this book. To expedite this challenging task, the publisher supported the team at every step. A small team of assistant editors was also appointed to further simplify the editing procedure and attain best results for the readers.

Apart from the editorial board, the designing team has also invested a significant amount of their time in understanding the subject and creating the most relevant covers. They scrutinized every image to scout for the most suitable representation of the subject and create an appropriate cover for the book.

The publishing team has been an ardent support to the editorial, designing and production team. Their endless efforts to recruit the best for this project, has resulted in the accomplishment of this book. They are a veteran in the field of academics and their pool of knowledge is as vast as their experience in printing. Their expertise and guidance has proved useful at every step. Their uncompromising quality standards have made this book an exceptional effort. Their encouragement from time to time has been an inspiration for everyone.

The publisher and the editorial board hope that this book will prove to be a valuable piece of knowledge for researchers, students, practitioners and scholars across the globe.

List of Contributors

Ayelet Machtei
Neonatal Intensive Care Unit, Schneider Children's Medical Center of Israel, 14 Kaplan Street, 49202 Petah Tikva, Israel

Gil Klinger and Lea Sirota
Neonatal Intensive Care Unit, Schneider Children's Medical Center of Israel, 14 Kaplan Street, 49202 Petah Tikva, Israel
The Sackler School of Medicine, Tel Aviv University, Tel Aviv, Israel

Rivka Shapiro
The Sackler School of Medicine, Tel Aviv University, Tel Aviv, Israel
Institute of Gastroenterology, Nutrition and Liver Diseases, Schneider Children's Medical Center of Israel, Petah Tikva, Israel

Osnat Konen
The Sackler School of Medicine, Tel Aviv University, Tel Aviv, Israel
Radiology Department, Schneider Children's Medical Center of Israel, Petah Tikva, Israel

M. Fröhlich-Gildhoff, C. Berhold, U. Ketterer, S. Kische and H. Ince
Department of Cardiology and Intensive Care Medicine, Vivantes Klinikum im Friedrichshain, Landsberger Allee 49, 10249 Berlin, Germany

W. J. Jabs and M. K. Kuhlmann
Department of Nephrology, Vivantes Klinikum im Friedrichshain, Landsberger Allee 49, 10249 Berlin, Germany

Julia Park, Josh Tan, Sylvia Krzeminski and Meghana Bandlamuri
Department of Medicine, Maricopa Medical Center, Phoenix, AZ, USA

Maryam Hazeghazam
Department of Psychiatry, Maricopa Medical Center, Phoenix, AZ, USA

Richard W. Carlson
Department of Medicine, Maricopa Medical Center, Phoenix, AZ, USA
College of Medicine, University of Arizona, Phoenix, AZ, USA
College of Medicine, Mayo Clinic, Scottsdale, AZ, USA

Pablo Lucero
Hospital Británico de Buenos Aires, Intensive Care Services, Argentina

Sebastián Chapela
Hospital Británico de Buenos Aires, Intensive Care Services, Argentina
Universidad de Buenos Aires, Facultad de Medicina, Departamento de Bicquimica Humana, Argentina

Alejandro Sanchez-Nadales, Miguel Treminio-Quezada, Hasan Abad, Jessica Navarro-Motta and Pamela Contreras-Chavez
Department of Medicine, Advocate Illinois Masonic Medical Center, Chicago, IL 60657, USA

Anil Kachru and Chae Chu
Department of Medicine, Advocate Illinois Masonic Medical Center, Chicago, IL 60657, USA
Department of Pulmonology and Critical Care Medicine, Advocate Illinois Masonic Medical Center, Chicago, IL 60657, USA

Hiromi Ihoriya, Tetsuya Yumoto, Noritomo Fujisaki, Takaaki Osako, Hiromichi Naito and Atsunori Nakao
Advanced Emergency and Critical Care Medical Center, Okayama University Hospital, Japan

Masaya Iwamuro
Department of Gastroenterology and Hepatology, Okayama University Graduate School of Medicine, Dentistry, and Pharmaceutical Sciences, Japan

Ashish Lal Shrestha
Department of Pediatric Surgery, Grande International Hospital, Tokha Road, Kathmandu, Nepal

Santosh Maharjan
Department of Radiodiagnosis, Grande International Hospital, Tokha Road, Kathmandu, Nepal

Anil Dev Pant and Pankaj Bahadur Nepali
Department of Pathology, Grande International Hospital, Tokha Road, Kathmandu, Nepal

Priti Gandre, Julien Nguekam, Alanna Wall, ShiYu Ong, Abdul N. Karuppamakkantakath, Konstantinos Tasopoulos and Jeronimo M. Cuesta
Critical Care Unit, North Middlesex University, Hospital NHS Trust, Sterling Way, London N18 1QX, UK

Farook Ahmad
Critical Care Unit, North Middlesex University, Hospital NHS Trust, Sterling Way, London N18 1QX, UK
Cardiology Unit, Medical Department of Universiti Teknologi MARA (UiTM) Sungai Buloh, Malaysia

Sazzli Kasim
Cardiology Unit, Medical Department of Universiti Teknologi MARA (UiTM) Sungai Buloh, Malaysia

Muhammad Athar Sadiq
Cardiology Unit, Department of Medicine, Sultan Qaboos University, Muscat 123, Oman

Shruti Hegde, Gemini Yesodharan and Alena Goldman
Division of Cardiovascular Medicine, Department of Medicine, St. Elizabeth's Medical Center, Tufts University School of Medicine, USA

John Tedrow
Division of Pulmonary and Critical Care Medicine, Department of Medicine, St. Elizabeth's Medical Center, Tufts University School of Medicine, USA

Karama Bouchaala, Mabrouk Bahloul, Sabrine Bradii, Hela Kallel, Kamilia Chtara and Mounir Bouaziz
Department of Intensive Care, HabibBourguiba University Hospital, Sfax, Tunisia

Thibault Lebreton, Fréderic Aubrun, Laurent Heyer and Camille Perrin
Hospices Civils de Lyon, Hôpital de la Croix-Rousse, Service d'Anesthésie Réanimation, 103 Grande Rue de la Croix-Rousse, 69004 Lyon Cedex, France

Jean-Yves Mabrut
Hospices Civils de Lyon, Hôpital de la Croix-Rousse, Service de Chirurgie Générale, Digestive et Transplantation Hépatique et Intestinale, 103 Grande Rue de la Croix-Rousse, 69004 Lyon Cedex, France

Ashani Ratnayake, Prabhashini Kumarihamy, Sujeewa Gunaratne, Hiranya Abeysinghe, Sahan Perera and Shirley Ekanayake
District Base Hospital, Teldeniya, Sri Lanka

Héctor Acosta, Paul Pilares and Jordi Colomina
Hospital Universitari de Santa Maria, 25198 Lleida, Spain

Pau Forcada, Marta Bonjorn and Amer Mustafa
Hospital Universitari Arnau de Vilanova, 25198 Lleida, Spain

Mirko Di Capua and Stefano Paglia
Emergency Department, "Maggiore" Hospital of Lodi, Largo Donatori del Sangue, 1, 26900 Lodi, Italy

Michela Tonani
Emergency Department, "Guglielmo da Saliceto" Hospital of Piacenza, Via Giuseppe Taverna, 49, 29121 Piacenza, Italy

Edward Hamaty Jr
Department of Medicine, AtlantiCare Regional Medical Center, Atlantic City, NJ, USA
Department of Critical Care, AtlantiCare Regional Medical Center, Atlantic City, NJ, USA

Saif Faiek, Minesh Nandi and Hari Kandukuri
Department of Medicine, AtlantiCare Regional Medical Center, Atlantic City, NJ, USA

David Stidd
Division of Neuroscience, AtlantiCare Regional Medical Center, Atlantic City, NJ, USA
Department of Neurological Surgery, Thomas Jefferson University and Jefferson Hospital for Neuroscience, Philadelphia, PA, USA

Manish Trivedi
Division of Infectious Disease, Atlanti Care Regional Medical Center, Atlantic City, NJ, USA

Giorgio Berlot, Giulia Moratelli, Martina Tarchini, Katiuscia Battaglia and Paolo Grassi
Department of Anesthesia and Intensive Care, University of Trieste, Italy

Nadia Zarrillo and Vincenzo Colella
Department of Anesthesia and Intensive Care, Azienda Ospedaliera Sant'Anna e San Sebastiano di Caserta, Italy

Rossana Bussani
Department of Pathology, University of Trieste, Italy

Anusha Ganapati Bhat
Department of Internal Medicine, Baystate Medical Center, University of Massachusetts Medical School, Springfield, MA, USA

Armand Golchin
Division of Critical Care Medicine, Baystate Medical Center, University of Massachusetts Medical School, Springfield, MA, USA

Deepak Kumar Pasupula
Department of Internal Medicine, University of Pittsburgh Medical Center, Pittsburgh, PA, USA

Jaime A. Hernandez-Montfort
Division of Cardiology, The University of Texas Medical Branch, Galveston, TX, USA

Amit Toor, Anika Toor and Mahesh Krishnamurthy
Department of Internal Medicine, Easton Hospital, Easton, Pennsylvania, USA

Lauren Doig and Kevin Solverson
Department of Critical Care Medicine, Cumming School of Medicine, University of Calgary, Calgary, Alberta, Canada

John A. Cuenca, María P Reyes, Joseph L. Nates and Gregory H. Botz
Department of Critical Care & Respiratory Care, Division of Anesthesiology, Critical Care and Pain Medicine, The University of Texas MD Anderson Cancer Center, Houston, TX, USA

Andres Laserna
Department of Anesthesiology and Perioperative Medicine, The University of Rochester, Rochester, New York, NY, USA

Fatemeh Vafapour and Moslem Sedaghattalab
Department of Internal Medicine, Yasuj University of Medical Sciences, Yasuj, Iran

Nishant Sharma, Si Li, Metlapalli Venkata Sravanthi, Dan Kazmierski and Yichen Wang
The Wright Center for Graduate Medical Education, 501 South Washington Avenue, Scranton, PA 18505, USA

Amit Sharma and Pragya Dhaubhadel
Geisinger Community Medical Center, 1800 Mulberry Street, Scranton, PA 18510, USA

Haneen Abdalhadi and Yazan Fahmawi
Department of Internal Medicine, University of South Alabama, Mobile, AL, USA

Abhijin Das
Department of Internal Medicine, University of South Alabama, Mobile, AL, USA
Division of Nephrology, University of South Alabama, Mobile, AL, USA

Brian Fouty
Department of Internal Medicine, University of South Alabama, Mobile, AL, USA
Division of Pulmonary and Critical Care, University of South Alabama, Mobile, AL, USA

Habiba Hussain
Department of Internal Medicine, University of Illinois College of Medicine at Peoria, Peoria, IL, USA

Matthew Sehring and Bhagat Singh Aulakh
Department of Pulmonary & Critical Care Medicine, University of Illinois College of Medicine at Peoria, Peoria, IL, USA

Sarah E. Gardner Yelton, Rajeev S. Wadia and Sean S. Barnes
Department of Anesthesia and Critical Care Medicine, Charlotte R. Bloomberg Children's Center, Johns Hopkins University School of Medicine, Baltimore, Maryland, USA

James B. Leonard
Maryland Poison Center, Baltimore, Maryland, USA

Caridad M. de la Uz
Department of Pediatrics, Division of Pediatric Cardiology, Charlotte R. Bloomberg Children's Center, Johns Hopkins University School of Medicine, Baltimore, Maryland, USA

Johnny F. Jaber and Matthew Standley
Division of Internal Medicine, University of Florida College of Medicine, Gainesville, FL, USA

Raju Reddy
Division of Pulmonary, Critical Care and Sleep Medicine, University of Florida College of Medicine, Gainesville, FL, USA

Curtis Converse, Atish Dey and Sarkis Arabian
Department of Internal Medicine, Arrowhead Regional Medical Center, Colton, CA, USA

Samuel Decker and Michael Neeki
Department of Emergency Medicine, Arrowhead Regional Medical Center, Colton, CA, USA

C. Laivier and J. Devos
Department of Intensive Care, Centre Hospitalier de Mouscron, 7700 Mouscron, Belgium

M.-O. Bleuze
Department of Pneumology, Centre Hospitalier de Mouscron, 7700 Mouscron, Belgium

P. Hantson
Department of Intensive Care, Cliniques St-Luc, Université catholique de Louvain, 1200 Brussels, Belgium

Lauren Howdershelt
Department of Family Medicine, West Virginia University, 1 Medical Center Dr, Morgantown WV 26506, USA

Michael J. Forte and Rahul G. Sangani
Department of Medicine, Section of Pulmonary, Critical Care and Sleep Medicine, West Virginia University, 1 Medical Center Dr, Morgantown WV 26506, USA

Jessica D. Workum
Department of Clinical Pharmacology, Radboud University Medical Center, Geert Grooteplein Zuid 10, 6525 GA, Nijmegen, Netherlands
Department of Intensive Care, Radboud University Medical Center, Geert Grooteplein Zuid 10, 6525 GA, Nijmegen, Netherlands

Stephanie H.V. Janssen
Department of Intensive Care, Radboud University Medical Center, Geert Grooteplein Zuid 10, 6525 GA, Nijmegen, Netherlands
Department of Anaesthesiology, Radboud University Medical Center, Geert Grooteplein Zuid 10, 6525 GA, Nijmegen, Netherlands

Hugo R.W. Touw
Department of Intensive Care, Radboud University Medical Center, Geert Grooteplein Zuid 10, 6525 GA, Nijmegen, Netherlands

Joshua Twito, Syeda Sahra, Abdullah Jahangir and Neville Mobarakai
Staten Island University Hospital, Staten Island, NY 10305, USA

Christopher R. Newey and Stephen Hantus
Cerebrovascular Center, Neurological Institute, Cleveland Clinic, 9500 Euclid Avenue, Cleveland, OH 44195, USA
Epilepsy Center, Neurological Institute, Cleveland Clinic, 9500 Euclid Avenue, Cleveland, OH 44195, USA

Naresh Mullaguri and Pravin George
Cerebrovascular Center, Neurological Institute, Cleveland Clinic, 9500 Euclid Avenue, Cleveland, OH 44195, USA

Vineet Punia
Epilepsy Center, Neurological Institute, Cleveland Clinic, 9500 Euclid Avenue, Cleveland, OH 44195, USA

Anusha Ganapati Bhat
Department of Internal Medicine, Baystate Medical Center, University of Massachusetts Medical School, Springfield, MA, USA

Armand Golchin
Division of Critical Care Medicine, Baystate Medical Center, University of Massachusetts Medical School, Springfield, MA, USA

Deepak Kumar Pasupula
Department of Internal Medicine, University of Pittsburgh Medical Center, Pittsburgh, PA, USA

Jaime A. Hernandez-Montfort
Division of Cardiology, The University of Texas Medical Branch, Galveston, TX, USA

Niclas Lundström, Malin Jonsson Fagerlund and Johan Petersson
Function Perioperative Medicine and Intensive Care (PMI), Karolinska University Hospital, Sweden

Gert Henriksson
Department of ENT Surgery, Karolinska University Hospital, Sweden

Ola Börjesson
Department of Rheumatology, Karolinska University Hospital, Sweden

Matthew R. Watson and Ceressa T. Ward
Pharmaceutical Services, Emory University Hospital Midtown, Atlanta, Georgia, USA

Amit Prabhakar, Babar Fiza and Vanessa Moll
Department of Anesthesiology, Emory Center of Critical Care, Emory School of Medicine, Atlanta, Georgia, USA

Sandra Iskandar
University of California-Riverside Medical Student, Riverside, CA, USA

Marina Souto Martins
School of Medicine, University of Fortaleza, Brazil SA

Andrew Hudson, Jason G. Hirsch and Jonathan S. Jahr
David Geffen School of Medicine at UCLA, USA

Kia Nikoomanesh Julian Choi and Sarkis Arabian
Department of Critical Care Medicine, Arrowhead Regional Medical Center, Colton, CA 92324, USA
California University of Science and Medicine, Colton, CA 92324, USA

Alexander T. Phan
California University of Science and Medicine, Colton, CA 92324, USA
Department of Internal Medicine, Arrowhead Regional Medical Center, Colton, CA 92324, USA

Michael M. Neeki
California University of Science and Medicine, Colton, CA 92324, USA
Department of Emergency Medicine, Arrowhead Regional Medical Center, Colton, CA 92324, USA

Ravinder Datt Bhanot
Department of Internal Medicine, Wayne State University, Detroit, MI, USA
Division of Pulmonary and Critical Care, St Mary's Of Michigan Medical Center Saginaw, MI, USA

Jasleen Kaur and Kendall Bell
Department of Internal Medicine, Wayne State University, Detroit, MI, USA

Shitiz Sriwastawa and Kushak Suchdev
Department of Neurology, Wayne State University, Detroit, MI, USA

Rashmi Mishra
Department of Medicine, Penn Highlands Healthcare, PA, USA

Harish Patel
Division of the Gastroenterology, Bronx Care Health System, NY, USA
Department of Medicine, Bronx Care Health System, NY, USA

Bindu Goel
Mercy Medical Center, IA, USA

Trupti Vakde
Department of Medicine, Bronx Care Health System, NY, USA
Division of the Pulmonary and Critical care Medicine, Bronx Care Health System, NY, USA

Kieran P. Nunn, Murray J. Blackstock and Alastair Morgan
Intensive Care Unit, Western General Hospital, Crewe Road South, Edinburgh EH4 2XU, UK
Intensive Care Unit, Royal Infirmary of Edinburgh, 51 Little France Crescent, Edinburgh EH16 4SA, UK

Ryan Ellis and Gauhar Sheikh
Intensive Care Unit, Western General Hospital, Crewe Road South, Edinburgh EH4 2XU, UK

Jonathan K. J. Rhodes
Intensive Care Unit, Western General Hospital, Crewe Road South, Edinburgh EH4 2XU, UK
Intensive Care Unit, Royal Infirmary of Edinburgh, 51 Little France Crescent, Edinburgh EH16 4SA, UK
Edinburgh Critical Care Research Group (ECCRG), The University of Edinburgh, The Royal Infirmary of Edinburgh, 51 Little France Cres, Edinburgh EH16 4SA, UK

Abdulaziz Alolayan and Azzah Alkhayrat
Pharmacy Department, Prince Sultan Military Medical City, Saudi Arabia

Abdullah S. Aldamegh
Pediatrics Department, Unaizah College of Medicine and Medical Sciences, Al-Qassim University, Saudi Arabia

Jacob Lowry
Department of General Surgery, Atrium Health Navicent, 777 Hemlock St, Macon, GA 31201, USA

Edva Noel
Department of Nephrology, Temple University Hospital, 3440 N. Broad Street, Kresge West, Suite 100, PA 19004, USA

Zouheir Ibrahim Bitar, Tamer Mohamed Zaalouk, Ossama Sajeh Maadarani and Ragab Desouky Elshabasy
Critical Care Unit, Ahmadi Hospital, Kuwait Oil Company, P.O. Box 46468, 64015 Fahaheel, Kuwait

Index

A

Abdominal Pain, 13-14, 27, 29, 31, 35, 37, 50-52, 69-72, 80, 90, 130, 134, 205

Acidosis, 13-15, 17-18, 27, 32, 35, 50-51, 70, 80, 96-97, 99-100, 104, 119, 121-122, 131, 146, 157-158, 182-185, 205

Acute Renal Failure, 56, 91, 93, 130, 132-133, 172

Adenocarcinoma, 96-97, 134-136

Aminotransferase, 22, 47, 51-52, 54, 100, 146

Amoebic Meningoencephalitis, 73, 76-78

Ampules, 90-91

Anticoagulation, 20-21, 47-49, 83, 87-88, 109-112, 141-142, 144, 153-154, 182, 199, 201-203

Antifungals, 64, 134

Arterial Blood Gas, 47, 58, 61, 70, 131, 157, 187

Arteriovenous Malformation, 177-178

Autonomic Dysfunction, 9-10, 103-105

B

Blood Pressure, 2, 5, 27, 35, 46, 51-52, 59-60, 64, 66, 69, 71, 75, 102-104, 106, 114, 125, 130, 142, 146, 157-159, 167-168, 183, 187, 196, 201, 205

C

Calcitonin, 135-136

Cardiopulmonary Bypass, 87, 89, 153, 155

Chronic Granulomatous Disease, 124

Circulatory Collapse, 156-158

Cirrhosis, 3, 14, 86, 88, 90-92, 140, 152, 154, 184

Coagulopathy, 2-3, 25, 61, 63, 67, 88, 106, 109-111, 154, 201

Cocaine Abuse, 15, 90

Coccidioidomycosis, 124-129

Corrosives, 29, 37

D

Diabetes, 5, 13-15, 17-19, 21, 24-25, 29, 37, 50, 52-53, 59-60, 89-90, 92, 96-98, 106, 119, 122, 124, 126, 130, 134, 155-156, 161-166, 182-185, 205-206

Diabetic Ketoacidosis, 13-15, 17-18, 50, 52-53, 96-97, 119, 122-126

Dyspnea, 5-6, 86, 94, 100, 124, 126-127, 130, 152, 205, 207

E

Endocrine, 18, 92, 96, 98, 122, 134-136

Erythrocytes, 6, 74

Euglycemia, 101, 119, 121-122, 162-164

F

Fibrinogen, 40, 47-48, 80, 82, 110-111, 183, 196, 201

Flecainide Toxicity, 113-114, 116-118

Fluoroquinolones, 161-165

G

Gastric Emphysema, 27, 29-30, 35, 37-38

Gastric Necrosis, 27, 29, 35, 37

Gastrointestinal Hemorrhage, 88, 154

Glycogenolysis, 13, 90-91

H

Hyperinflation, 156-160

Hypertension, 11, 14, 19, 25, 59-60, 103-104, 106, 156, 158, 168, 177, 180, 182, 205

Hypoglycemia, 2-3, 90-92, 161-165, 182, 184-185

Hypokalemia, 118, 131-132, 161

Hyponatremia, 27, 31-32, 35, 131-132

Hypoxaemia, 58-63

I

Immunoglobulins, 1, 80

Insulin Pump, 15, 119

Insulin Secretion, 163, 165, 184

Intubation, 6, 20-21, 39, 45, 51, 59, 76, 103, 106, 137, 146, 157, 160, 182-183, 186-187, 189-192, 194

J

Jaundice, 31, 54, 56

L

Lactate Level, 65, 131, 184-185

Legionella Infection, 131-133

Levofloxacin, 161-165

Linezolid Toxicity, 182, 184-185

Liver Dysfunction, 1, 133, 182

Lung Cancer, 96, 98, 134-136

M

Malnutrition, 27, 29, 35, 37, 91-92, 201

Metformin, 14, 125, 184-185

Methylprednisolone, 59, 106-107, 146, 196

Mortality Rates, 64, 72, 119, 121

Mucosa, 27, 32, 35, 46, 74, 84, 100, 127

Muscle Spasms, 102-104

N

Nasogastric Tube, 28-30, 36-38, 87, 146, 153

Nausea, 50, 74, 96-97, 99-100, 119, 124, 134, 205

Neonatal Hemochromatosis, 1, 4

O

Octreotide Therapy, 161, 163

Oxygenation, 5-6, 19-20, 22, 24, 40, 45, 48, 61, 86-87, 89, 107, 110, 152-153, 155, 158, 187, 190, 193-194

P

Pancreatitis, 18, 50-53, 80, 116, 182, 185

Paraneoplastic Diarrhea, 134, 136

Parenteral Nutrition, 53, 130-131

Pneumonia, 6, 10-11, 20, 22, 25, 28, 36, 39, 43, 45-46, 48-49, 58, 61-63, 93, 106-107, 109-110, 112, 125-126, 128, 130-133, 138, 141, 143, 162, 190-191, 193-194

Pulmonary Embolism, 12, 19-21, 23, 40-41, 45, 48-49, 86, 89, 111-112, 141, 143-144, 152, 155, 157

R

Respiratory Failure, 12, 19-20, 28-29, 36-37, 39-41, 45, 58, 86, 93, 102, 104, 106, 109, 129, 152, 158, 186-187, 189, 191, 193-194

Respiratory Rate, 5, 27, 35, 40, 46, 51-52, 59, 99, 102, 104, 109, 111, 125, 131, 158, 187, 194

Rhabdomyolysis, 11, 130-133, 172

S

Sepsis, 2-3, 5, 10, 13-15, 31, 33-34, 53, 64, 67, 79-82, 84-85, 90-91, 97, 106, 109-110, 124, 126, 128-129, 134, 182-187, 196-197, 199, 201-202, 205, 207

Somatostatin, 163

Sulfonylureas, 162-165

Symmetrical Peripheral Gangrene, 64, 66-68

T

Thromboplastin, 87-88, 100, 142-143, 153-154

Tocilizumab, 20, 22, 25, 40, 59, 62, 110

Tracheobronchomalacia, 156-157, 159-160

U

Urinary Tract Infection, 10, 144, 199

V

Vancomycin, 6, 10, 20, 28, 36, 75-76, 80, 103, 106-108, 125, 142-143, 145, 182-184, 196

W

Warfarin, 162, 182-185